Surgical Management of Strabismus

Saurabh Jain
Editor

Surgical Management of Strabismus

Springer

Editor
Saurabh Jain
Royal Free Hospital and UCL Medical School
London, UK

ISBN 978-3-031-80632-2 ISBN 978-3-031-80633-9 (eBook)
https://doi.org/10.1007/978-3-031-80633-9

This Springer imprint is published by the registered company Springer Nature Switzerland AG
The registered company address is: Gewerbestrasse 11, 6330 Cham, Switzerland

Contents

Introduction

Saurabh Jain

Strabismus surgery is often described as an art rather than a science, and no one has mastered this art better than our illustrious list of contributors. Their exceptional skills and profound knowledge have shaped this book, which attempts to distil the clinical acumen gained through countless hours of experience both in the clinics and the operating theatre into a readable text. Our aim is to create a comprehensive and practical guide for those practicing in the field, offering valuable insights and techniques that can only come from extensive, hands-on experience.

We are fortunate to have received input from some of the top experts in the field at this moment. These individuals are not only pioneers in the area of strabsimus but also dedicated educators who have graciously shared their expertise to help shape the future of strabismus surgery.

This book is divided into several sections to maximize its utility. It begins with the fundamentals of surgery, laying a solid foundation of essential principles and techniques. Following this, we delve into the orthoptic assessment, a crucial step in planning any surgical procedure. This section provides detailed guidance on evaluating patients, ensuring that practitioners can make informed decisions tailored to each unique case.

Subsequent chapters focus on various conditions related to strabismus, offering in-depth discussions and practical tips on when and how to operate, as well as scenarios where surgery may not be the best option. This structured approach ensures that readers can easily find relevant information and apply it effectively in their practice. It also features a section on how best to train the next generation of strabismus surgeons using both simulation as well as operating theatre experience.

Supplementary Information The online version contains supplementary material available at https://doi.org/10.1007/978-3-031-80633-9_1.

S. Jain (✉)
Royal Free Hospital, London, UK
e-mail: Saurabh.jain@nhs.net

S. Jain (ed.), *Surgical Management of Strabismus*,
https://doi.org/10.1007/978-3-031-80633-9_1

By necessity, a book of this kind will reflect slight variations in the style of its diverse group of authors. However, I feel this diversity enriches the text, making it more individualized and engaging to read. Each contributor brings their unique perspective and expertise, providing a well-rounded view of the subject matter.

I extend my heartfelt gratitude to all my contributors for their time, patience, and expertise. Their willingness to share their knowledge and experience has been invaluable in creating this book. I take full responsibility for any errors that may have inadvertently crept in during the editing process.

I hope you find reading this book as enjoyable as I found editing it. May it provide you with valuable insights and food for thought for your own practice, inspiring you to continue mastering the art of strabismus surgery.

Orthoptic Assessment

Liz Tomlin

Abstract This chapter delves into the significance of orthoptic reports in guiding ophthalmologists to achieve successful surgical outcomes for patients with strabismus. It explores the critical questions that need answering to ensure optimal results, distinguishing between functional (binocular single vision—BSV) and cosmetic outcomes. Understanding orthoptic reports is pivotal in confirming diagnoses, assessing binocularity, and determining the extent of strabismus, all of which are crucial for effective management, including surgical intervention.

Keywords Orthoptic report · Cover test · Ocular movement assessment · Diagnosis · Binocular vision · Post op diplopia · Surgical planning

An orthoptic report is an essential part of giving an ophthalmologist all the information they need to plan squint surgery. This should include:

- the diagnosis of strabismus, or the plan to further investigate the squint, to reach a diagnosis e.g. investigations for myasthenia gravis or a forced duction test to confirm a mechanical problem.
- The size of the deviation, in all positions of gaze.
- whether the squint has a Concomitant or Incomitant pattern. Concomitant means the angle of deviation is the same in all positions of gaze and fixing with either eye. Incomitant is where the angle of squint changes in different positions of gaze
- an assessment of whether the patient has binocular vision or potential binocular vision and if so, to what degree?

Orthoptic assessment should also consider the following patient attributes.

Observations can be made as the patient enters the clinic, e.g. gait (these can give important clues to the patient's general health) and abnormal head postures should be observed.

L. Tomlin (✉)
Guy's and St Thomas' Hospital, London, UK
e-mail: Liz.Tomlin@nhs.net

S. Jain (ed.), *Surgical Management of Strabismus*,
https://doi.org/10.1007/978-3-031-80633-9_2

1 Anomalous Head Postures

Head postures can be adopted for several reasons which may be ocular or non ocular.

Ocular causes

- To obtain binocular single vision e.g. Face turn to the right in a right lateral rectus sixth nerve palsy or Duanes syndrome, or Head tilt to the left in a right superior oblique or fourth nerve palsy. It is important to ask the patient if they are aware of their head posture. Patients with a longstanding problem are often unaware of their head postures. In acquired deviations the patients are usually very aware that moving their head and neck into a particular position which results in binocular single vision.
- Abnormal Head posture to obtain single vision. Occasionally patients may use an abnormal head posture to get single vision when binocular single vision cannot be achieved, this is rare but can be common in examination situations!
- To obtain better vision e.g. nystagmus patient using a null point; or a patient with bilateral ptosis using a chin elevation; uncorrected astigmatism, or a patient with a visual field defect centralising their visual field with a face turn.

Non Ocular Causes

- The most common head posture adopted for non ocular causes are due to:
- Deafness
- Shyness
- Torticollis
- Neck surgery.

2 Presenting Complaints

2.1 Squint

A patient can present with a variety of signs and symptoms to the strabismus clinic.

Longstanding or childhood squint which have become a psychosocial problem and may require surgery. These patients may present with unusual symptoms of pain and diplopia as they wish their problem to be taken very seriously as it effects every social interaction they have. If the clinician explains they can improve the appearance of the squint but do nothing for the alleged pain and other symptoms, often a patient with a true cosmetic squint is very happy.

2.2 *Diplopia*

Often acquired squints will be symptomatic with diplopia or double vision. Sudden onset of diplopia is often pinpointed by the patient and this can then be attributed to the preceding trauma or vascular incident. Gradual onset of diplopia or increasing prism power to treat the double vision should be investigated as it can indicate a slow increase in deviation which may be associated with a slow growing tumour.

Diplopia should be noted, carefully asking the patient to describe if its horizontal, vertical and/or torsional in nature and if its variable with position of gaze or time of day. Often asking the patient to draw what they see can be very useful.

Third nerve palsies often have vertical and horizontal diplopia which changes with direction of gaze, or no diplopia if the ptosis is complete.

Fourth nerve palsies usually complain of vertical diplopia which is also twisted or torsional when they look down and stairs may be particularly difficult.

Sixth nerve palsies get horizontal diplopia which increases in the distance and towards the side of the palsy.

With blurred vision in peripheral gaze consider INO (Internuclear Ophthalmoplegia), a gaze palsy, or Doral Midbrain Syndrome.

3 Previous Ocular History

A full previous ocular history is very important. There may well be a history of childhood squint with previous, glasses, occlusion, exercises, prisms or surgery. These should be fully explored. The morphology and timing of onset of the deviation may give important clues to the aetiology.

Congenital esotropia that occurs in the first six months of life, and this may lead to DVD (dissociated vertical deviation) MLN (manifest latent nystagmus) often later in life.

If a squint occurs at around two and half years if may be that this has an accommodative element associated with hypermetropia such as in fully or partially accommodative esotropia or convergence excess esotropia.

Often squint such as distance exotropia are not spotted until slightly later in childhood, often around 7 or 8 years.

Remember that small early onset squint can lead to suboptimal forms of BSV such as abnormal retinal correspondence with lower forms of fusion and stereopsis, but the patient will have an easily disrupted form of binocular vision with a small squint present.

Take note of glasses and refractive error present. It is also important to question the patient fully on this as more and more people now have corrective surgery, so a previously − 10 ds patient may present with no refractive correction but have distance esotropia associated with high myopia.

Use of bifocals as a child is an indicator that convergence excess esotropia was present with a high AC/A ratio.

3.1 Childhood Strabismus

Many people may be unaware whether they have had a squint as a child so asking the following questions can help

- Did you ever have a squint as a child?
- Did you ever wear glasses or a patch as child (amblyopia treatment)?
- Did you perform eye exercises in the past, did you ever put lions in cages (synoptophore exercises)! Exercises are often remembered by the patient if given. A history of this usually infers that the patient, has a small angle less that 20^ squint and possibly binocular vision.
- Did you ever have any previous eye surgery?
- Some patient don't count refractive eye surgery as a procedure so asking what the patient's previous refractive error was can be very helpful e.g. when seeing a distance esotropia who has no glasses or contact lenses but was previously −10.00 before clear lens extractions.

3.2 Acquired Strabismus with pre-existing squint

Longstanding squint patients that then develop an acquired squint can present in a very different way to the normal population. Some examples include:

- an adult who has previously had an esotropia as a child, may not get horizontal diplopia when they develop a lateral rectus palsy but others may notice an increase in esotropia or a change in eye movement.
- an adult with Duanes who develops a lateral rectus palsy may just realize they have an increase in their face turn (abnormal head posture).
- an adult who has had a childhood squint who then has an INO (Internuclear Ophthalmoplegia) will not develop abducting nystagmus, but will present as a MR palsy.

3.3 Medical History

The past medical history is very important and may contain clues to the aetiology of both acute and longstanding squint. Specific questions on Hypertension, Diabetes, past cerebrovascular incidents, dyslipidemia, abnormal thyroid function, and previous suspicion or investigations for myasthenia gravis can be very helpful.

3.4 Social History

Prior to treatment of strabismus a knowledge of the patient's profession is very useful. A hedge fund manager or accountant with many computer screens may experience symptoms due to an alphabetical pattern as may a darts or snooker player, drop-handle bar bike cyclist or boxer in upgaze. Recent travel to areas where tick bites are common, can be helpful in the diagnosis of sixth nerve palsy due to Lyme disease.

3.5 Birth History

This can give an indication of general health and specific conditions associated with strabismus such as dragged disc seen following retinopathy of prematurity, cerebral palsy or periventricular leukomalacia causing visual field defects etc.

4 Examination

4.1 Visual Acuity

Testing of visual acuity must be bespoke to age and abilities of the patient. This may include observation of visual behavior in young children. Some tests used are:

- Forced Choice preferential looking cards
- Cardiff cards
- Kays pictures singles and linear
- Sheridan Gardiner singles and linear
- LogMar vision or Snellen.

Sub-normal vision should be examined with a pinhole to see if there is improvement indicative of refractive error. Failure of improvement with pinhole is an indicator of amblyopia or organic disease. Eye poking or pressing and only looking at bright overhead lights may be a sign of poor vision in a young child (oculodigital syndrome) [1].

In a patient with 0.2 or 6/9 vision in one eye and 0.0 or 6.6 vision in the other consider the presence of a microtropia and sub normal binocular vision.

A refraction in all patients is very useful as it may give clues to the underlying etiology e.g. distance esotropia in myopes, small esotropia in hypermetropes etc. Use of a cycloplegic is especially important in children and patients with suspected convergence and accommodative spasm.

4.2 Cover Test

The Cover Test assesses the fixation and the type of deviation and should be described and measured under the following conditions:

- Near and distance
- With and without abnormal head posture
- With and without glasses
- With and without accommodation
- ***Manifest deviation should be assessed with an on off cover test (Video 1.1)***
- Note whether the size of the strabismus is the same fixing either eye (concomitant) or different fixing either eye (incomitant)
- If the cover test fails, this may be due to very poor vision in one eye or a mechanical limitation of the eye so it is unable to fix
- ***Latent deviations are best assessed with an alternate cover test***.

Remember this gives the full angle of the squint as some manifest squints also have a latent component. During the alternate cover test, points worth noting include

- ***The rate of recovery***
- When an alternate cover test is used to see the extent of the phoria it is very useful to assess how quickly the eye returns to its normal position and BSV resumed, when the occluder is finally removed. If this is quick, it is an indicator of good BSV and a well compensated phoria. A recovery following a blink is an indicator that some effort and refocusing need to be used to obtain BSV. Failure of recovery shows weak BSV and these are the most symptomatic patients. When this is suspected, a Controlled Binocular Visual Acuity (CBVA) often can give a numerical value to the control of the deviation. This is carried out by asking the patient to read down a vision chart and noting the level of vision at which spontaneous decompensation occurs. This is particularly useful in cases of decompensating tropia.
- Presence of ***DVD and MLN***
- ***Size of deviation***.

This should be measured carefully with a prism cover test in which the prisms are increased until the reverse movement is seen then reduced to the previous prism power. This should be measured in all nine positions of gaze, either in free space or on a synoptophore (Video 1.2: Prism cover test in esotropia).

4.3 Hess Charts

Hess charts can be very useful and should be repeated at each orthoptic appointment. This enables the patient to see progress with time and pre- and post operatively. An adaptor while plotting the Hess chart (or synoptophore) may allow measurement of torsion. If there is a history of trauma and a vertical squint; inferior oblique overaction and/or superior oblique underaction it is very important to assess this.

Top tip: Measurement of more than 10° intorsion in 15° of depression is a very strong indicator of bilateral fourth nerve palsy and the patient may well need a Fells modification of the Harado-Ito method rather than an inferior oblique recession.

4.4 *Simultaneous Prism Cover Test (SPCT)*

In a patient with a tropia (with a suspected underlying phoria), it may be useful to measure the degree of deviation in real life or without dissociation. This can be determined using a simultaneous prism cover test. This involves placing a prism of varying strength, oriented to match the deviation, over the eye that isn't fixating. At the same time, an occluder covers the fixating or preferred eye. The prism's strength is adjusted until there's no further shift in fixation or until the deviation is corrected.

This test is usually used for measuring small angle tropias to prevent patient dissociation and to avoid revealing an underlying phoria (a latent deviation). It's important to keep eye occlusion brief during a single cover test. Prolonged occlusion may disrupt binocular fusion and cause patient dissociation, potentially exaggerating the deviation by imposing a phoria.

4.5 *Fixation*

If the patient has very poor vision and can not fixate a light then PRT or Krimsky is very useful. Remember if vision is very low that there is no true fixation point or it is wandering then assessment with a light and prism may be the best form of measurement. A post operative diplopia test is still very useful in these patients as it can simulate the effect of surgery and can indicate if a preoperative toxin injection would be needed. Alternation is a good indicator that the vision is equal in either eye in longstanding squint this goes with alternating suppression.

5 Ocular Movements

This is an essential part of the orthoptic examination. It should be performed without the patient's glasses and a light is useful to assess the full extent of the version in each eye and ensure fixation with the corneal reflection being seen by the examiner.

Sometimes facial features make it challenging to obtain a full assessment of ocular movement. The examiner should perform a cover test in the primary position and then compare this result in all nine positions of gaze.

If the deviation is the same size in all positions, then the squint can be considered concomitant. If the size changes in different positions of gaze then if should be considered whether this is a limitation (or under action) or whether an overaction is present.

Limitations are often associated with mechanical problems such as orbital disease or trauma, thyroid eye disease and myositis etc. These are characterised by only having the primary limitation and the overaction of the contralateral synergist and no other muscle sequalae present. In contrast under action secondary to cranial nerve palsies may demonstrate a full range of sequelae. Overactions are secondary to under action than this pattern can be considered to find the under action which is usually the primary problem.

It is very important to perform horizontal movements and consider the workings of the medial and lateral rectus. This should align with any history of previous squint surgery. When examining horizontal movements consider mechanical, neurogenic, INO (Intranuclear Ophthalmoplegia) and lesions on the PPRF (Parapontine Reticuar Formation) resulting in a gaze palsy.

Overactions of vertical muscles such as the inferior oblique can be seen on lateral gaze, or downdrifts associated with Duanes or Browns syndrome.

Routine testing of ocular movements should include comparison of the deviation in elevation and depression. This ensures the present of an alphabetical pattern (such as A V X Y) is not missed.

Vertical movements should look at the limitations such as TED and Browns syndrome, orbital disease. The function of the third and fourth nerves, of the riMLF vertical centre and/or the presence of dorsal midbrain syndrome, can be seen in elevation.

Variability and non-repeatable movements should always make the clinician think of Myasthenia Gravis.

5.1 BHTT and supine CT (Wong Test)

When a vertical squint is seen the following protocol can be very useful

- Assess the squint in the primary position together with a vertical fusion range. An enlargement of the vertical fusion range above the normal value of 2^ Base Up and 2^ Base down may indicate a longstanding or gradual onset vertical deviation such as a longstanding fourth nerve palsy, orbital tumour or TED.
- Consider the ocular movements and if there is an IO overaction seen on lateral gaze, which would fit with a fourth nerve palsy.
- This can then be confirmed with a Bielchowsky Head Tilt test at 3 m.
- The patient fixates an object at 3 m and puts their ear on their shoulder to each side in turn. An alternate cover test is performed and compared with the vertical deviation in the primary position. If a fourth nerve palsy is present then the deviation increases to the side of the palsy.

- If there is a vertical deviation is concomitant then a concomitant skew may be considered. A skew can be confirmed 80% of the time by performing a supine cover test at 1/3 m. So, the patient lies down or puts their head back fully and a cover test is performed. In 80% of skew deviations the angle reduces but not for other types of vertical squints [2].
- Measurements can be taken on 9 gaze (app), PCT, PRT Hess and synoptophore to build up a full picture of eye movements. This can include torsion with the adapter on the Hess chart and on the synoptophore.

5.2 *Lids*

Palpebral apertures should be carefully inspected and if there is narrowing on adduction and on abduction then the presence of a Duanes retraction syndrome should be excluded. If there is the reverse of this pattern (this can be a sign of primary aberrant regeneration or acquired ocular motor misdirection syndrome) with widening on adduction and even a very small suggestion of third nerve weakness, then cavernous sinus pathology due to an aneurysm or a meningioma should be suspected. Eye lid movements can help detect small vertical deviations.

5.3 *Saccades*

Just as you can carefully and gently examine a faulty electrical circuit, by gently turning on a rheostat, or you can blast the circuit by the flip of a switch, Saccadic testing blasts the extra ocular system, so INOs become very visible as does a gaze palsy.

Slow saccadic movements can be identified associated with weak muscles or gaze palsies.

5.4 *Vestibular Testing of Eye Movements*

Vestibular eye movement testing is essential in supra nuclear problems. Moving the patients head whilst they maintain straight ahead fixation produces an eye movement that bypasses the supranuclear eye movement centers. So, if this is the only way they can generate a movement to the left it is indicative of a left gaze palsy. If they can follow a light to the left, but have left absent saccades and full vestibular movement this is indicative of a partial left gaze palsy. E.g. a patient may present with a complete failure of elevation on smooth pursuit and duction and version testing. No elevation is also seen on saccadic testing. When the patient fixates the examiners eye and depresses their chin the elevation may be perfectly normal demonstrating a complete superior gaze palsy.

5.5 *OKN Drum*

This is particularly useful in cases of gaze palsy, dorsal midbrain syndrome and, congenital esotropias where uniocular nasal to temporal OKN is absent.

5.6 *Convergence*

Assessment of convergence is important and can give clues to how the rest of the orthoptic investigation can be tackled. Convergence should be binocular and smooth to 6 cms indicating NRC (Normal Retinal Correspondence). Alternatively, a small squint with convergence would indicate ARC (Abnormal Retinal correspondence) and this may also be present in a microtropia.

If the patient converges reflexly and then diverges at the intersection of the visual axes then this is suggestive of a lack of retinal correspondence.

A jittery convergence can be an indication of dorsal midbrain syndrome and convergence in elevation can often then demonstrate convergence retraction nystagmus.

6 Assessment of Binocular Single Vision

Binocular single vision (BSV) is the ability to use both eyes together to achieve a single fused percept, even in the presence of disparity of the image seen by each eye. It is divided into five grades: simultaneous perception, superimposition, sensory fusion, motor fusion, and stereopsis [3].

Superimposition is demonstrated by Bagolini glasses or Worth's 4 lights. This is one of the lowest levels of binocular vision of being able to see two images and appreciate that they are one.

Fusion is probably the most important form of BSV. It is measured by determining both horizontal and vertical fusion ranges so that the patient can appreciate single vision through a range of eye positions. It is often useful to do this with a Baglioni glasses control so that the patient can recognize easily when they have binocular vision, diplopia or suppression. A normal fusion range is 20^ BO and 14^ BI horizontally and 2^ BD and 2^ BU vertically.

Patients who have a traumatic loss of fusion are usually very symptomatic as they may be able to superimpose images but even their heart beat can disturb their fusion leading to diplopia. Every patient should have their fusion considered with their deviation. So if a patient with a relatively small exophoria of 8^ has only 4^ BO convergent fusion range they may well be very symptomatic with asthenopia and diplopia and be much happier post orthoptic exercises or with the addition of prisms. If the same 8^ BI exophoria patient has a prism fusion range of 25^ BO they will be very well compensated and asymptomatic.

Stereopsis is Worth's third grade of binocular vision. It can be measured with:

- TNO,
- Frisby,
- or demonstrated with the Lang two pen test, for patients with poor stereopsis or only having peripheral fusion or a very weak form of BSV.

Suppression

A patient may be able to demonstrate good binocular vision on testing but a patient who has a childhood squint may be very amblyopic or have dense suppression in one eye and only use one eye even in the presence or absence of strabismus. Remember some patients use alternating suppression.

The density of suppression can be measured with a Bagolini filter bar or with a Sbiza bar. The patient fixates on the light with both eyes. The filter is put over the non-suppressing eye which is seen as red or faded. As the filter is increased an additional white light is seen when the filter equals or is greater than the suppression. Generally, if the suppression is under 8 in a Sbiza bar it is considered light and over 8 it is considered as dense.

7 Prism Adaptation Test

The prism adaptation test is a diagnostic procedure used to evaluate and quantify a patient's ability to adapt to changes in visual alignment induced by prismatic lenses. It is primarily utilized in cases of heterophoria or small angle strabismus.

Initially, the patient's ocular alignment is assessed using methods such as the cover-uncover test or the alternate cover test. This establishes the baseline deviation or phoria. Prismatic lenses are then placed on the glasses in the form of Fresnel prisms inducing a correction of the deviation. The direction and strength of the prisms are selected based on the patient's deviation pattern and the purpose of the test. The patient is then asked to use these glasses for a period of time that may vary from a few hours to a few days and the deviation re measured.

The angle of deviation may remain unchanged or the patient may have "eaten up the prisms" and shows a persistent deviation even with the correct Fresnel prisms in place. The prisms are then increased and the test re performed after a few hours or days and this is repeated until there is no further increase in the deviation.

Thus this test can help uncover the true amount of strabismus and provide valuable information about the patient's binocular control and adaptive mechanisms, aiding in the diagnosis and management of binocular vision disorders such as heterophoria and small angle strabismus.

8 Post Operative Diplopia Test

If there is no detectable binocular vision present then it is very important to perform a post-op diplopia test regardless of how poor the vision may be.

The patient fixates on a light and reports how many lights they see. For example, if no diplopia is appreciated initially on using a small BI prism in an exotrope, the prisms are increased to correct the full amount of deviation. Then they are increased further to see if the patient experiences diplopia when they are made esotropic. This gives the surgeon a good idea if the patient can be over corrected to a small cosmetically good esotropia. It is important that the patient doesn't use fast alternation to experience diplopia. But, if the result is positive for diplopia or inconclusive, then it is prudent to do a pre-operative toxin injection to simulate the surgical result and see if they can cope with surgical correction.

9 Field of Binocular Single Vision

Plotting a field of binocular single vision (BSV) for patients with incomitant squints can be important as it shows the extent to which they can fuse and may be useful to demonstrate improvement with intervention pr the passage of time. This is an essential part of the orthoptic examination as patients with binocular vision should be able to achieve a functional and good cosmetic result (Fig. 1).

10 Using orthoptic measurements in planning strabismus surgery

- Patients with good fusion do well with strabismus surgery and the fusion range may guide surgical dosage. For example, myopic esotropes with a normal BO range for near can cope with full correction or even a small overcorrection. Some patients can demonstrate Binocular vision when their squint is corrected with either the synoptophore or prisms. Patients with this usually had binocular vision during the developmental critical period for vision
- In patients who demonstrate a lack of binocular vision and/or suppression, the ophthalmologist will aim to give the patient a good cosmetic result while trying to avoid diplopia. For example, in a case of secondary exotropia, the surgeon will usually want to achieve a small cosmetically acceptable esotropia to buy some

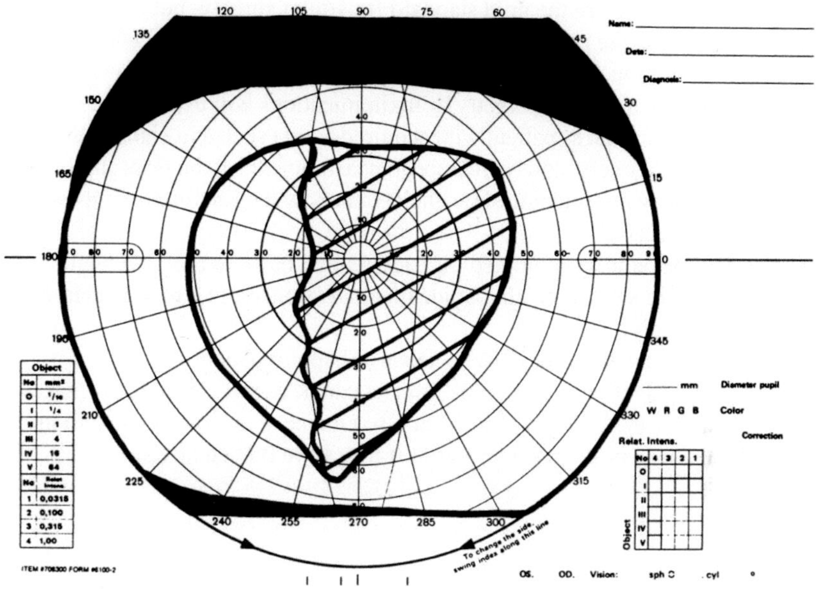

Fig. 1 Field of binocular single vision

time before the eye starts to diverge again. Pre-op assessment of post-operative diplopia with prisms and the use of toxin if this is positive is essential in assessment of these patients.

- With the angles assessed in all positions and the presence of absence of binocular vision the surgeon has the information to help them make their surgical plan. Concomitant squints when the angle is the same in all positions of gaze are easier to plan for. Incomitant squints may need consideration of difference in deviation in different gazes, attempting to correct this as part of the procedure, e.g. advancing a muscle which has previously been recessed and has given the patient a limitation of eye movement with a larger deviation in the direction of action of the weakened muscle. If the deviation can not be corrected in all directions of gaze, the primary gaze and reading positions are the most important to aim for.
- Previous squint surgery may require forced duction tests and exploration. A careful history of ocular surgery is very useful especially when put together with ocular movements to ensure that the limitation or under actions seen concur with the surgery performed. This can then be built into any further surgical plan e.g. a history of inferior oblique recession or myectomy and a clear over action of the eye in adducted elevation may lead to inferior oblique exploration for a dual insertion. The history of a recession of the Medial rectus (MR) and a limitation of ocular movements on adduction may lead to an exploration of the MR and an advancement to obtain full ocular movements.

- Adjustable sutures are the gold standard for squint surgery, but it is important to discuss this with the patient to see if they can cope with this procedure. A patient who will allow touching the anesthetized conjunctiva with a cotton bud in clinic, undergone applanation tonometry or toxin injections will usually cope well.
- Charting progression as patient with acquired squint such as a diabetic third nerve palsy can recover very slowly and repeat measurements of the Hess chart and field of BSV are very important to show the patient how they are improving over a few weeks or months.
- No surgery should be attempted on patients that have an unstable angle and the surgeon should seek three almost identical Hess charts two month apart prior to planning surgery.
- Under promising and over delivery leads to happier patients
- Using post op duction and version exercises can be useful, this not only makes sure the patient has the best movement but also enables their fusion range to increase to make the best of the residual squint if they have binocular vision

References

1. Yoganathan S, Kumar M, John D, Danda S, Oommen SP, Umakant SB, Thomas M. Oculodigital sign: a clinical clue for diagnosis. Ann Indian Acad Neurol. 2022;25(3):560–1.
2. Wong AM, Colpa L, Chandrakumar M. Ability of an upright-supine test to differentiate skew deviation from other vertical strabismus causes. Arch Ophthalmol. 2011;129(12):1570–5.
3. Piano MEF, O'Connor A. The effect of degrading binocular single vision on fine visuomotor skill task performance. Invest Ophthalmol Vis Sci. 2013;54(13):8204–13.

Basics of Strabismus Surgery

Saurabh Jain and Alasdair Kennedy

Abstract Strabismus surgery, like most surgical procedures, demands thorough preparation and meticulous attention to detail to ensure optimal outcomes. This discussion encompasses peri-operative considerations and the operative process, building on the pre-operative assessment and planning detailed in earlier chapters. A fundamental understanding of the extraocular muscles and their anatomical relationships is crucial for strabismus surgeons. Establishing patient expectations through a detailed history is vital in formulating a surgical plan. The primary goal in cases of diplopia is to restore single vision in primary and downgaze positions, while patients with aesthetic concerns but no binocular vision require positioning that ensures a straight appearance and long-term surgical stability. Managing patient expectations is essential, particularly in complex strabismus cases where compromises may be necessary. Anticipating and discussing such outcomes with patients can prevent postoperative dissatisfaction. Strabismus surgery principles emphasize the need for stable orthoptic findings, delaying re-do surgeries until deviations stabilize, and conducting pre-operative forced duction tests. Specific surgical guidelines include careful handling of conjunctival tissues, limiting medial rectus recession to 6.5 mm and lateral rectus recession to 8 mm, with supramaximal recessions for larger deviations potentially leading to muscle action limitations. Recessions for the inferior and superior rectus muscles should not exceed 5 mm and 10 mm, respectively. These principles and guidelines aim to optimize surgical outcomes while minimizing complications and ensuring patient satisfaction.

Supplementary Information The online version contains supplementary material available at https://doi.org/10.1007/978-3-031-80633-9_3.

S. Jain
Royal Free Hospital, London, UK

A. Kennedy (✉)
Moorfields Eye Hospital, London, UK
e-mail: alasdairkennedy@nhs.net

S. Jain (ed.), *Surgical Management of Strabismus*,
https://doi.org/10.1007/978-3-031-80633-9_3

1 Introduction

Like most surgical procedures, strabismus surgery requires careful preparation and meticulous attention to detail to ensure the best results. Section 2 covers the pre-operative assessment and planning in detail and here we will discuss the peri-operative considerations and operative process.

2 Pre-operative Considerations

2.1 Patient Expectations

A thorough history is essential when making a surgical plan for strabismus surgery. Addressing the patient's symptoms and desired outcome will dictate what the surgical aim will be.

In cases of diplopia, the priority is to restore single vision in primary position and downgaze. This may be all that is achievable in complex strabismus such as in thyroid eye disease or cranial neuropathies. On the other hand, in patients with no binocularity but an aesthetically unacceptable deviation the aim should be to position the eyes so that they appear straight but also to ensure the longevity of the surgery, for example slightly overcorrecting cases of secondary exotropia.

Establishing the patient's desired outcome and managing their expectations accordingly is essential. In complex strabismus, there is often compromise. For example, medial rectus recession in cases of type 1 Duane syndrome to improve head posture may result in limited adduction of the eye. Anticipating and discussing these potential outcomes with patients will avoid surprises and prevent any disappointment later down the line.

2.2 General Rules of Strabismus Surgery

There are certain principles which should be followed when planning surgery for a patient. However, due to the nature of complex strabismus, exceptions often have to be made:

- Surgery is not indicated if orthoptic findings are unstable.
- Re-do surgery should only be carried out several weeks after the most recent surgery to ensure the orthoptic findings are stable except in emergencies such as a suspected slipped muscle. The post-operative deviation can take 6–12 months to stabilize.
- Patients with underlying medical conditions which may be causing their strabismus, such as hyperthyroidism, should be first managed medically and their

strabismus measurements stable for at least 6-12 months prior to considering surgery.

- Any orbital surgery should take place before strabismus surgery as it may change the strabismus deviation and motility. Similarly, strabismus surgery can alter the eyelid position and should take place prior to eyelid surgery.

2.3 *Calculating the Amount of Surgery to Perform*

There are many surgical tables available that try to estimate the amount of recession or resection to be carried out for a given deviation. An example of such a table is presented in Table 1. A few principles are helpful to keep in mind while deciding on these values:

- On average, a recession is more effective than a resection.
- Procedures on the MR are more effective than those on the LR. Surgery on the MR corrects between 3–4 PD/mm and LR 2–3 PD/mm.
- When a recession and resection are carried out on the same eye, there is an additive effect of 25%. For example, carrying out a 5 mm MR recession and 7 mm LR resection as in the example below will give an approximate correction of 36.25 PD ($5 \times 3 = 15 + 7 \times 2 = 14 + 25\%$ of $29 = 7.25$).
- Excessive amounts of surgery on any of the recti can lead to limitations of ocular rotation due to mechanical effects. A large recession can place the insertion of the muscle behind the equator resulting in a significant reduction in its action. Similarly, an over enthusiastic resection can convert the muscle to an inelastic tether.
- The medial rectus should only be recessed to a maximum of 6.5 mm. The lateral rectus 8 mm. Therefore, the maximum horizontal deviation that can be corrected by surgery in one eye is about 50 PD and anything larger than that needs three muscle surgery or supramaximal surgery.
- Supramaximal recession of the medial rectus is usually 8–10 mm and of the lateral rectus is 9–10 mm. This may be indicated in larger deviations but may results in limitation of the field of action of that muscle.
- For vertical rectus muscle surgery, usually 1 mm corrects around 2–3 PD. The inferior rectus should only be recessed up to 5 mm. The superior rectus can be recessed up to 10 mm. In both cases, it is important to isolate the muscle from the lid retractors (or elevators) to prevent a suboptimal cosmetic outcome such as lower lid retraction.

Table 1 Surgical dose response tables

Binocular surgery				
	Esotropia		Exotropia	
Deviation in prism dioptres	Surgery in mm			
	MR OU recession	LR OU resection	LR OU recession	MR OU resection
15	3.0	3.5	4.0	3.0
20	3.5	4.5	5.0	4.0
25	4.0	5.5	6.0	5.0
30	4.5	6.0	7.0	5.5
35	5.0	6.5	7.5	6.0
40	5.5	7.0	8.0	6.5
50	6.0	7.5	9.0	
60	6.5			
70	7.0			
Monocular surgery				
Deviation in prism dioptres	Surgery in mm			
	Esotropia		Exotropia	
	MR recession	LR resection	LR recession	MR resection
15	3.0	3.5	4.0	3.0
20	3.5	4.0	5.0	4.0
25	4.0	5.0	6.0	4.5
30	4.5	5.5	6.5	5.0
35	5.0	6.0	7.0	5.5
40	5.5	6.5	7.5	6.0
50	6.0	7.0	8.5	6.5
60	6.5	7.5		
70	7.0	8.0		

From Kenneth Wright. Color Atlas of Strabismus Surgery. 3rd ed. Springer 2015—Rights obtained

2.4 *Anaesthesia*

In the vast majority of cases, a general anaesthetic (GA) is the anaesthesia of choice in strabismus surgery. It offers the advantage of patient immobility for the surgeon and adequate analgesia for the patient. If immediate post-operative adjustment isn't indicated, no modification is required to the anaesthetist's usual GA protocol. However, in complex strabismus, adjustment is often indicated and therefore full anti-emetic protocols and avoiding the use of muscle relaxants is recommended.

Although patients can tolerate procedures such as cataract surgery under local anaesthetic, strabismus surgery may be uncomfortable due to the length of procedures and the unpleasant symptoms caused by the oculo-cardiac reflex. However, the use of sedation and a good local anaesthetic block can give the patient a comfortable experience. Indications include patients who are unfit for a GA and do not require adjustment on the same day. Following a local anaesthetic block, same-day adjustment is usually not possible due the persisting effects of the anaesthetic on ocular mobility.

A peri-bulbar block may be preferable to a sub-Tenon's anaesthetic which may cause bleeding around the surgical site. However, peri-bulbar blocks are associated with complications such as retrobulbar haemorrhages or injection into the optic nerve sheath.

2.5 *Strabismus Set*

It is essential to have a strabismus set with the basic instruments readily available.

2.6 *Suture Selection*

It is important to plan which sutures will be required as this may change depending on the type of surgery. For example, a non-absorbable suture may be required for a re-do operation or after revision of a stretch scar. The list below is a guide and, as always with strabismus surgery, there will be exceptions

(1) Stay sutures: these tend to be non-absorbable such as 5′0 silk or 6′0 ethibond with either a spatulated (minimal risk of perforation) or reverse cutting (better episcleral bite) needle.
(2) Muscle sutures: most operations only require a 6′0 vicryl suture. However, in redo surgery, superior oblique tucks, thyroid eye disease and other restrictive pathology, for example, some surgeons may prefer to use a non-absorbable suture such as ethibond or mersiline. These have the advantage of providing more resistance and security during adjustment and possibly reduce the risk of slippage but may erode through the conjunctiva with time. Tucking the free suture ends beneath the muscle at the end of the procedure may reduce the risk of this.
(3) Conjunctival sutures: the suture of choice tends to be 8′0 vicryl (rapide if available) but the remaining 6′0 vicryl can also be used

2.7 *Optical Devices*

Many surgeons tend to use loupes or similar magnification devices to carry out strabismus surgery as they provide maximum flexibility of positioning during the surgery with many surgeons choosing to sit opposite the muscle they are operating on. However, microscope assisted strabismus surgery offers considerable advantages: The magnification can be adjusted during the procedure, the surgeons benefit from a more ergonomic position and the surgery can be easily recorded. Using the microscope makes it easier to train residents and perform complex surgeries such as retrieval of lost muscles and redo procedures. The disadvantage is a small reduction in the field of vision but, with appropriate magnification, this can be easily overcome.

3 Preparation of the Patient

3.1 Positioning and Draping

The patient is positioned as for cataract surgery with the forehead and the chin in the same plane to allow for optimal surgical access. The skin surrounding the eye should be cleaned with a disinfectant such as povidone-iodine or chlorhexidine. The authors prefer to use a phaco drape that allows the lashes to be kept away from the surgical field but any drape with a round opening can also be used.

3.2 Drops

Anaesthetic drops should be instilled, even though the patient is under GA, followed by an disinfectant such as topical povidone-iodine ophthalmic solution.

Vasoconstrictor drops can be instilled into the fornix preoperatively to assist haemostasis during the operation. The choices include dilute adrenaline, phenylephrine 2.5% and apraclonidine. These may also blur the vision by dilating the pupil which should be taken into consideration if postoperative adjustment is planned. The cornea can be protected with a dispersive viscoelastic.

3.3 Speculum

The palpebral aperture increases nearly 50% in width and 20% in height between infancy and adulthood and an appropriately sized speculum thus needs to be used. The authors prefer the Clarks speculum, named after the American ophthalmologist Dr. Edwin Clark, which has the advantage of being adjustable and having a lock. Each strabismus set should have a right and left sided Clarks speculum, the side being determined by the position of the locking knob which should be superior. Clarkes speculum allows the widest separation of the lids for good surgical exposure but alternatively a mechanical speculum can be used. The authors drape a wet gauze over

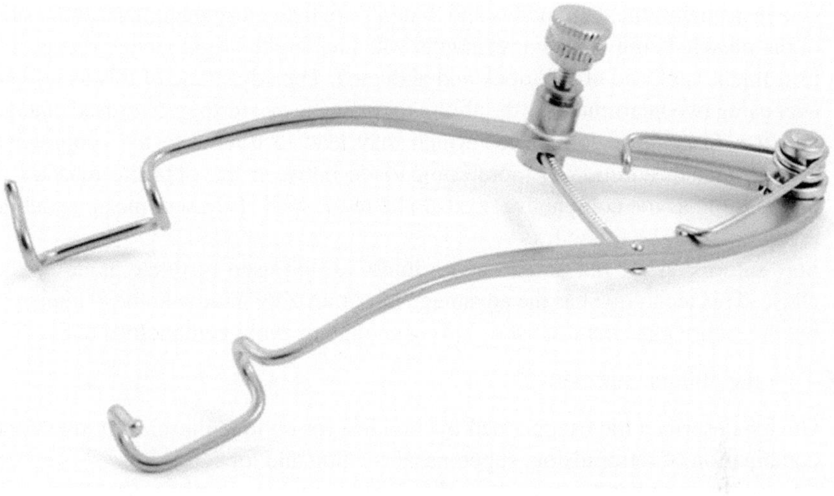

Fig. 1 Clarkes speculum

the hinge mechanism of the speculum which prevents the suture getting entangled during the operation (Fig. 1).

4 Forced Duction Test

Once the patient is anaesthetised, a forced duction test (FDT) should be carried out. The FDT is an essential part of strabismus surgery, especially in complex strabismus. The aim is to establish the presence of mechanical restrictions to globe rotation or muscle laxity prior to starting surgery. The results of an FDT can alter the surgical plan and the amount of restriction or laxity felt can be graded. As a rule, a tight muscle should be recessed in the first instance.

The surgeon can use toothed forceps which have the advantage of giving a good grip but may cause tears in the conjunctiva. This can cause bleeding, discomfort and may interfere with the site of the planned stay sutures. Alternatively, non-toothed forceps or the stay sutures can be used. One or two instruments can be used. Both eyes can be tested one after the other which may help pick up subtle differences.

FDT for rectus muscles

- Two instruments: the conjunctival and underlying Tenon's are held close to the limbus at 12 and 6 o'clock. To test the medial rectus, the globe is rotated away from the medial rectus and into abduction. The globe can then be rotated into adduction to test the lateral rectus. The conjunctiva and Tenon's are then grasped at 3 and 9 o'clock. Depression of the eye will test the superior rectus and elevation the inferior.

- One instrument: the conjunctiva and Tenon's are held close the limbus at the side of the muscle being tests. For example, when testing the right medial rectus, the instrument is placed at 3 o'clock and abducted. The advantage of this technique over using two instruments is the ability to rotate the eye further. The disadvantage is that a firmer grip is required which may lead to trauma to the conjunctiva and cornea. In addition, a rapid comparison between the opposite muscles is not possible as the conjunctiva needs to be re-grasped elsewhere meaning subtle restriction may be missed.
- Stay sutures: After placement, stay sutures can be used to rotate as described above. This technique has the advantage of minimizing trauma to the conjunctiva but the suture placement must be strong enough to avoid conjunctival tears.

FDT for the oblique muscles

- Guyten described the exaggerated traction test for oblique muscles. It involves a combination of retropulsion, superonasal rotation and torsion [1].
- Practically and intra-operatively, a simplified technique involves retropulsion of the globe and supero-nasal rotation as only a relative impression is required (for example before and after a tuck). This can be achieved by holding the globe at 10 and 4 o'clock in the right eye or 2 and 8 o'clock in the left. Alternatively, one instrument can be used by holding the globe at 7 o'clock in the right eye or 5 o'clock in the left or the stay suture can be used.

Video 1: Forced duction testing

5 Stay/Traction/Bridle Sutures

Stay sutures are placed to rotate the eye and maximize the surgical field overlying the operated muscle. They provide tension during conjunctival dissection and hooking of the muscle.

As described previously, a non-absorbable suture, such as 6′0 or 5′0 ethibond or silk, and spatulated or reverse cutting needles can be used.

As well as a conjunctival and tenon's capsule bite, it is important to involve episclera in the stay suture to increase its strength, resistance to tension and to avoid conjunctival tears. This can be achieved by grasping these structure 1–2 mm from the limbus with toothed forceps and lifting up, away from the globe. The needle can then be passed flatly under the forceps and parallel to the globe thus capturing some episclera and minimizing the risk of scleral perforation.

In horizontal rectus muscle surgery, stay sutures are placed at 12 and 6 o'clock except in fornix based surgery where the stay suture is placed infero-nasally for the medial rectus and infero-temporally for the lateral rectus. In vertical muscle surgery, one suture is placed at 12 o'clock for the superior rectus and superior oblique and 6 o'clock for the inferior rectus. A suture can be placed infero-temporally for inferior oblique surgery.

The sutures can then be grasped with artery clips and the globe rotated away from the muscle to be operated on. For the medial rectus, the globe is rotated into abduction. The same pattern follows for the other rectus muscles. For the inferior oblique, the globe is rotated supero-nasally and for the superior oblique, rotated inferiorly. Then, either the weight of the artery clips can provide the required tension or the surgical drape can be incorporated into the artery clips to provide further tension.

An alternative to sutures are Moody curved fixation forceps. These forceps provide a quick and atraumatic grasp of the required tissues with the weight of the instrument providing the tension. The forceps can be moved quickly and efficiently for example when moving from horizontal rectus surgery to inferior oblique surgery. In addition, they provide the ability to manipulate the eye and improve exposure during surgery (Fig. 2).

Some surgeons mark the 0 and 90 degree poles at the limbus to assess torsion of the eye, especially when operating on obliques (Fig. 3).

Video 2: Fixing and marking the eye for surgery

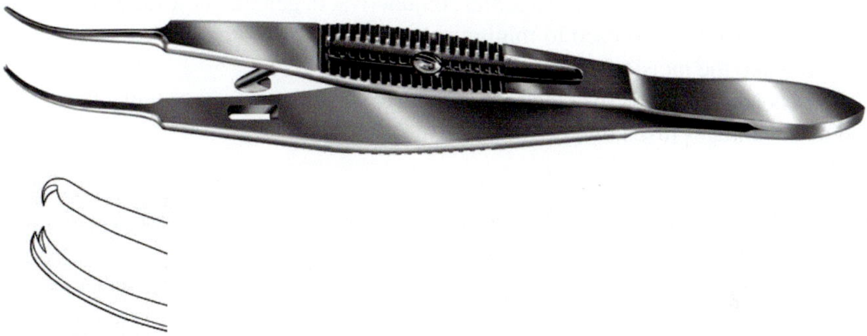

Fig. 2 Moody curved fixation forceps with 0.5 mm, 1 × 2 teeth

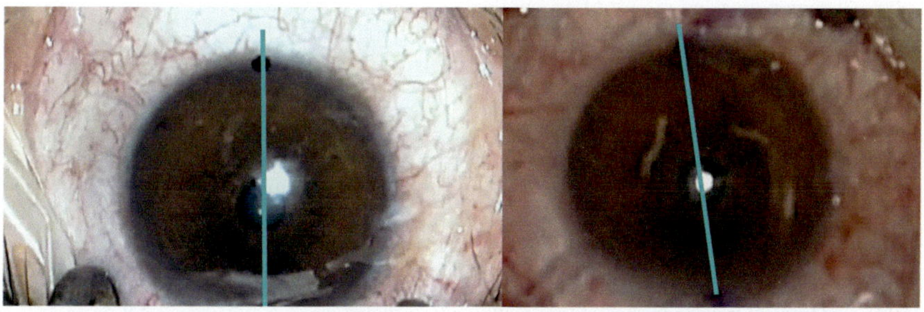

Fig. 3 A straight line joining the marks shows intorsion of the left eye following Harada-Ito surgery

6 The Conjunctival Incision and Other Relevant Anatomical Structures

The bulbar conjunctiva and the underlying Tenon's capsule cover the extraocular muscles and contain multiple arterioles and veins that contribute to the anterior ciliary circulation. The conjunctiva and Tenon's fuse firmly to the sclera at the limbus and form a fold medially called the plica semilunaris. The caruncle, covered with squamous epithelium, lies just medial to the plica. It is important to preserve the relationship of the plica and caruncle to each other as well to the palpebral fissure during any strabismus procedure as a laterally drawn plica is cosmetically unsightly and may detract from an otherwise perfect strabismus operation. A fat pad lies in the inferior fornix, 12–14 mm from the limbus, beneath the conjunctiva but outside the Tenon's capsule. Conjunctival incisions should therefore be placed to avoid this. A breach of the fat pad can cause increased scarring which at its worse is called adhesion syndrome. Incisions between 8 and 12 mm from the limbus avoid both the fused conjunctiva as well as the fat pad to reach bare sclera easily. No incisions should involve either the fornix or the palpebral conjunctiva. In general, non-toothed forceps, such as Moorfields, are used to minimize trauma to the tissues. Spring scissors are used to make the incision.

The choice of conjunctival incision is down to surgeon preference with advantages and disadvantages discussed below and listed in Table 2.

Table 2 The different types of conjunctival incisions used in strabismus surgery with their advantages and disadvantages

	Advantages	Disadvantages	Muscle
Limbal	Best exposure Good technique for teaching	Larger amount of surgery Most post-operative scarring Longer post-op recovery	Mostly horizontal recti
Fornix	Minimal trauma to the conjunctiva and scarring Less symptomatic post-op and fast recovery	More technically difficult Less surgical exposure	All muscles
Swan	Reasonable exposure Good for teaching Excellent for adjustments Mild scarring	Sutures in interpalpebral area therefore more symptomatic in post-operative period	All muscles except inferior oblique
MISS	Minimal trauma to the conjunctiva and scarring Less symptomatic post-op and fast recovery	More technically difficult Less surgical exposure	All muscles

6.1 Limbal Incision

A limbal incision is the most widely used incision in strabismus surgery and was initially described by Harm's in 1949, later popularized by Von Noorden. It offers excellent exposure of the muscle, prevents the need to carry out the procedure over the muscle belly and facilitates the use of adjustable sutures. It is usually used for horizontal rectus surgery but can be used for the vertical recti and superior oblique.

It involves a peritomy along the limbus with one or two radial conjunctival relaxing incisions. As the conjunctival incision involves the limbus, it can lead to significant post-operative discomfort and dellen formation in the initial few weeks as well as long term perilimbal scarring. This may present difficulties in reoperation when the peri-limbal conjunctiva is adherent to the sclera leading to conjunctival tearing and the formation of "button holes" during attempted dissection. In such cases, to avoid the scarring, rather than repeating the limbal incision, an alternative incision such as Swan or fornix can be used.

6.2 Fornix Incision

Parks described a fornix cul-de-sac incision that is usually placed in the lower fornix and is thus completely covered by the lids. The incision can also be placed in the superior fornix for the superior rectus muscle or if muscles are to be superiorly transposed. While this incision affords excellent cosmesis, it is hampered by difficulty of access to the extraocular muscles, the need to stretch the conjunctiva over the muscle insertion which is not always possible in older patients or reoperations, difficulty in placing the scleral sutures and a steeper learning curve. It is important not to place this incision too deeply in the fornix as that carries the risk of bleeding and increased difficulty in muscle exposure for no extra benefit.

There has been an effort to achieve the same goals through smaller incisions and techniques have been described by Velez who suggested a radial incision covered by the upper lid and Santiago who advocated a paralimbal approach between the limbus and muscle insertion (Figs. 4 and 5).

6.3 Swan Incision

Swan described a transconjunctival incision over the rectus muscle insertion, followed by a radial incision of Tenon's capsule over the bulk of the muscle. This incision is now seldom used due the associated risks of intraoperative hemorrhage from the muscular vessels and of postoperative scarring over the muscle. A modification of this incision where the incision site is just anterior to the muscle insertion

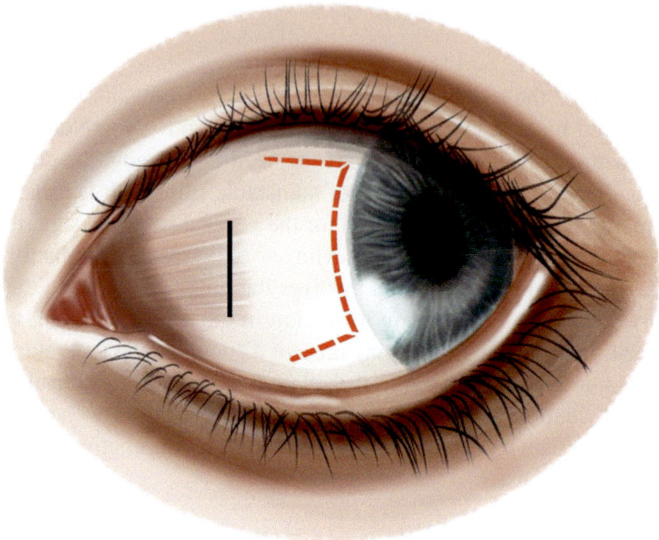

Fig. 4 Diagram depicting the limbal incision (red) and Swann's incision (black). From Jain S. *Simplifying strabismus*. 1 ed. Cham: Springer Nature, 2019

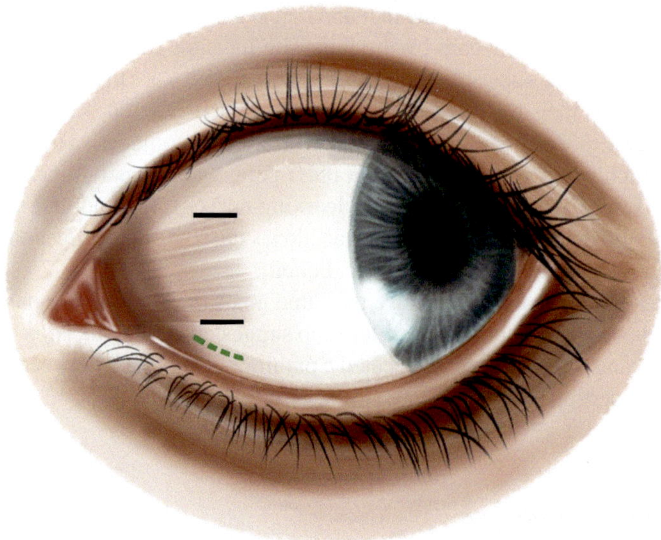

Fig. 5 Diagram depicting an inferior fornix incision (green) and paired minimally invasive surgery incisions (black). From Jain S. *Simplifying strabismus*. 1 ed. Cham: Springer Nature, 2019

can be used. The advantage of this technique is that access to the muscle is easy and it provides excellent exposure of the muscle during post-operative adjustment.

6.4 Minimally Invasive Strabismus Surgery (MISS)

Minimally invasive strabismus surgery is a term introduced to encompass strabismus surgery techniques that minimize tissue disruption and improve postoperative comfort and cosmesis. This is achieved by creating several small keyhole openings through the conjunctiva through which the procedure is performed instead of a usual large conjunctival opening. Due to the nature of the incisions the view of the extraocular muscles is limited and if necessary, tunnels can be created between these incisions to facilitate ease of maneuver and carry out further surgical steps. Most types of strabismus surgeries can be carried out in this manner including rectus muscle recession, resection, plication, advancement, transposition and retroequatorial myopexy and oblique muscle recession, myectomy or plication (Table 2).

6.5 Conjunctival Closure

Careful conjunctival closure is a crucial aspect of strabismus surgery. Careless closure may cause increased scarring, making re-do surgery more challenging, and may result in complications such as Tenon's capsule prolapse which can be painful. Careful suture placement and cutting the suture ends as short as possible may reduce post-operative discomfort. A buried suture technique may reduce symptoms further.

The conjunctiva should be closed using a reef knot with normal anatomy restored. As has been previously mentioned, 8′0 vicryl with a spatulated needle is frequently used but some surgeons prefer to use the remaining 6′0 vicryl which can be buried effectively, or tucked under the eyelid if using a fornix incision.

In fornix, MISS and Swan incisions, the conjunctiva which requires apposing is easy to visualize. Care should be taken to identify the edges of the conjunctival incision. This can be achieved by massaging the conjunctiva with the forceps.

In order to easily visualize the conjunctiva that requires closure, a marker pen can be used prior to making the incision to mark the conjunctiva and the incision made at the centre of the mark. Once the muscle surgery is complete, the marks are identified and sutured together. Alternatively, a suture can be passed through the incised edge of the conjunctiva at the start of surgery indicating the edge of the conjunctiva to be re-opposed at the end of surgery.

Care should also be taken to avoid incarcerating Tenon's capsule in the wound which can be achieved by tenting the conjunctiva upwards once the sutures are in place and prior to tying the knot.

In limbal incisions, the conjunctiva is often recessed once the muscle surgery has been completed. Care must be taken to carefully massage the conjunctiva back towards the limbus until the incision edge is visualized. In medial rectus surgery, the surgeon must be careful not to drag the plica semilunaris temporally. If the plica appears excessively dragged, the conjunctiva may need to be recessed rather than fully re-opposed to its original location. Two sutures are required to the inferior and superior angles of the incision with a further two sutures often required to close the radial incisions.

6.6 Re-do Considerations in Conjunctival Closure

In re-do surgery, the conjunctiva will have variable amounts of scarring depending on the original incision used and the scarring response from the patient. The surgeon may therefore need to improvise and use an alternative incision to their habitual one. Care must be taken to minimize conjunctival tearing and button holes. When closing a conjunctival incision that has torn, the first conjunctival suture is placed to divide the torn and non-torn conjunctiva. The conjunctiva can then be closed conventionally. In cases of conjunctival loss or if the surgeon is unable to appose the incision borders due to excessive tension, it may be acceptable to tack the conjunctival to an episcleral bite with care taken to ensure the muscle is covered. This will leave bare sclera to epithelize which usually poses no problem so long as the extraocular muscle is covered. A symblepharon may develop if both opposing surfaces lack epithelium.

6.7 Tenon's Capsule

This a fibrous structure that envelops the extraocular muscles and is much more complex than previously realized. The anterior Tenon's capsule is the vestigial remains of the capsulopalpebral heads of the extraocular muscles and encases the anterior half to two thirds of the muscles. The posterior Tenon's is composed of the fibrous sheaths of the rectus muscles as well as the intermuscular membrane. These two structures fuse together 15–20 cm behind the insertion of the rectus muscles to hold back the intraconal fat. The posterior Tenon's also forms the muscle capsule and the intermuscular septae which join to form a ring around the globe and the muscle pulleys which serve as its functional origins.

Care should be taken to dissect this structure off the extraocular muscle to as limited an extent as possible.

6.8 Muscle Pulleys

These are a relatively new concept and one that explains the movement and relative stability of the posterior rectus muscles to the globe due to extraocular fibrous tissue

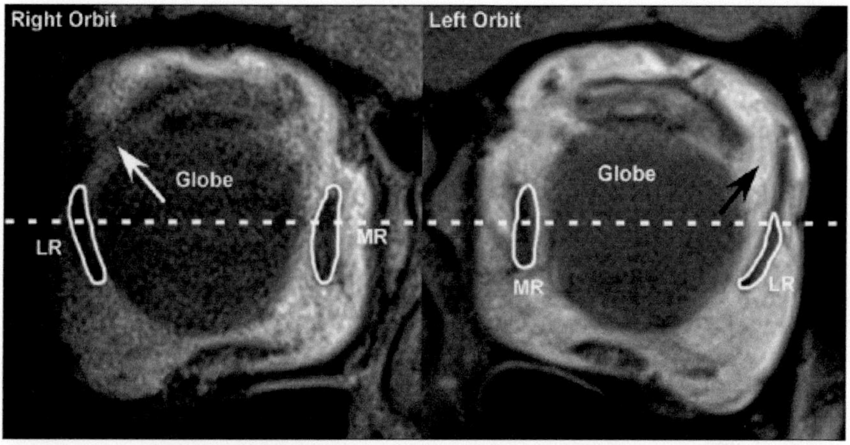

Fig. 6 Coronal magnetic resonance imaging near the equator of the globe in an elderly patient with age-related divergence insufficiency esotropia shows an intact lateral rectus-superior rectus band in the right orbit (white arrow) with a normal lateral rectus pulley position and a dehisced lateral rectus-superior rectus band in the left orbit (black arrow) with an inferiorly displaced lateral rectus pulley. *MR* Medial rectus, *LR* Lateral rectus from Clark RA. The Role of Extraocular Muscle Pulleys in Incomitant Non-Paralytic Strabismus. Middle East Afr J Ophthalmol. 2015 Jul-Sep;22(3):279–85. Under the terms of the Creative Commons Attribution-Noncommercial-Share Alike 3.0 Unported, which permits unrestricted use, distribution, and reproduction in any medium, provided the original work is properly cited

condensations that form connective tissue sleeves. It was initially thought that these were passive pulleys, elastically stabilized relative to the orbital wall and that the extraocular muscles slide freely through them. With further development in understanding of eye movements, a dynamic pulley model has been proposed. The pulleys are now thought to be attached to the orbital wall as well as the globe underneath with the orbital portion of the extraocular rectus muscles directly inserting onto their own pulleys. Surgically, the location of pulleys can be important to define and they may be involved in craniosynostosis, connective tissue disorders (e.g., Marfan syndrome), globe size disorders (e.g., high myopia), senile degeneration (e.g., sagging eye syndrome) and trauma (e.g., orbital fracture or postsurgical). New techniques such as equatorial myopexy for sagging eye syndrome have been described that correct the ocular deviation by restoring the location of the pulley of the inferiorly displaced LR by a single suture at the equator (Fig. 6).

6.9 *Lockwood Ligament*

The suspensory ligament, as described by Lockwood, consists of a blending of the sheaths of the inferior oblique and inferior rectus muscles to form a special thickening of the fascial structure. The lateral expansion of this sheath extends upward laterally

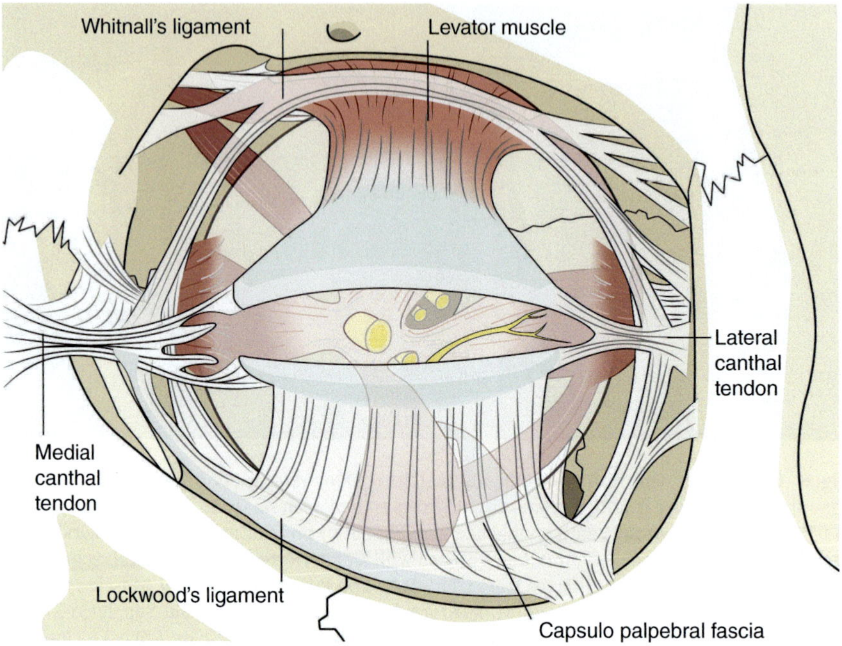

Fig. 7 Diagram depicting the fascial structure that supports the extraocular muscles

and medially to join the sheaths of the lateral and medial rectus muscles, thereby gaining indirect attachment to the orbital margin. This forms a 0.1 inch (0.25 mm) thick continuous band beneath the globe which supports it like a hammock. It is important to divide this when recessing the inferior rectus to prevent retraction of the lower lid (Fig. 7).

7 Rectus Muscles

The rectus muscles all arise from the bony orbit and insert at different distances from the limbus as shown in Fig. 8 and Table 3. Each rectus muscle is about 10 mm wide at insertion and 40 mm long. They are inserted onto the sclera in the shape of a spiral (of Tillaux) and are separated from each other by 10 mm.

Due to the considerable variability in the insertion distances from the limbus and the effect of the differential elongation of the posterior pole of the eye after infancy, some surgeons prefer to measure recession distances from a fixed anatomical point such as the limbus rather than the muscle insertion.

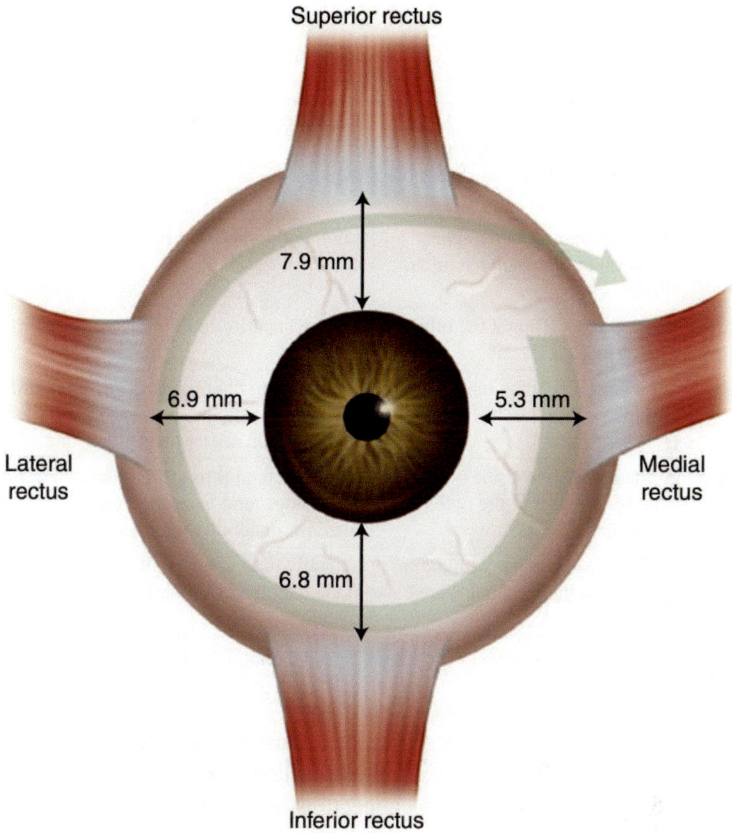

Fig. 8 Attachments of extra ocular muscles forming the spiral of Tillaux. From Strabismus Surgery and its complications—David Coats—Rights obtained

7.1 Hooking and Dissecting the Muscle

Following a limbal, Swan or MISS conjunctival incision, two pockets are made into the sub-Tenon's space either side of the muscle. A round bodied squint hook is passed through one pocket, under the muscle and out the other. To avoid inadvertently hooking the inferior oblique, the lateral rectus can be hooked through the superior pocket.

The posterior edge of the conjunctival incision is then tented up and the tenon's capsule dissected from the muscle until the muscle is exposed taking care to clear the inferior and superior border as well. Any tissues fibres extending from to muscle vertically to the conjunctiva are safe to dissect.

Some surgeons prefer to use scissors for sharp dissection and others use a cotton tip for blunt dissection or a combination of both.

Table 3 Action and innervation of the extra ocular muscles

Extraocular muscle	Origin	Insertion	Innervation
Medial rectus	Both the upper and the lower parts of the common ring tendon and from the sheath of the optic nerve	5.5 mm from the limbus	Third nerve
Lateral rectus	Lateral part of the annular tendon or common tendinous ring	7 mm temporal to the limbus	Sixth nerve
Superior rectus	Annulus of Zinn at the orbital apex	7.5 mm superior to the limbus	Third nerve
Inferior rectus	Lower limb of the tendinous ring	6.5 mm from the limbus in an arc, convex side forward, with the nasal side nearer the limbus	Third nerve
Superior oblique	Sphenoid bone at the orbital apex, superior to the optic foremen	Into the scleral through a wide diaphanous tendon on the outer posterior quadrant of the eyeball	Fourth nerve
Inferior oblique	Orbital surface of the maxilla, lateral to the lacrimal groove	Laterally onto the eyeball, deep to the lateral rectus overlying the macula	Third nerve

From Jain S. *Simplifying strabismus*. 1 ed. Cham: Springer Nature, 2019

When operating on the inferior rectus, care must be taken to dissect the muscle from the lower lid retractors to avoid lid malposition. Similarly, the superior rectus must be carefully dissected from its connections with the levator complex and the underlying superior oblique. A Chavasse hook, especially designed to spread the muscle and facilitate suturing, is then passed to replace the round bodied hook. In cases where the muscle is particularly tight or for teaching purposes, a Wright hook, which contains a central groove, can be passed instead.

8 Rectus Muscle Weakening Techniques

Recession is the process of weakening the effect of a muscle by disinserting it and moving it away from the limbus, thus decreasing the arc of contact and the power of the muscle.

The muscle is disinserted from its original attachment and placed posteriorly by a pre-determined amount. It may be sutured directly to the sclera or anchored to the original insertion in a hang back fashion. Direct scleral sutures have the advantage of precisely placing the muscle at the intended recession location and firmly tacking the muscle down to the sclera. A hang back recession has the advantage of a lower rate of scleral perforation as the suturing is carried out anteriorly with better access and visibility. An alternative technique is the anchored hangback with a superficial scleral bite posteriorly at the intended recession location and the surgical knot placed at the insertion following deeper scleral bites (Fig. 9).

Myectomy is the process of disinserting a muscle. It is allowed to retract into its capsule and is not attached at a specific point on the sclera, reducing the risk of perforation and therefore advantageous when training. It is only really used in Inferior oblique weakening procedures. Rarely, a LR myectomy is performed in a third nerve palsy where the muscle is attached to the periosteum.

Myotomy is the weakening of a muscle by partial division of the muscle fibres or removing a portion of the tendon. It tends to have a non-predictable effect and is not commonly used.

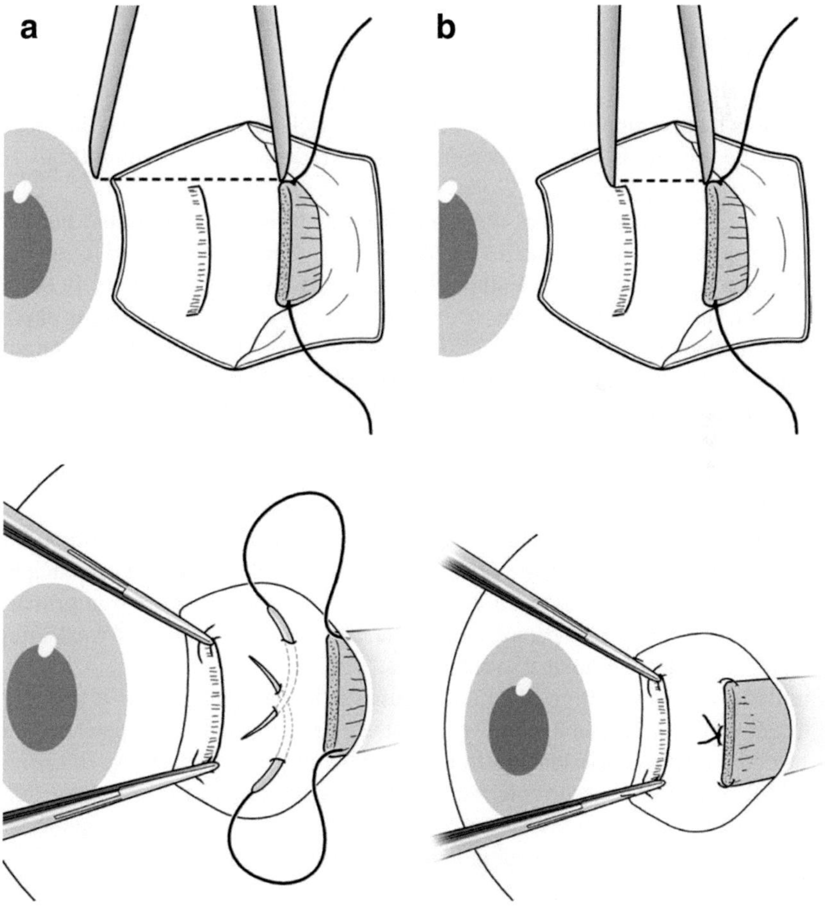

Fig. 9 Marking the sclera for the rectus muscle recession. **a** Measurement from the limbus, or **b** measurement from the original insertion site. **c** Passage of the needles in the sclera using the "crossed swords" technique. **d** The muscle has been pulled up to its new insertion and the sutures have been tied and cut (rights obtained)

Partial tenotomy—central, temporal and nasal.

There has been a growing interest in partial tenotomy of extraocular muscles, especially with the recognition that due to compartmental innovation, different parts of the rectus muscles may work differently.

Kenneth Wright [2] described a central tenotomy in which the vertical or horizontal rectus muscle tendon is incised 3–4 mm in its central part through the conjunctiva as an outpatient procedure. The authors use this to correct small angle deviations up to 2 to 3 PD.

Chang et al. have described using a combination of temporal and nasal tenotomies to correct small angle, vertical and cyclotorsional presentations of strabismus [3].

9 Rectus Muscle Tightening Procedures

Resection is a tightening procedure wherein the muscle is shortened and then reattached to the original insertion thus simulating a strengthening procedure (Figs. 10 and 11).

Plication or tucking achieves the same result as resection without the need to detach the muscle and thus preserves the blood supply. It may be indicated in patients at risk of anterior segment ischaemia. Plication is attaching the muscle belly to the sclera at the insertion while a tuck is attaching the muscle to itself thereby shortening the tendon. These techniques also possess the advantage of being potentially reversible by dividing the fixing sutures. However, some surgeons feel they is not quite as effective as resection and so surgical dosages may need to be increased (Fig. 12).

While performing a recession or resection, it is important to be aware of their secondary effects as they might have unintended consequences.

After a recession, the effect of a muscle is diminished in primary position but is even further diminished in the direction of action of the muscle. For example, following a right MR recession for esotropia, the deviation is corrected in primary position. However, when the person looks to the left, there is an enhanced weakening effect potentially leading to an exotropia in left gaze.

Similarly, after a resection, the muscle behaves like a tight leash as it has been shortened. When the patient looks away from the muscle that has been operated there is a potential bridle action leading to an enhanced effect. For example, following a right LR resection for esotropia, the deviation is corrected in primary position. However, when the person looks to the left, there is an enhanced effect due to the pull of a tight LR, potentially leading to an exotropia in left gaze.

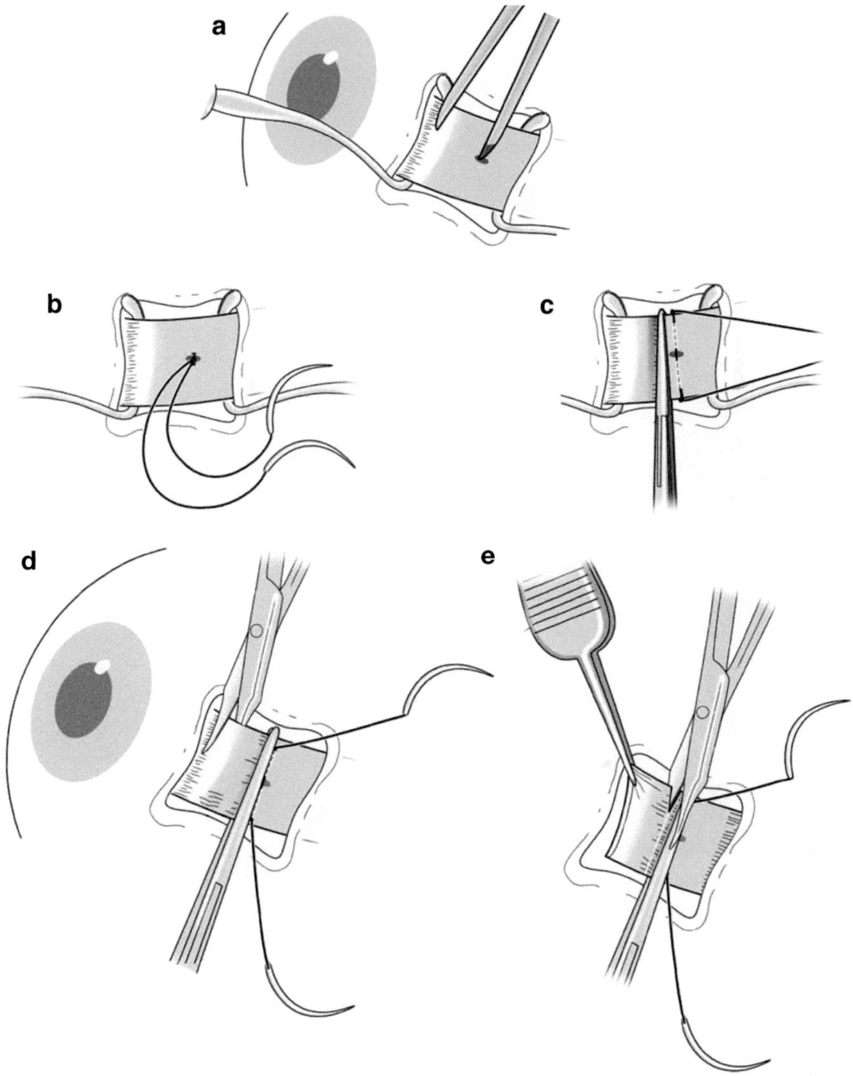

Fig. 10 Measuring and marking the resection: **a** after coating the tip of the caliber with ink from a sterile gentian violet skin-marking pen or ink pad, a caliber is used to mark the resection position on the muscle, **b** a central knot is placed at this site, and **c** transverse passes and locking bites are placed in the muscle and a hemostat is placed anterior to the sutures. Detachment and resection of the muscle: **d** the muscle is detached from the globe at its insertion and **e** the distal portion of the muscle is excised. Rights obtained from Strabismus surgery and its complications, Coats, David and Olitsky Scott

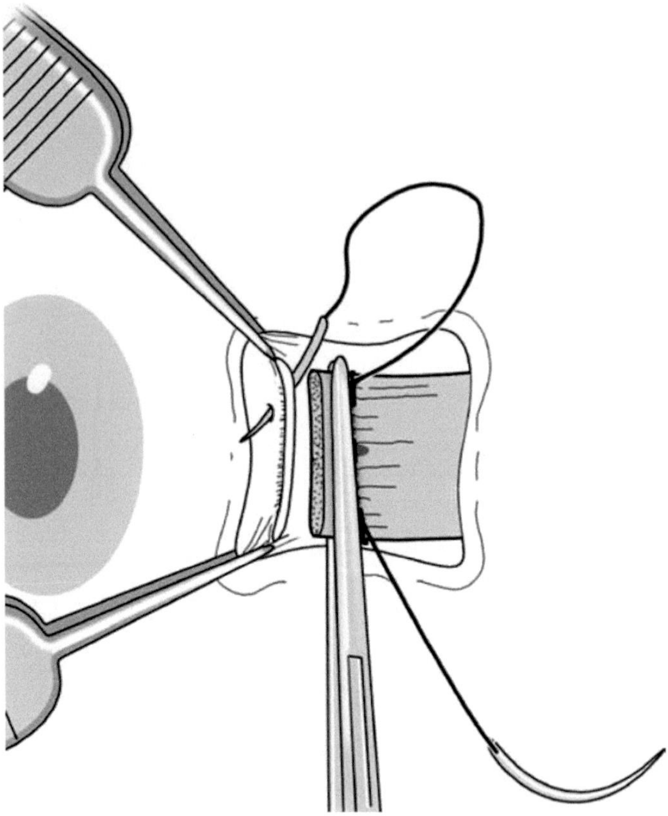

Fig. 11 Reattachment of the rectus muscle. The assistant may place anterior traction on the hemostat to place the muscle in apposition to the insertion site. Rights obtained from Strabismus surgery and its complications, Coats, David and Olitsky Scott

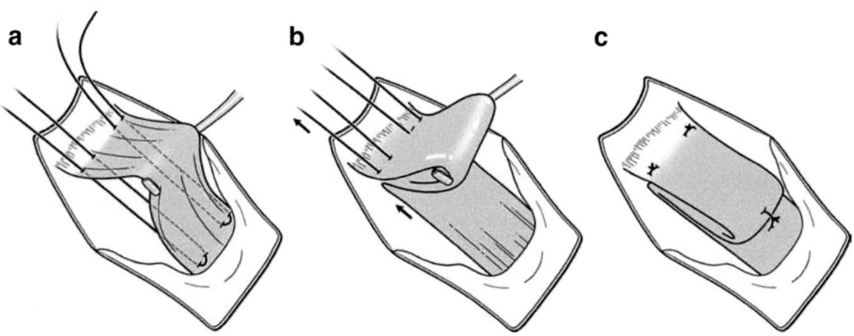

Fig. 12 Plication of rectus muscle. **a** After placement of two double-armed suture in the muscle posterior to the insertion, the sutures are passed into the sclera adjacent to the muscle insertion or through the muscle insertion. **b** The sutures are tied, **c** creating a tuck of the anterior portion of the muscle. Rights obtained from Strabismus surgery and its complications, Coats, David and Olitsky Scott

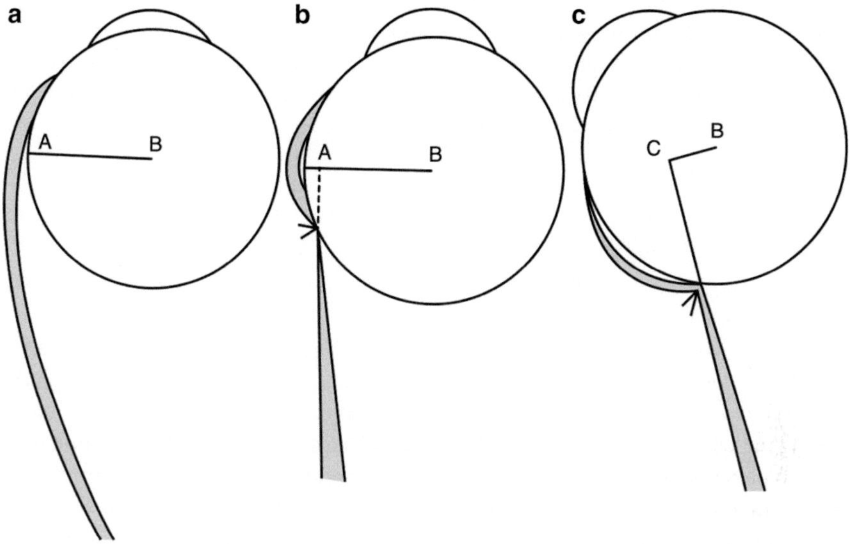

Fig. 13 **a** The drawing shows the normal length of the moment arm when the eye is in the primary position (A-B), **b** A faden pinning the rectus muscle 12 mm posterior to the muscles insertion leaves the moment arm unchanged in the primary position (A-B), **c** When the eye rotates towards the fadened muscle, the moment arm is significantly shortened (C-B) leading to a reduced rotational force. K. W. Wright, YNJ Strube. Color Atlas of Strabismus Surgery. Rights obtained

9.1 *Retroequatorial Myopexy (Faden's Procedure)*

In this technique, the muscle is fixed to the sclera posterior to the equator. As a result, the lever arm is shortened with consequent reduced force generation but only when the muscle is used. There is no effect in primary position but a reduction in movement in the direction of action of the muscle. This can be used very effectively in incomitant strabismus where there is a deviation in particular direction of gaze but none in primary gaze (Fig. 13).

9.2 *Scotts Procedure*

This combined recession-resection procedure can be used as an alternative to Faden's procedure. It is similar in that it induces no change in the primary position, but a selective weakening of the operated muscle in its direction of gaze. It also offers the additional advantage of being adjustable as opposed to a Faden's procedure. It can also be modified to take into account a small amount of primary deviation.

There are various guidelines for the way to calculate the amount of recession and resection. Cruz and Roper Hall used a technique where the appropriate single rectus muscle was first resected and then recessed. Resection amounts were approximately 50% of the recession amounts [4]. The amount of recession was determined for the deviation in the maximum position according to standard surgical tables for the particular muscle or slightly less at the surgeon's discretion, if there was an increased risk of overcorrection in primary gaze (Fig. 14).

9.3 Transpositions

There are occasions where a muscle has no power to carry out its designated action e.g. LR following a complete sixth nerve palsy. Resecting such a muscle is rarely useful as it has no action that can be strengthened. A neighbouring muscle can be recruited to assist in the action of the paralysed muscle. This can be done by either moving the whole muscle or part of the tendon. The latter emerged as an option in an effort to preserve the blood supply of the anterior segment. The extraocular muscles are supplied by the muscular branches of the ciliary artery that gets disrupted when the muscle is detached. Vessel sparing procedures or partial tendon transposition can help avoid anterior segment ischaemia by preserving the blood supply. Further details on these more complex procedures are detailed in later chapters.

Some examples include:

- Full tendon
- Partial tendon
- Hummelscheim Procedure
- Jensens Procedure
- Lateral transposition of the SR and IR to the LR in sixth nerve palsy
- Lateral transposition of the SR the LR in sixth nerve palsy with an augmentation suture between the two muscles that potentiates the effect (Crouch's procedure) [5] (Fig. 15)
- The modified Nishida procedure where no tenotomy or splitting is required [6] (Fig. 16)
- Split lateral rectus transposition to the medial rectus in third nerve palsy

9.4 Yokoyama's Procedure

Heavy Eye syndrome or strabismus fixus is a condition where there is progressive development of hypotropia and esotropia in a highly myopic eye. It has been demonstrated that the posterior pole of the large globe prolapses between the SR and the LR displacing them nasally and inferiorly respectively. The loop myopexy procedure was first described by Yokoyama for the treatment of this condition [7]. The LR and SR muscle bellies are sutured together around 10 mm posterior to their insertion to reform the muscle cone without involving the sclera or splitting the muscles with good results (Fig. 17).

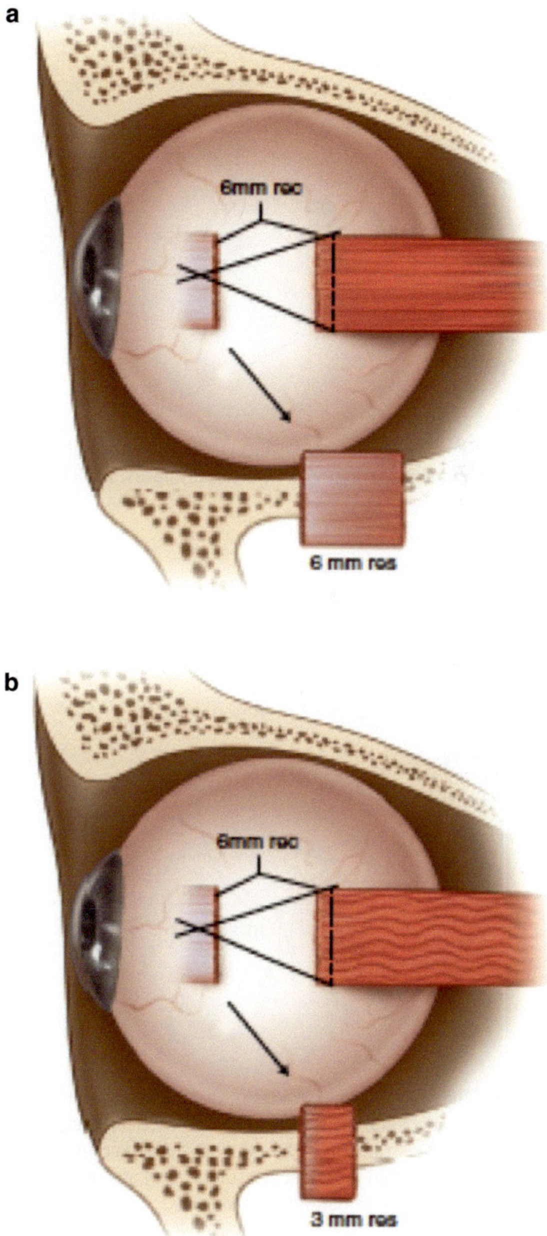

Fig. 14 Scotts procedure: A combined recession-resection on the same muscle has the effect of a Faden's procedure but can be adjusted postoperatively. **a** To have no effect on the primary position, the amount of recession equals the amount of resection (6 mm), and no shortening occurs to the sarcomeres in the muscle. **b** To get an effect on the primary position, the recession (6 mm) exceeds the resection (3 mm), thus creating some shortening of the sarcomeres in the muscle. Strabismus—Burton Kushner—Rights obtained

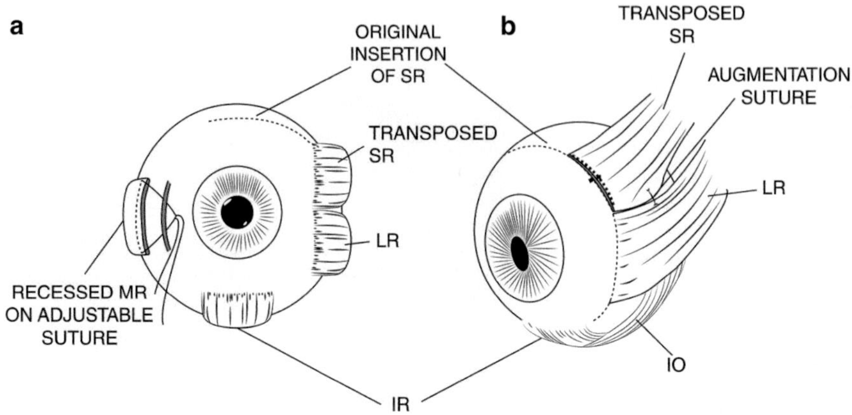

Fig. 15 Superior rectus transposition (SRT) plus medial rectus recession procedure demonstrating. **a** Medial rectus recession with adjustable sutures; **b** SRT technique with augmentation suture

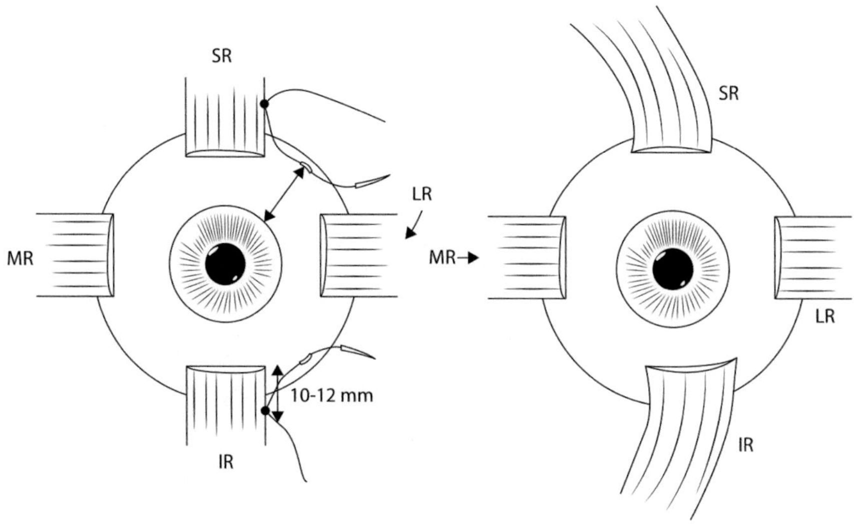

Fig. 16 The modified muscle transposition procedure of Nishida and associates, where a 6–0 or 5–0 nonabsorbable suture is inserted through each temporal margin of vertical recti at approximately one third of the width from the edge at a distance of 8–10 mm behind the insertion. The same suture also is inserted through each scleral wall at a distance of 10–12 mm behind the limbus at the superotemporal or inferotemporal quadrant

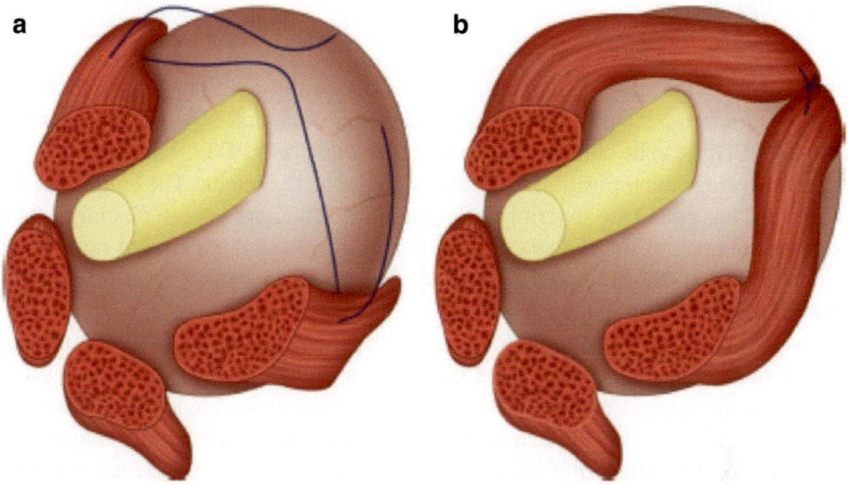

Fig. 17 Heavy eye syndrome. **a** Artist's depiction of the heavy eye syndrome OD viewd from posterior. The lateral rectus muscle (LR) is inferiorly displaced and the superior rectus muscle (SR) nasally displaced. **b** For the Yokoyama prpcedure, sutures are passed through the edges of the muscles. From Jain S. *Simplifying strabismus*. 1 ed. Cham: Springer Nature, 2019

10 Superior Oblique

The superior oblique muscle has a muscular portion and a tendinous portion, both of which are approximately 30 mm long. It originates superiorly and temporally to the ligament of Zinn at the apex of the orbit and becomes tendinous 10 mm before reaching the trochlea located at the junction of the medial and superior orbital rim. The trochlea acts as a pulley redirecting the course of the superior oblique tendon. The tendinous portion of the superior oblique goes through the trochlea and then courses posteriorly and temporally passing beneath the superior rectus and inserts near the lateral border of the superior rectus. That portion of the superior oblique tendon passing beneath the superior rectus muscle is attached to the under surface of this muscle through the sheath of the superior rectus muscle. Therefore, to obtain an effective large recession of the superior rectus muscle, it is necessary to completely free it from the superior oblique tendon. The hang-loose superior rectus recession will not accomplish the intended retroplacement of the superior rectus muscle unless the superior oblique-superior rectus attachment is freed.

The insertion of the superior oblique is broad and diaphanous, measuring an average of 10.7 mm and can be difficult to visualise. This may be made even more difficult because it may insert at varying distances from the limbus.

10.1 SO Tuck

This is a procedure carried out in treatment of superior oblique palsies (SOP), when the deviation is more in downgaze, and specially in congenital SOP associated with a lax tendon. This can be confirmed by a forced duction test (FDT). The globe is fixed in a downwards facing position using a stay suture at 12 o'clock. The conjunctiva is incised just anterior to the superior rectus tendon. The authors suggest placing a small mark on the apex of the L-shaped incision and then extend the wound posteriorly as that helps put the conjunctiva back together again. Once the superior rectus is hooked, the superior oblique can be isolated.

The authors suggest using an iris spatula or phaco chopper 'second instrument' to help identify the anterior fibres of the superior oblique. If this is not successful, the SO can be hooked medial to the SR tendon as here the tendon is much more prominent and easier to define, and a suture passed underneath it. The suture ends can be pulled through to the lateral aspect of the superior rectus which can help identify the SO insertion.

Once the SO is identified and hooked, the loose tendon is stretched up, away from the globe to estimate the amount of tuck needed. A double ended non-absorbable suture is passed through the anterior and posterior aspects of the tendon and placed on a bowtie, similar to that for an adjustable recession. The SR is unhooked and the stay suture removed to repeat the forced duction test. Correctly performed, the inferior limbus should just clear a line formed by joining the two canthi as shown in Fig. 18. Too lax a tuck will need further surgery in the future and too tight a tuck can induce a troublesome iatrogenic Brown syndrome. Once the appropriate amount of tuck has been achieved, the bowtie can be converted to a locking knot and conjunctiva replaced.

Some surgeons prefer to use a tendon tucker for this purpose, which helps quantify the exact amount of tuck, but we feel that this can be accomplished using a simple squint hook as well.

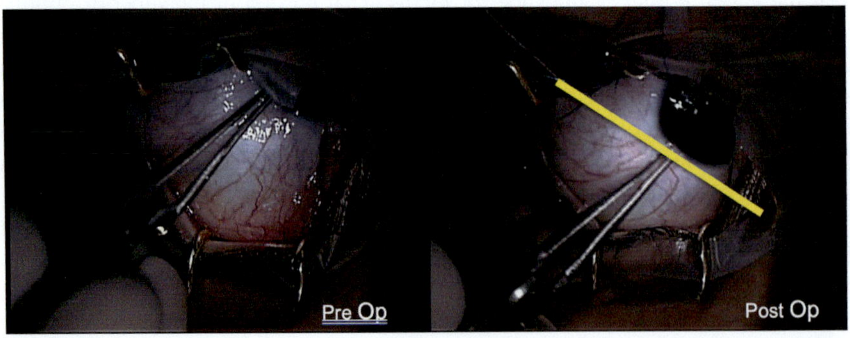

Fig. 18 The appropriate amount of SO tuck will mean the lower limbus just clears a line formed by joining the two canthi (yellow line)

10.2 Tendon Spacer

A tendon spacer can be used in cases of Brown syndrome where a tight inelastic SO tendon is lengthened to help improve the motility in up-gaze and adduction.

A silicon expander (retinal band number 240) is the most commonly used spacer material and is cut to about 6 mm in length and placed between the two ends of the tendon nasally. Note that as the SO is hooked nasally; the tendon is easier to visualise than the temporal SO tendon [8] (Fig. 19).

Due to concerns about long-term risks of extrusion of the silicon band, many surgeons prefer to use a chicken wire technique where the tendon is elongated, using a non-absorbable mattress suture. This also carries the advantage of being

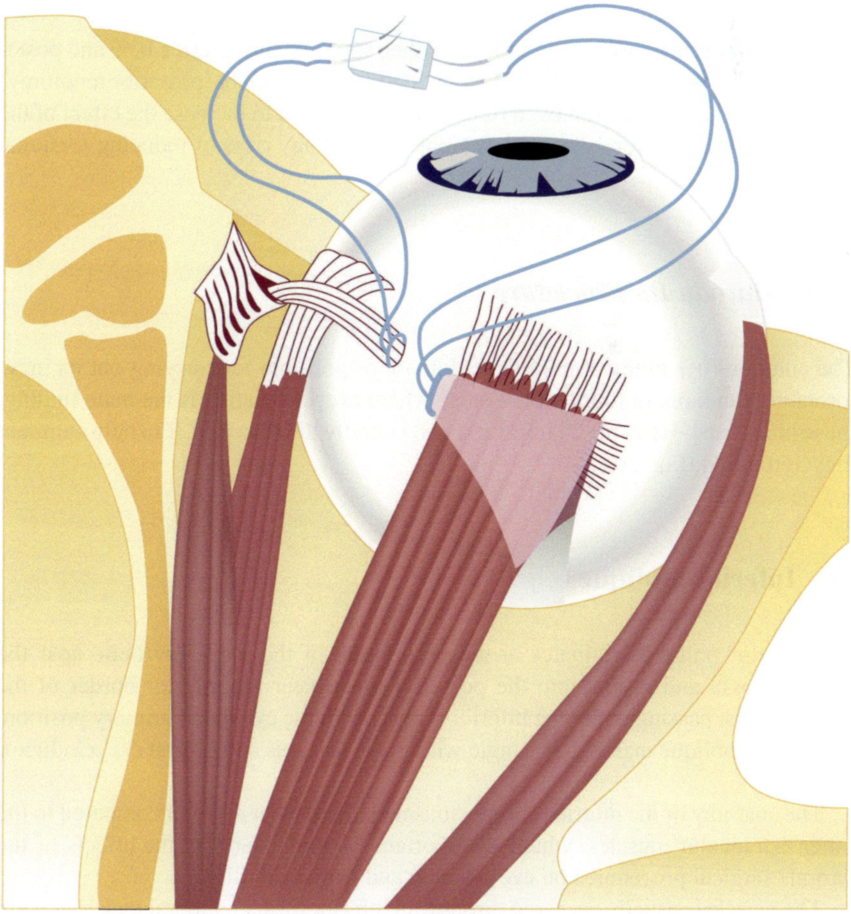

Fig. 19 Silicone tendon expander procedure: Diagram shows a segment of silicone 240 retinal band being sewn to cut ends of superior oblique tendon. A tenotomy and placement of silicone implant is done 3 mm nasal to the superior rectus muscle

potentially adjustable [9]. Furthermore, some surgeons elect to simply disinsert the SO from its insertion and recess it under the SR nasally. This technique is effectively a combination of a recession and myectomy. The advantage is that it is quick and simple but disadvantaged by the fact that it cannot be adjusted, although this is not commonly required when treating a Brown syndrome, or easily reversed.

10.3 Posterior Tenotomy

The posterior 90% of the superior oblique muscle contributes to the depression of the eye and may need to be weakened in cases of an A-pattern. In this condition, bilateral overaction of the SO leads to increased deviation in downgaze causing an A pattern with associated difficulties in reading.

The SO muscle is isolated as above and then split into the anterior 10% and posterior 90%. The posterior fibres are then divided from the sclera (posterior tenotomy) and can even be partially removed (tenectomy) in a block to increase the effect of the procedure. The anterior 10% are left alone to avoid any risks of inducing torsional effects.

10.4 Harada Ito Procedure

The anterior 10% fibres of the SO tendon are responsible for carrying out its incylorotating function. In fourth nerve palsy where excyclorotation is the main finding, these fibres can be transposed inferiorly and laterally towards the LR to help augment incyclorotation (Fig. 20).

11 Inferior Oblique

The inferior oblique originates at the periosteum of the maxillary bone near the lacrimal fossa and inserts into the posterior globe near the inferior border of the lateral rectus, passing under the inferior rectus. With the eye in the primary position, the inferior oblique makes a 51° angle with the visual axis and acts an excycloductor [10].

The anatomy of the inferior oblique muscle is somewhat atypical compared to the other extraocular muscles, which is important for understanding the effects of the various surgical procedures on eye position and ocular motility.

The muscle is usually accessed through an inferior fornix temporal incision, 8mm from the limbus between the IR and LR. The conjunctiva and Tenon's are incised to reach bare sclera and then the Tenon's is advanced in a "hand over hand" manner to aid exposure of the muscle. Once the superior border of the muscle becomes visible

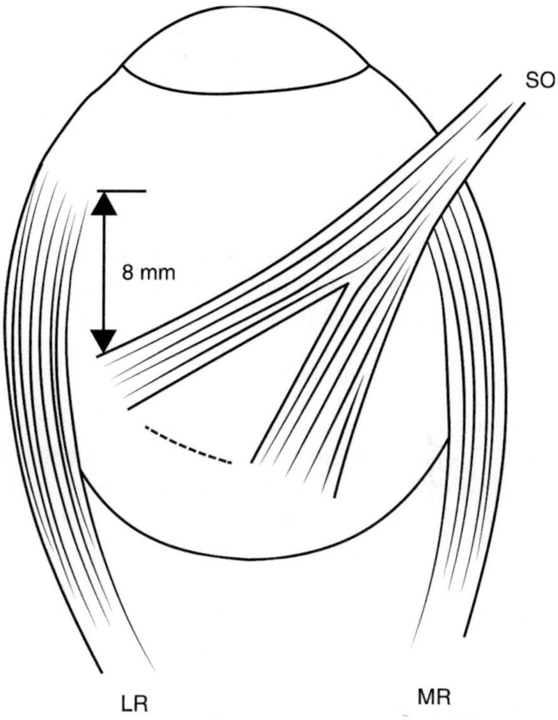

Fig. 20 Harada-Ito technique, the anterior fibres of the superior oblique tendon are sutured, then disinserted and moved anteriorly and laterally, to be secured to sclera at a point 8 mm posterior to the superior border of the lateral rectus insertion. Lateralizing the anterior fibres intorts the eye, thus correcting extorsion

an incision is made in the superior muscle sheath to expose the muscle belly. The muscle is further advanced until the posterior edge becomes visible as well as the Tenon's beyond it, forming a "white triangle". The muscle is then hooked from the white triangle with the tip of the hook directed upwards to appear in the previously made incision thus ensuring the whole muscle is hooked. Care must be taken to avoid opening the fat pad, which can lead to adhesion syndrome, or damaging the vortex vein which can cause significant bleeding obscuring the surgical view. It is essential to hook the entire muscle as any remaining fibres will lead to a recurrence of the IO overaction. This is particularly important in an IO with two or three heads of insertion.

Primary inferior oblique overaction commonly develops in individuals with infantile esotropia, often after surgical treatment of the original horizontal strabismus, as well as in some children with accommodative esotropia or intermittent exotropia [11]. Secondary inferior oblique over-action occurs in patients with superior oblique palsy. It may also be seen in Duane syndrome with up-shoots in adduction.

Surgery on the inferior oblique in most cases is carried out with the intention of weakening the muscle. The various techniques described include:

(1) Myectomy

This procedure involves isolating the IO as above on two surgical hooks and the removal of a segment of muscle measuring around 2.5 cm or 1 inch, between the neurofibrovascular bundle (NFVB) and the insertion of the muscle. It is faster than a recession and there is less risk of surgical intraoperative complications because there is no scleral pass required to reattach the muscle. The disadvantage is the possibility that the muscle may reattach and lead to recurrent overaction. There may also be variable results due to the variability in the site of reattachment [12].

(2) Recession

The inferior oblique muscle can be recessed along its anatomical path by as much as 14 mm and is usually placed at Parks point 3 mm posterior and 2 mm superior to the lateral border of IR [13].

(3) Anterior transposition

This technique first described by Elliot and Nankin, converts the inferior oblique muscle from an elevator to a depressor on attempted elevation. Innervation of the muscle occurs through the NFVB, which attaches midway between the origin and the insertion 2 mm temporal to the inferior rectus muscle [14]. After anterior transposition of the muscle, the NFVB ligament will mechanically act as the muscle's new origin [15]. Anterior transposition is a more powerful operation, especially in larger vertical deviations or in cases of significant inferior oblique over-action.

There are various techniques described which vary in where the IO is attached, but there seems to be consensus that it should not be anterior to the temporal border of the IR. The muscle is isolated as above and is clamped as close to the insertion as possible. The muscle is then divided from the sclera and the cut end attached just temporal to the lateral border of the IR. It is essential to ensure that the cut ends are bunched together to minimise the risk of inducing an antielevation syndrome (AES). Despite taking these steps, patients can still experience limitation of up-gaze which usually wears off with time. AES manifests as a significant limitation of up-gaze worse in abduction resulting in an apparent inferior oblique overaction in the contralateral eye, often accompanied with Y-pattern exodeviation.

In severe cases, the surgeon should consider reversing the surgery early; revising inferior oblique procedures, specifically isolating the muscle from the inferior rectus, can be challenging once scarring has settled in.

Anterior transpositions can also cause a fullness to the lower lid which can be permanent (Fig. 21).

12 Adjustable Strabismus Surgery

Adjustable sutures can be used to fine tune the results of the strabismus surgery when the patient has regained consciousness, and the fusion mechanisms are active. This is usually performed on the same day but can be performed several days later. The patient should be fully awake and encouraged to move their eyes to stimulate the muscles and allow them to settle into their new position.

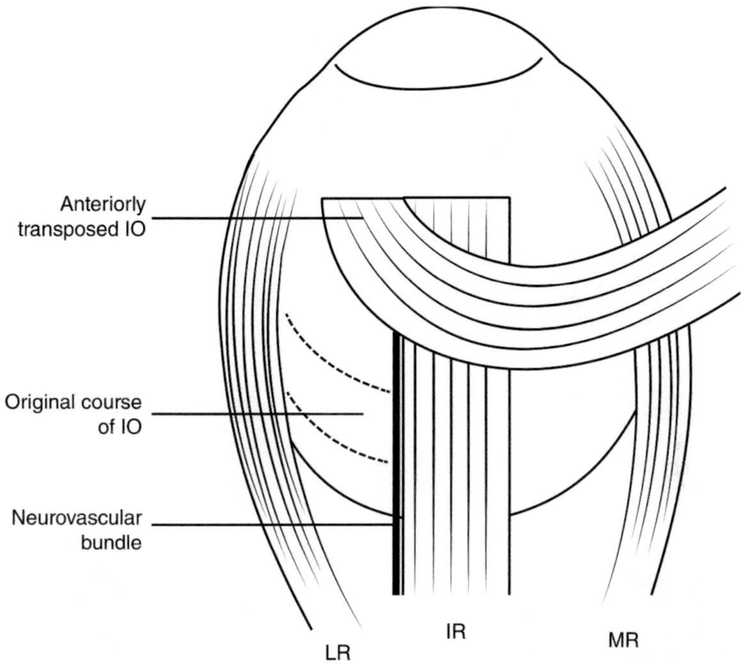

Fig. 21 Inferior oblique anteriorisation where the IO is moved away from its original path to be reinserted just lateral to the lateral border of the IR

Some surgeons also perform an intraoperative adjustment, gauging the position of the eyes under general anaesthesia.

There are two main techniques in use:

(1) Bow tie: The recessed (and sometimes the resected) muscles are placed on a hangback suture with an adjustable securing knot as below. The long ends of the suture can be brought out of the conjunctival incision and taped to the cheek and secured with micropore. This enables easy access to the sutures to perform the adjustment. Some surgeons prefer to bury the sutures under the conjunctiva which carries the advantage of avoiding any further manipulation if the desired effect is achieved but may increase the chance of developing a suture granuloma. If the correction of the deviation is thought to be non-ideal, the bow tie is undone and the muscle moved to try and achieve the desired correction. It thus serves as way to optimise surgical results avoiding further surgery. It is usually helpful to recess more than planned when using an adjustable suture as it is easier to pull the muscle up than to let it out. This can be done in stages, tying a bow tie prior to each subsequent measurement.

If more recession is needed, the bow tie is untied, and a closed Moorfields forceps is placed underneath the knot. The bladed of the forceps are then separated that loosens the knot and another bow tie can then be tied on to secure

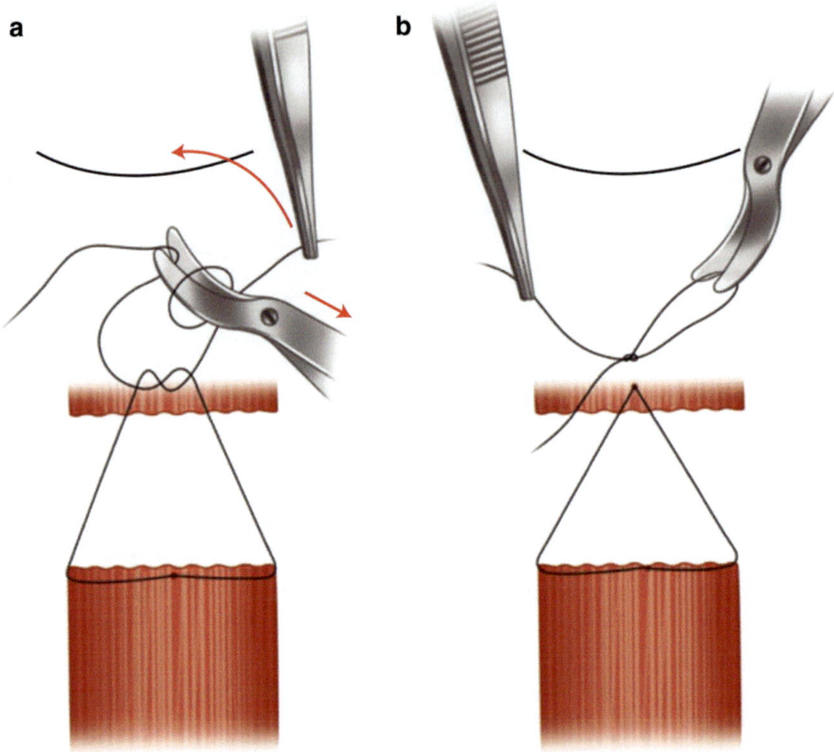

Fig. 22 Hangback recession on an adjustable slipknot. From Jain S. *Simplifying strabismus*. 1 ed. Cham: Springer Nature, 2019

the new suture position. Care must be taken when handling vicryl as it can be friable and snap. Using a non-traumatic instrument such as a needle holder or fingers is recommended.

Once the surgeon and patient are happy with the result, the bow tie can be finally undone and two locking knots put on top using single throws and the suture ends trimmed that will retract back into the conjunctival opening. If necessary, the conjunctiva can then be sutured close (Fig. 22).

Video 12: The use of a hang back adjustable suture on a bow tie while carrying out a LR recession

(2) Sliding noose technique: Alternatively, the suture can be used to adjust the muscle position as shown in Fig. 23. The muscle is secured on a hangback suture as above but a second suture is tied around the first allowing it to be slid up and down the length of the original suture. This allows easy adjustment of the amount of recession depending on the postoperative deviation.

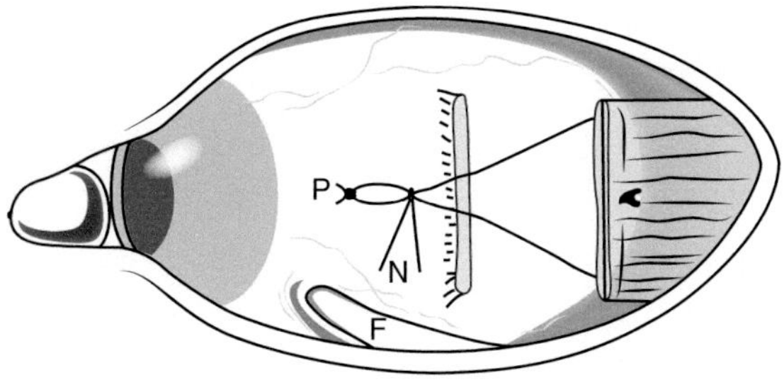

Fig. 23 Short tag noose technique

References

1. Guyton DL. Exaggerated traction test for the oblique muscles. Ophthalmology. 1981;88(10):1035–40. https://doi.org/10.1016/s0161-6420(81)80033-4. PMID: 7335306.
2. Wright KW. Mini-tenotomy procedure to correct diplopia associated with small-angle strabismus. Trans Am Ophthalmol Soc. 2009;107:97–102.
3. Chang MY, Pineles SL, Velez FG. Adjustable small-incision selective tenotomy and plication for correction of incomitant vertical strabismus and torsion. J AAPOS. 2015;19(5):410–6.
4. Roper-Hall G, Cruz OA. Results of combined resection-recession on a single rectus muscle for incomitant deviations-an alternative to the posterior fixation suture. J AAPOS. 2017;21(2):89–93.
5. Mehendale RA, Dagi LR, Wu C, Ledoux D, Johnston S, Hunter DG. Superior rectus transposition and medial rectus recession for Duane syndrome and sixth nerve palsy. Arch Ophthalmol. 2012;130(2):195–201.
6. Nishida Y, Hayashi O, Oda S, et al. A simple muscle transposition procedure for abducens palsy without tenotomy or splitting muscles. Jpn J Ophthalmol. 2005;49(2):179–80.
7. Yamaguchi M, Yokoyama T, Shiraki K. Surgical procedure for correcting globe dislocation in highly myopic strabismus. Am J Ophthalmol. 2010;149(2):341–6.
8. Wright KW. Brown's syndrome: diagnosis and management. Trans Am Ophthalmol Soc. 1999;97:1023–109.
9. Suh DW, Guyton DL, Hunter DG. An adjustable superior oblique tendon spacer with the use of nonabsorbable suture. J AAPOS. 2001;5(3):164–71.
10. Stager Jr D, Dao LM, Felius J. Uses of the Inferior Oblique Muscle in Strabismus Surgery. Middle East Afr J Ophthalmol. 2015;22(3):292–7.
11. Basic and Clinical Science Course. San Francisco: American Academy of Ophthalmology;2010. American Academy of Ophthalmology. Pediatric Ophthalmology and Strabismus.
12. Toosi SH, von Noorden GK. Effect of isolated inferior oblique muscle myectomy in the management of superior oblique muscle palsy. Am J Ophthalmol. 1979;88:602–8.
13. Parks MM. The weakening surgical procedures for eliminating overaction of the inferior oblique muscle. Am J Ophthalmol. 1972;73(1):107–22.
14. Elliott RL, Nankin SJ. Anterior transposition of the inferior oblique. J Pediatr Ophthalmol Strabismus. 1981;18(3):35–8.
15. Stager DR, Weakley DR, Jr, Stager D. Anterior transposition of the inferior oblique. Anatomic assessment of the neurovascular bundle. Arch Ophthalmol. 1992;110:360–2.

Management of Exotropia

Manoj Parulekar, Nervine Elmeshad, and Sanil Shah

Abstract This chapter discusses the management of comitant exotropia (XT) both surgical and non-surgical, as well as the principles of pre-operative assessment and surgical planning. Intermittent Exotropia [X(T)] is by far the most common type of exodeviation encountered in practice and will be the primary focus in this chapter. Evaluation of the level of motor and sensory control, careful pre-operative assessment to avoid re operation, and managing over and under corrections are vital to the success of surgery. Associations such as AHP (abnormal head posture), various alphabetical patterns and DVD/DHD (Dissociated vertical deviation/ Dissociated horizontal deviation) need to be addressed and managed accordingly. Other forms of exotropia will be briefly covered at the end of the chapter.

Keywords Exotropia · Divergent strabismus · Intermittent exotropia · Bilateral or unilateral lateral rectus recession · Medial rectus resection and lateral rectus recession · Overcorrection · Under correction

1 Introduction

Exotropia is a common misalignment of the eye, where the eye deviates outward. The most common type of exotropia seen in practice is intermittent exotropia [1]. Careful history, clinical evaluation of motor control and sensory status are important in decision making [2]. Distance-near disparity can pose a challenge in surgical

M. Parulekar (✉) · N. Elmeshad · S. Shah
Oxford Eye Hospital, Oxford, UK
e-mail: manoj.parulekar@nhs.net

N. Elmeshad
e-mail: nervine.elmeshad@ouh.nhs.uk

S. Shah
e-mail: sanil.shah@ouh.nhs.uk

S. Jain (ed.), *Surgical Management of Strabismus*,
https://doi.org/10.1007/978-3-031-80633-9_4

management and should be an integral part of the assessment [3]. Associated head posture and patterns should be evaluated and addressed. It is important to be aware of potential short and long term complications such as double vision (usually seen with surgical overcorrection).

2 Clinical Evaluation

Presenting Features

- Patients with exotropia usually present with concerns about their appearance or with double vision.
- Eye strain after visual activity or towards the end of the day and intermittent monocular closure particularly in bright sunlight are other common symptoms.
- Rarely, patients complain of micropsia possibly due to the myopic shift resulting from use of accommodative convergence to control exotropia.
- Children are usually asymptomatic, and absence of symptoms may suggest well-developed suppression mechanisms.

Assessment

- Observing the patient before the eyes are dissociated for visual acuity testing provides useful information about control of the squint under normal viewing conditions.

Assessing Home Control:

- Enquire about home control and any change over time. Maintaining a diary of how often the eyes deviate in a day as a percentage or score out of 10 is useful.
- Often parents notice control of the squint worsens in the evening, while tired, daydreaming or when the child is systemically unwell.
- The squint may be more frequently noticed as the child grows and the child and/or parents become more aware of it, or draws comments at school.

Clinic assessment of control:

- Control for distance and near fixation with and without abnormal head posture should be noted.
- It is useful to observe if the child spontaneously manifests the squint, and speed of recovery and effect of blinking on hastening recovery.

Revised Newcastle control score:

- Revised Newcastle control score [4] (Table 1) is one of the many different grading systems proposed to provide objective evaluation of control and help monitor over time.
- A score of 3 or worse is likely to benefit from surgery, while a score of less than 3 is likely to indicate good control and can be observed.

Table 1 The revised Newcastle control score

	Score
Home control	
XT or monocular eye closure seen	
Never	0
< 50% of time fixing in distance	1
> 50% of time fixing in distance	2
> 50% of time fixing in distance + seen at near	3
Clinic control	
Near	
Immediate realignment after dissociation	0
Realignment with aid of blink or re-fixation	1
Remains manifest after dissociation/prolonged fixation	2
Manifest spontaneously	3
Distance	
Immediate realignment after dissociation	0
Realignment with aid of blink or re-fixation	1
Remains manifest after dissociation/prolonged fixation	2
Manifest spontaneously	3
Total NCS: Home + Near + Distance	

- There may however be a bias introduced by parental assessment of home control.

2. *Abnormal head posture:*
   - An abnormal head posture usually indicates an alphabetical pattern in children with X(T), with the head posture aiding control of the deviation.
   - Chin up head posture will aid control of V pattern exotropia, and chin down posture may be seen with A pattern X(T) to control the squint.
   - Abnormal head posture can also be due to incomitant strabismus, nystagmus or non-ocular reasons like neck or spine pathology.

3. *Sensory evaluation*:
   - Patients with Intermittent exotropia usually have some level of binocular vision, and the ability to fuse two images (peripheral fusion with or without central fusion) with a variable level of stereopsis.
   - Binocular vision may be lost if control of the squint deteriorates or if the squint becomes manifest. Surgery can help preserve binocular vision. This is particularly applicable to young children with large angle, largely manifest XT with very poor control [5].
   - Patients with exotropia often have well developed suppression mechanisms, and rarely report diplopia.

- In order to assess the level of binocular vision accurately, the sequence of tests should be arranged so that the least dissociative tests are done first, followed more dissociative tests.

4. *Visual Acuity:*

   - Divergent squints rarely result in amblyopia and visual acuity is usually normal [5]. If amblyopia is at all present, it is usually associated with anisometropia which needs to be treated and could subsequently improve the control of the squint. Conversely, poor vision in one or both eyes can result in a divergent squint. This usually occurs in children over 2 years and adults. Poor vision early in life is more likely to result in a convergent squint.

5. *Motor evaluation*:

   - The angle of deviation should be evaluated using alternate prism cover test, for distance and near fixation in primary position and various positions of gaze. Large differences between distance and near deviations will identify near distance disparity. The near deviation must also be measured with + 3 lenses in front of both eyes to negate the effect of accommodative convergence and differentiate between true and simulated divergence excess (Fig. 1). Measuring the near point of convergence will identify convergence insufficiency. Measurements in lateral gaze will identify lateral incomitance, particularly limitation of adduction. Measuring the distance deviation in up and downgaze will identify A, V or Y patterns.
   - Assessment of control is important. The control of the exodeviation can vary depending on fixation distance, position of gaze (up or downgaze) and degree of tiredness. The speed of recovery of alignment after dissociating the two eyes to make the squint manifest is a useful parameter. As a rule of thumb, inability to regain control beyond 2 blinks indicates poor control. Another useful test is checking ability to regain control in up gaze- the physiological V pattern can accentuate the exodeviation and make it harder to regain control, and might explain some of the patient's symptoms e.g. difficulty with the whiteboard at school.
   - It is important to record the maximum angle when planning surgery to minimise surgical under correction

   Underestimation of angle of deviation can be minimised by:

1. Use of 6 m or far distance target rather than 3 m mirrored target for measurements to reduce the effect of proximal convergence.
2. Prolonged occlusion test with 30–40 min of monocular occlusion helps disrupt fusion and assists measurement of the maximum angle of exodeviation for distance fixation.
3. Measuring the angle of deviation later in the day when the subject is tired.

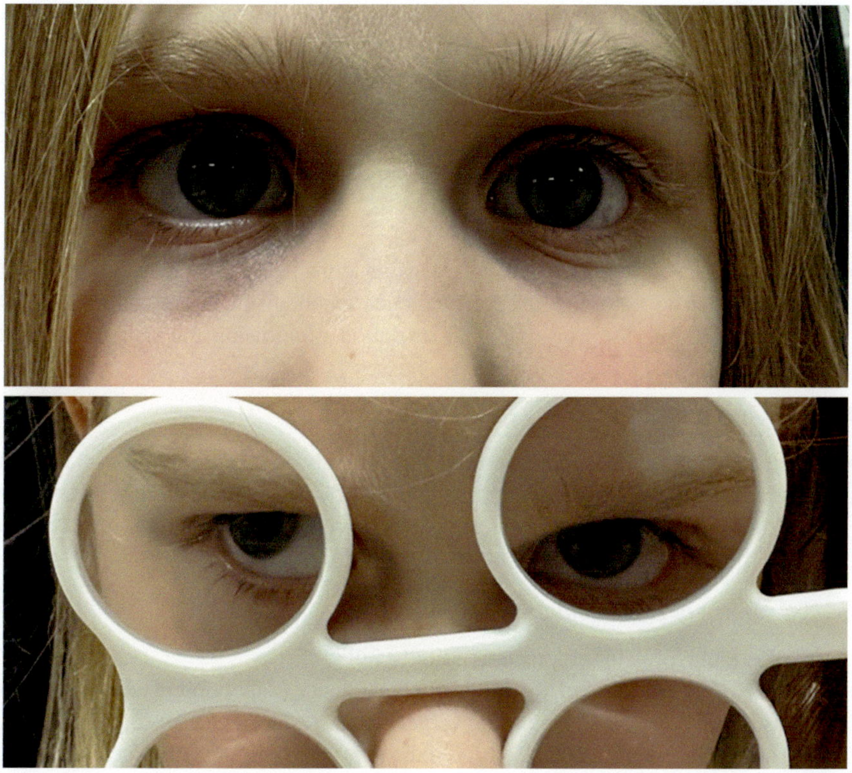

Fig. 1 Assessing the deviation with and without + 3.0 D lenses to negate the effect of accommodative convergence

4. Asking patients/parents to send photographs obtained later in the day to demonstrate the maximum deviation.
5. Care should be taken to hold the near fixation target level with the eyes and avoid holding it in downgaze to avoid interference from any A/V pattern.

Distance-near disparity Exotropia:

- A difference of greater than 10PD between distance and near measurements is considered significant. If the near angle is greater, it is due to convergence insufficiency. When the distance angle is greater, it is referred to as divergence excess. Some individuals use accommodative convergence to control the near deviation, resulting in a smaller angle for near. This is referred to as simulated divergence excess. Measuring the deviation with + 3 dioptre lenses for near fixation helps uncover the true near angle in such cases.

- Several classification systems (e.g. Burian, Kushner) been proposed to help understand the underlying mechanism and plan management [6].
- The patch test and measurement with + 3D lens are useful in assessment. The + 3D test involves placing + 3D lenses (often a flipper as in Fig. 1) to remove the accommodative influence when measuring the near deviation- this helps differentiate between true and simulated divergence excess exotropia.

Prism adaptation test:

- Some patients have mismatch between the objective and subjective angle of deviation due to a strong fusional vergence mechanism. Prism adaptation test can help uncover the true extent of deviation minimising the risk of surgical undercorrection.

Krimsky or modified Krimsky test:

- Prism cover test cannot be performed when the vision is poor in one eye. In such cases, the angle of deviation can be measured by Krimsky or modified Krimsky test (the prism is placed in front of the fixing eye to deviate the light reflex into a central position in the deviating eye) [7].

6. *Assessment of Extra-ocular movements*:
   - The range of ocular motility is usually full.
   - It is important to check the range of convergence (near point of convergence is usually 10 cm) as deficient convergence can result in near distance disparity (convergence insufficiency type exotropia). It is important when planning surgery e.g. greater amount of surgery on medial recti in cases of convergence insufficiency.
   - It is not uncommon for A and V alphabet patterns to be associated with exotropia.
   - The alphabet patterns may be associated with superior oblique (A pattern) or inferior oblique (V pattern) overaction. Y pattern is common among patients with exodeviation; An increase in exotropia in down gaze by > 10PD (A pattern) and in up gaze by 15PD (V or Y pattern) is considered significant.
   - In cases with freely alternating exotropia, it is useful to note the eye that drifts out in up gaze. It is usually the non-dominant eye that drifts which can help decide which eye to operate on.
   - Poor control in up gaze can cause difficulty in viewing the white board at school and indicate the need for surgical correction.

3 Treatment

- Although prognosis for surgery is usually very good for intermittent exotropia, non-surgical measures can be adequate when control is good, or in very young children.

1. **Non-surgical Management**:

   – Non-surgical measures are usually recommended when control of the exotropia is good, particularly in children under the age of visual maturity (6–7 years). This is due to the risk of surgical overcorrection which can result in amblyopia, loss of binocular vision or development of monofixation. Such cases can be observed infrequently in clinic, with patient/parent monitoring control at home.
   – **Observation**: Most cases will be suitable for this approach. The natural history of exotropia is very variable, and some cases will improve with time. There is no urgency to treat in most cases as the risk of amblyopia is minimal, and rapid degradation of binocular vision is unusual. Observation over time can provide valuable information about degree of control, improvement, worsening or stability of the exotropia.
   – **Refractive correction**: Blurred vision related to uncorrected refractive error can affect ability to fuse two images and fusional vergences. All patients with intermittent exotropia should be refracted appropriately.

     Myopic overcorrection (− 1 or − 2D lenses) induces accommodation and accommodative convergence and can be used to temporise, particularly in very young children [8, 9].
     Children usually accept myopic overcorrection better than adults who complain of asthenopia.
     Prisms: Prisms are poorly tolerated and not needed in most cases [10].
     Orthoptic exercises: There is a role for convergence exercises in older children and adults with convergence insufficiency type intermittent exotropia and when the angle of deviation is small.

   – **Botulinum toxin**: has also been tried in the management of exotropia but the benefit lasts a few months. It is usually reserved for symptomatic patients with small deviations who cannot or do not wish to undergo surgery or anaesthesia.
   – **Alternate eye patching**: has been tried to preserve binocular vision and prevent development of amblyopia but there is limited evidence of long term success.

2. **Surgical management**:

   a. **Indications**:

      - The commonest indication for surgery is deterioration in control, evidenced by increasing frequency of manifest deviation (tropia). The Newcastle control score can be helpful.
      - The aims of surgery may be to preserve/ improve binocular vision, relieve double vision, reduce asthenopia and/or to restore normal appearance.

b. **Target angle for surgery**:

- Several studies report residual exotropia following surgery is more common than overcorrection. Many authors recommend initial overcorrection anticipating gradual improvement within the first few months after the surgery.
- However, overcorrection can be associated with bothersome double vision lasting weeks to months, affecting activities such as driving in adults. Overcorrection in children can result in amblyopia and loss of binocular vision.
- Surgery is usually avoided in very young children due to the risk of overcorrection and consecutive esotropia, except in cases with very large deviation or poor control. In such cases the desired outcome is a small undercorrection [11].
- The risk of overcorrection in adults can be minimised with the use of adjustable sutures. These could be fully adjustable on a hang-back suture, or semi adjustable when the recessed muscle is attached with the sclera on a fixed suture and a suture is passed between the original insertion and the central part of the recessed muscle to allow advancement. Both the resected and recessed muscle could be placed on adjustable/semi-adjustable sutures permitting advancement of the recessed muscle or recession of the resected muscle in the event of an overcorrection. Use of adjustable sutures maximises the options for reversal of overcorrection and enables the surgeon to aim for maximum correction without the worry of overcorrection and postoperative diplopia.

4 Types of Surgical Procedures

Lateral rectus weakening procedures

- Recession
- Central tenotomy
- Faden
- Resect-recess procedure or Adjustable faden.

Medial rectus tightening procedures:

- Resection
- Advancement
- Plication
- Central plication.

- The choice of muscles to be operated is determined by the angle of deviation for distance and near fixation. The lateral rectus is most active for distance fixation,

Table 2 Suggested surgical treatment options for Exotropia

Feature of exotropia	Suggested surgical procedure	Principle
Basic exotropia or simulated divergence excess-comitant without true distance-near disparity	LR recession with MR resection/plication	Tight MR possibly act as a leash and reduces risk of recurrence/under correction
True divergence excess	Bilateral lateral rectus recession or asymmetric recess/resect with larger recession of LR	Larger LR recession would correct distance angle more than the near angle
Ture convergence insufficiency	Asymmetric recess/resect with larger MR resection/ plication or bilateral MR resection	MR resection would correct angle for near fixation more

and the medial rectus for near. It therefore follows that lateral rectus recession will have a greater effect on the distance angle and medial rectus resection will have a greater effect for near.

- The safe maximum recession for the lateral rectus is to the equator i.e. 16 mm from the limbus in adults, and slightly smaller in young children. Recessions beyond the equator can result in limitation of abduction and lateral incomitance.
- While there is no consensus on the maximum amount of medial rectus resection/ plication, it is recognised that a large medial rectus resection or plication greater than 7–8 mm reduces the risk of postoperative exotropic drift. The tightened medial rectus can however act as a leash, limiting the range of abduction [12].

Several surgical strategies for various types of exotropia are discussed below. Our preferred approach is summarised in Table 2.

5 Basic and Simulated Divergence Excess Exotropia

- Two randomised controlled trials [13, 14] suggest that unilateral recession-resection procedures have a higher success rate than bilateral lateral rectus recessions, possibly because of the tightened medial rectus muscle acting as a leash and preventing recurrence of exotropia [15].

1. The advantages of unilateral recess resect procedures include easier postoperative care (easier for parents to instill drops in one eye rather than both), equal correction of distance and near angle by dividing the surgery between distance dominant lateral rectus and near dominant medial rectus and restricting any serious risks e.g. scleral perforation to one eye only. Arguably, the biggest benefit is leaving the other eye unoperated in case a further procedure is needed. In the

event of recurrent/residual exotropia following bilateral lateral rectus recession, the only subsequent procedure possible is resection of one or both medial recti. The residual exotropia is often greater for distance, and mechanistically, further surgery should ideally include lateral rectus recession which is not possible in such cases. Bilateral medial rectus resections can also result in considerable restriction of abduction and lateral incomitance. Unilateral recess resect leaves the option of a subsequent procedure on the fellow eye especially lateral rectus recession which improves the chance of full correction.

- The drawbacks of unilateral recess-resect surgery particularly with larger amounts of surgery are limitation of abduction, with diplopia on lateral gaze that improves within weeks, palpebral fissure narrowing and enophthalmos. The risk of overcorrection is greater with a unilateral recess resect procedure than bilateral lateral rectus recession.
- Bilateral lateral rectus recessions are less likely to result in overcorrection, and work well when precise measurements are difficult to obtain e.g. very young children with very large and variable angle exodeviations, or children with developmental delay.
- The authors prefer a unilateral recess resect procedure in most cases of basic and simulated divergence excess exotropia.

6 True Divergence Excess Exotropia

- Bilateral lateral rectus recession is usually considered to be more successful with lower risk of overcorrection.
- Asymmetric recess-resect procedures with higher amounts of lateral rectus recession can also be useful when the difference between Distance and near angle is not very large.
- The risk of overcorrection and consecutive esotropia for near is very low. In the unlikely event of an overcorrection, the medial rectus can be recessed later. Retro-equatorial myopexy (Faden operation) and medial rectus pulley fixation have been tried with variable success.

7 Convergence Insufficiency Type Exotropia

- Orthoptics exercises can be tried before considering surgical options particularly when angle of deviation is not very large.
- Some form of medial rectus tightening procedure is preferred for this type of exotropia.

- Options include unilateral or bilateral medial rectus resection with or without slanting (greater resection of lower half of medial rectus), conventional recession-resection procedure or improved unilateral recession-resection procedure (MR resection based on larger near angle and LR recession based on smaller distance angle).

8 Alphabet Patterns

- Common patterns are V, Y or X patterns.
- Less than 15PD of V pattern and < 10PD of A pattern is usually considered to be insignificant.
- Significant V or Y pattern with inferior oblique overaction is treated with simultaneous bilateral inferior oblique recession.
- Significant A pattern with superior oblique overaction can be treated with bilateral superior oblique weakening
- Alphabet patterns without oblique overaction are usually treated with vertical transposition or slanted recession of horizontal recti.
- Lateral rectus recession alone can correct small V, Y and X patterns too and MR resection can correct small A patterns.

9 Management of Over/Under Correction

Early undercorrection:

- A large angle under/overcorrection in the immediate postoperative period would raise suspicion of partial/complete slipped muscle.
- The patient should be assessed for limitation of ocular motility and re-operated soon for repair of the slipped muscle.

Delayed undercorrection (residual or recurrent exotropia):

- Small undercorrections should be observed initially.
- Overminus glasses or orthoptic exercises can be an option.
- It is not uncommon for the angle to increase over the time. Large angle residual exotropia usually needs repeat surgery.
- Surgical strategies depend on what procedure has been performed previously. If previous surgical records are unavailable, ocular motility patterns e.g. restrictions, and slit lamp examination for conjunctival surgical scars and blood vessel configuration often provide useful clues.
- If previous surgery was unilateral recess-resect, the subsequent procedure is usually considered on the fellow eye to allow maximum room for lateral rectus recession. However, if the deviating eye has poor vision, the patient may prefer

further surgery on the same eye due to the small but serious risks such as ocular perforation. This would involve exploring and further recessing the lateral rectus to the equator (usually 9 mm from the insertion or 16 mm from the limbus) and medial rectus resection/plication/advancement depending on intra-operative findings. If the lateral rectus is maximally recessed, central tenectomy of the lateral rectus can further weaken (lengthen) the lateral rectus without altering the point of contact of the muscle, avoiding recession beyond the equator and risk of inducing limitation of abduction The use of adjustable sutures is advisable in such cases. There is some risk of inducing lateral incomitance from repeat surgery on a previously operated eye, but this is rarely problematic.

- If the previous procedure involved bilateral lateral rectus recession, the surgical options include exploring and further recessing the lateral rectus to maximum (usually 9 mm from the insertion or 16 mm from the limbus) or a central tenectomy, along with medial rectus resection/plication on the deviating eye. An alternative is unilateral/bilateral medial rectus resection/plication and avoiding further surgery on the lateral rectus. The authors prefer the former approach.

Over-correction:

- Many surgeons consider 8–10PD of consecutive esotropia as the target in the immediate postoperative period.
- Overcorrections are commonly associated with double vision. Spontaneous recovery of even large angle consecutive esotropia is not uncommon within a few days to weeks, especially with unilateral recess resect surgery as the resected medial rectus stretches.
- Most cases can be managed conservatively. Full hyperopic correction, monocular occlusion (typically patching the two eyes alternately) or Fresnel prisms can help.
- If spontaneous improvement is not seen, repeat surgery (usually after 6 months except in very young children when early correction of consecutive esotropia can preserve binocular vision) in the form of medial rectus recession or lateral rectus advancement may be necessary.

10 Other Forms of Concomitant Exotropia

Congenital (Infantile) Exotropia

- Congenital (infantile) exotropia is rare and often associated with other pathology such as craniofacial anomalies, hypoxic ischaemic encephalopathy (cerebral palsy) or ocular albinism [16].
- In contrast to normal variable small angle exotropia seen in newborns (neonatal ocular misalignments), congenital exotropia presents with a large angle misalignment. The angle may be constant or maximally manifest but variable. Amblyopia is common (Fig. 2).

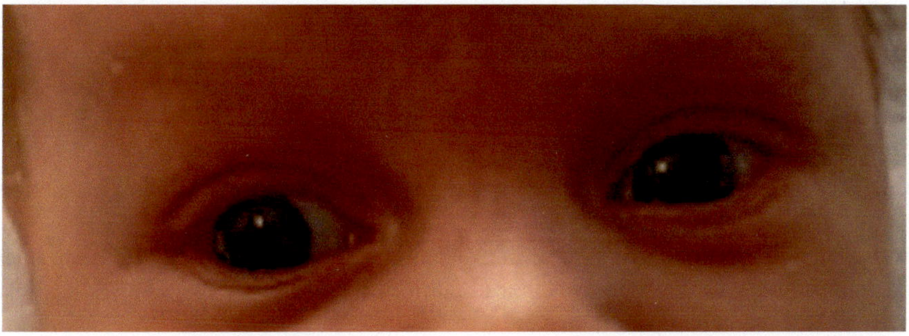

Fig. 2 Infantile exotropia (large angle)

- Surgical correction in the form of bilateral lateral rectus muscle recession or recession of the lateral rectus and resection of the medial rectus improves cosmesis and can maximise the chances of developing binocular vision. The authors prefer bilateral lateral rectus recessions if the angle is highly variable to minimise the risk of overcorrection. If there is a large angle constant deviation, a unilateral recess resect procedure is preferred to leave the other eye unoperated should a subsequent operation for residual/recurrent exotropia become necessary.

11 Dissociated Horizontal Deviation (DHD)

DHD is a type of intermittent exotropia of the non-fixing eye, often associated with latent nystagmus possibly due to microtropia and can be controlled by convergence dampening [17].

- The expression of DHD depends on the fixation, visual acuity, and the level of nystagmus in the dominant eye in relation to the other eye.
- Although more commonly associated with esotropia, DHD can be seen in exotropia, particularly after surgical correction of infantile esotropia.
- There may be associated Dissociated vertical deviation (DVD).
- DHD, if cosmetically significant, can be improved with a lateral rectus weakening procedure on the affected eye. Medial rectus resection should be avoided in DHD as there is a significant risk of overcorrection and consecutive esotropia for near.

Sensory Exotropia

- Sensory exotropia is secondary to poor vision in one/both eyes and consequently reduced fusion. Causes of reduced vision include refractive errors, corneal or lenticular opacities, aphakia, optic nerve, and retinal pathology. The incidence of sensory exotropia in children varies from 2.7 to 10.2%.
- Surgical correction in the form of lateral rectus recession and medial rectus resection is commonly aimed at correcting the cosmetic appearance.

- As there is usually no binocularity, the rate of recurrence can be high. Long term outcome studies suggest younger patients with larger preoperative deviation had a higher risk of recurrence [18].

Consecutive Exotropia

- Consecutive exotropia may result spontaneously or following surgical correction of esotropia.
- Spontaneous consecutive exotropia is usually associated with poor vision in one/both eyes due to underlying ocular conditions and/or amblyopia. Anisometropia is a common accompaniment.
- Consecutive exotropia following previous (typically childhood) strabismus surgery for infantile or accommodative esotropia often presents in childhood or early adulthood. Depending on whether the previous procedure involved unilateral recess resect surgery or bilateral medial rectus recession, there may be adduction deficit in one or both eyes. Several mechanisms have been proposed such as poor convergence, reduced AC:A ratio, stretching of the medial rectus scar, over-recession beyond the equator, and the viscous drag of the orbital tissues dragging the poorly sighted eye to line up with the long axis of the orbit which is at 23 degrees divergent from the sagittal plane.
- Assessment of horizontal saccades can help differentiate between a stretched medial rectus and a tight lateral rectus. A rapid adducting saccade with an abrupt termination usually indicates a tight lateral rectus. Slower floating adducting saccade which ends prematurely, followed by a small further adducting saccade often indicates a stretched medial rectus.
- Slit lamp examination may reveal a recessed caruncle suggesting a previously recessed medial rectus. Lack of the ciliary vessel pattern under the medial conjunctiva is also suggestive of a previously recessed medial rectus (Figs. 3 and 4).

- The maximum angle of deviation must be determined, often with measurements later in the day, and photos showing the maximum deviation provided by patients/parents.

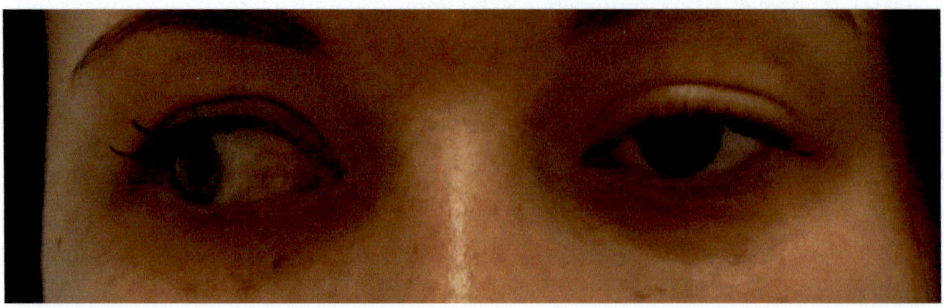

Fig. 3 Right consecutive exotropia-note the recessed caruncle following previous medial rectus recession

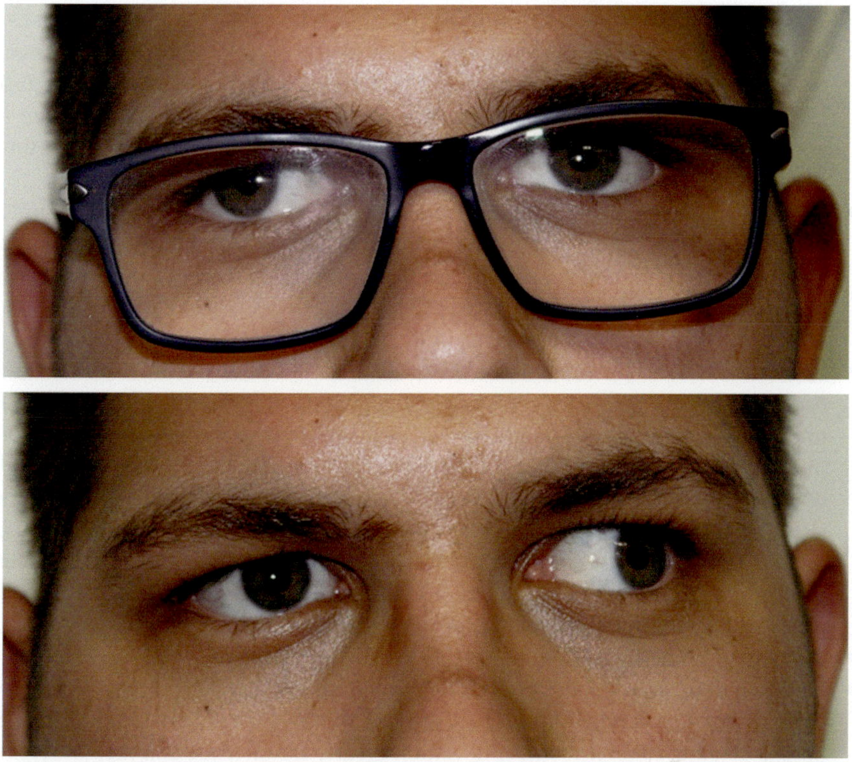

Fig. 4 A Right consecutive exotropia. B Right adduction deficit suggests recessed medial rectus ± tight lateral rectus

- Careful attention must be paid to incomitance. The deviation must be measured fixing with each eye. The incomitance is often due to asymmetric limitation of adduction in the two eyes. The deviating eye is often the eye with the greater adduction deficit. Occasionally, the fixing eye (usually with better vision) has a larger adduction deficit, and there is considerable incomitance. The mechanism here is the fixing eye must make a greater effort to achieve central position, creating fixation duress and greater innervation flowing to the contralateral lateral rectus (Hering's law) which results in a large secondary deviation.
- Surgical strategies must be directed to the deviating eye. If the fixing eye has better range of movement with fuller adduction, surgery can be performed on the deviating eye alone. The angle is usually large and requires surgery on two muscles.
- Surgical management involves forced duction test, particularly to look for a tight lateral rectus. This is followed by incisions over the original (native) site of muscle insertions, and exploration of (the previously operated) medial rectus, as well as the lateral rectus before deciding on the surgical dose.

- The medial rectus is often found to be recessed, with or without a stretched scar or pseudo tendon [19]. Care must be taken as the pseudo tendon can dehisce, resulting in slippage of the medial rectus muscle. We recommend a safety 6/0 Vicryl or similar suture through the muscle belly immediately after passing a hook under the recessed medial rectus before further manipulation to avoid this risk.
- If the lateral rectus is found to be previously resected, the inferior oblique muscle may be found drawn forward in some cases, adherent to the lateral rectus resection scar. The inferior oblique must be gently separated from the lateral rectus by interposing a squint hook between the two, or sharp dissection of the intermuscular septum before further manipulation of the lateral rectus.
- If the medial rectus is found to be recessed, it should be advanced to correct the exodeviation, and to improve the range of adduction, if it was deficient. Recessed muscles do not remain slack and shorten over time to take up the slack. Advancement of a previously recessed (and therefore shortened) muscle is a very powerful operation, and can correct up to 4 prism dioptres per mm of advancement. This is because advancing the muscle insertion increases the mechanical advantage of the muscle, and advancing a previously recessed (therefore shortened) muscle further adds to the correction. In addition, the effect is greatest with the medial rectus as it has the shortest arc of contact with the globe.
- If the lateral rectus was tight on forced duction test, it should be recessed.
- For deviations upto 20 Prism dioptres, single muscle surgery may suffice. The choice of muscle would depend upon whether the deviation is greater for distance or near fixation (lateral rectus if deviation greater for distance and medial rectus if greater for near), any limitation of saccades on eye movement testing (slower adducting saccade would support medial rectus advancement while abrupt end to adducting saccade would support lateral rectus recession) and findings on forced duction test (finding a tight lateral rectus would support lateral rectus recession).
- For deviations greater than 20 prism dioptres, medial rectus advancement with lateral rectus recession, both on adjustable sutures is advisable.
- The aim is usually to leave the eyes slightly esotropic, anticipating an exotropic drift over time. However, some patients do not like the appearance of an esotropic eye, and prefer an undercorrection. It is important to have the discussion prior to surgery to ascertain the preference of the patient, so the surgeon can aim for the desired outcome.

References

1. Von Noorden GK, Campos EC. Binocular vision and ocular motility. 6th ed. St. Louis: Mosby; 2002. p. 367.
2. Burian HM. Exodeviations: their classification, diagnosis and treatment. Am Ophthalmol. 1966;62(6):1161–6.

3. Kushner BJ, Morton GV. Distance/near differences in intermittent exotropia. Arch Ophthalmol. 1998;116(4):478–86.
4. Buck D, Clarke MP, Haggerty H, et al. Grading the severity of intermittent distance exotropia: the revised Newcastle Control Score. Br J Ophthalmol. 2008;92(4):577.
5. Mohney BG. Common forms of childhood strabismus in an incidence cohort. Am J Ophthalmol. 2007;144:465–7.
6. Kushner BJ. Forty-five years of studying intermittent exotropia—what have I learned? The WSPOS keynote strabismus lecture, October 3, 2020. J Binocul Vis Ocul Motil. 2022;72(3):131–8. Epub 2022 Jul 12. Erratum in: J Binocul Vis Ocul Motil. 2022;72(4):248. PMID: 35819892.
7. Choi RY, Kushner BJ. The accuracy of experienced strabismologists using the Hirschberg and Krimsky tests. Ophthalmology. 1998;105:1301–6.
8. Caltrider N, Jampolsky A. Overcorrecting minus lens therapy for treatment of intermittent exotropia. Ophthalmology. 1983;90(10):1160–5.
9. Kushner BJ. Does overcorrecting minus lens therapy for intermittent exotropia cause myopia? Arch Ophthalmol. 1999;117(5):638–42.
10. Hardesty HH. Prisms in the management of intermittent exotropia. Am Orthopt J. 1972;22:22–30.
11. SY Suh et al. Outcomes of surgery in children with early-onset exotropia.ye (2013) 27, 836–840
12. Wright KW. Mini-tenotomy procedure to correct diplopia associated with small-angle strabismus. Trans Am Ophthalmol Soc. 2009;107:97–103.
13. Donahue SP, Chandler DL, et al. Pediatric eye disease investigator group. eight-year outcomes of bilateral lateral rectus recessions versus unilateral recession-resection in childhood basic-type intermittent exotropia. Ophthalmology. 2024;131(1):98–106.
14. Pediatric Eye Disease Investigator Group; Writing Committee; Donahue SP, Chandler DL, Holmes JM, Arthur BW, Paysse EA, Wallace DK, Petersen DB, Melia BM, Kraker RT, Miller AM. A randomized trial comparing bilateral lateral rectus recession versus unilateral recess and resect for basic-type intermittent exotropia. Ophthalmology. 2019;126(2):305–17.
15. Choi J, Chang JW, Kim SJ, Yu YS. The long-term survival analysis of bilateral lateral rectus recession versus unilateral recession-resection for intermittent exotropia. Am J Ophthalmol. 2012;153(2):343-351.e341.
16. Wan MJ, Chiu H, Shah AS, Hunter DG. Long-term surgical outcomes for large-angle infantile esotropia. Am J Ophthalmol. 2018;189:155–9.
17. Brodsky MC. Dissociated horizontal deviation: clinical spectrum, pathogenesis, evolutionary underpinnings, diagnosis, treatment, and potential role in the development of infantile esotropia (an American Ophthalmological Society thesis). Trans Am Ophthalmol Soc. 2007;105:272–93.
18. Varrone E, et al. Surgical outcomes in sensory exotropia. J AAPOS. 2023;27(147):e1-5.
19. Hatt SR, Leske DA, Jung JH, Holmes JM. Intraoperative findings in consecutive exotropia with and without adduction deficit. Ophthalmology. 2017;124(6):828–34.

Esotropia in Children

Robert Taylor

Abstract The management of childhood esotropia encompasses various presentations and requires a tailored approach for each case. Childhood esotropia, common especially below the age of five, presents in diverse forms such as intermittent, sudden onset, or constant esotropia. Accurate examination, including visual acuity measurement, alignment assessment, and cycloplegic refraction, is crucial for diagnosis and treatment planning. While some children may resist examination due to age or other factors, close follow-up is recommended to avoid missing significant refractive errors, a treatable cause of poor vision and esotropia. Treatment typically involves correcting refractive errors, addressing amblyopia if present, and considering alignment surgery to promote binocular vision or improve appearance. Surgical intervention aims to align the eyes, with early correction potentially enhancing binocular function and techniques vary based on factors like age, degree of deviation, and associated conditions like developmental delay. Patient/parent counselling is essential to discuss the benefits, risks, and potential need for repeat surgeries. Effective treatment involves a combination of refractive correction, amblyopia management, and surgical intervention tailored to each case's unique presentation and goals.

Keywords Childhood esotropia · Infantile · Sensory · Accommodative · Refraction

1 Introduction

Childhood esotropia is common particularly under the age of five. Some children present with an intermittent strabismus, with parents, carers or teachers observing a strabismus despite aligned eyes on examination. Some present with a sudden onset of esotropia and others have a constant esotropia. Patients with a pseudostrabismus need to be excluded.

R. Taylor (✉)
York Teaching Hospital, York, UK
e-mail: robert.taylor41@nhs.net

S. Jain (ed.), *Surgical Management of Strabismus*,
https://doi.org/10.1007/978-3-031-80633-9_5

Key examination findings include measurement of visual acuity in each eye, alignment, binocular vision, and control (if relevant), refractive error based on cycloplegia and a structural exam of each eye to confirm clear media and healthy posterior segment structures.

In some children accurate measurement is not possible because of their age, resistance to be examined, so close follow up is recommended. However, it is essential that a large refractive error is not missed as this is a cause of poor vision and esotropia and is eminently treatable. Cycloplegic refraction is mandatory.

Treat any refractive error, then treat any amblyopia, followed by alignment surgery. Surgery is indicated to promote binocular vision, or improve appearance, or both. It is not always possible to predict what will be needed at presentation, for example glasses alone might be sufficient to treat visual acuity, alignment and restore binocular vision. It is also not possible to predict for how long the child will require optical correction.

Consent for surgical correction requires a discussion of the benefits and risks.

2 Infantile Esotropia

Introduction

The primary aim of management is to align the eyes and promote binocular vision, reduce the prevalence of secondary adverse effects of poor binocular vision (latent nystagmus and dissociated vertical deviation) and normalise the child's life.

History

Presentation is often below 12 months of age but may be delayed due to a variety of reasons, including parental observation, false reassurance, referral, or system delays. The history is usually of large esotropia from before 6 months of life. Use of family photographs is very helpful. There is usually no family history and the presence of accommodative esotropia in the family history raises the possibility of accommodative esotropia with an early presentation. Developmental factors are important in guiding surgical management.

Prior Strabismus Surgery

Not present.

Examination

Visual acuity readings are dictated by age and cooperation. A search for any inequality in acuity is important to exclude a sensory issue that may be unilateral (e.g. optic nerve hypoplasia) or amblyopia. Amblyopia is rare due to cross fixation. Refractive error is commonly a low hypermetropia, normal for this age group. Demonstration of full abduction is desirable to exclude a sixth nerve or other motility disorder such as Duane Retraction syndrome. In the first year to 18 months of life, manifest/latent

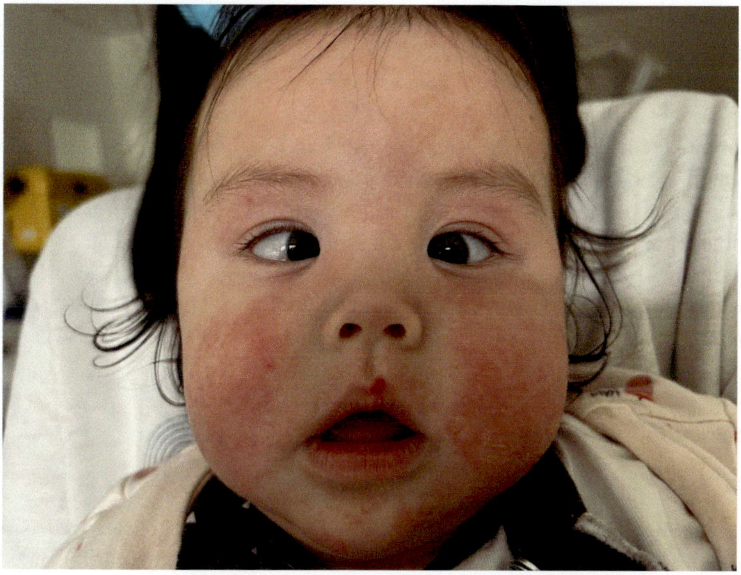

Fig. 1 Photograph of 1 year old with large angle esotropia. Note the displaced corneal reflexes

nystagmus is rare and its presence needs further enquiry. Measurement of the angle of deviation is difficult in this age group and use of prism reflection maybe the best guide to surgical dosage (Fig. 1).

Non Surgical Treatment

Children under 1 year are commonly hypermetropic and if more than 2.00 dioptres may be worth consideration of refractive correction. Any glasses trial may not help the alignment and needs to be viewed in the context of delay to surgical alignment.

Timing

Timing is important with data suggesting that early alignment may be rewarded with some binocular functions. Ideal surgical time is debated, the suggestion here is first surgery at 10–12 months aiming for alignment by 14 months of age [1].

Aim of Surgery

To align the eyes using toxin, surgery or both. A small under correction is desirable.

Surgical Dosage

Use of toxin alone will often require repeat or later surgery [2], with a non randomised prospective cohort study suggesting better results for surgery as compared to toxin, if the angle is larger than 30 prism dioptres [3].

Unilateral recess resect or bilateral medial rectus surgery are both in common practice. A review published in 2023 concluded there was no sound evidence to base this decision on, so this must remain a surgeon's preference [4].

For patients with angles above 55 prism diopters, options include a larger bilateral medial rectus recession, considering three horizontals (usually both medial recti and a unilateral lateral rectus resection) or augmenting standard bilateral medial rectus recession with botulinum toxin [5, 6]. Large surgical doses of bilateral medial rectus recession are associated with a high rate of consecutive exotropia [7].

Children with developmental delay may require a reduced surgical dose, [8] as they are prone to a large and sometimes intractable over corrections. These children are good candidates for toxin alone.

Adjustable

Not relevant.

Patient/Parent Counselling

The parents need to be educated about the wish to promote binocular vision, the lack of non surgical options and the ideal timing. Surgical complications need to be discussed, including the rate of repeat surgery [8].

Surgical Technique

Forced Duction

Forced ductions are usually normal, or a mild resistance to abduction.

Inspection

Normal conjunctiva and muscle anatomy.

Conjunctival Incision

Fornix or limbal incisions are commonly used.

Muscle Surgery

Medial rectus recession is complicated by difficult access in a small eye. A decision will need to be made as to how to re-attach the muscle to sclera. Commonly attachment is desired 10–11 mm back from the limbus. If passing a scleral bite is difficult, consider a modified hang back [9]. In general, avoid hang backs anchored only at the original insertion due to the concern about poor attachment and late over correction.

Adjustable

Not appropriate.

Closure

Conjunctival closure can be with 8/0 vicryl (polyglactin) or, in the case of fornix incisions, left alone. This is followed by a drop of broad spectrum antibiotic.

Local Anaesthesia

A small bolus of 1% lignocaine can be made in the tenons capsule around the operated muscles. This can be delivered using a blunt cannula (e.g. lacrimal cannula) avoiding the risk of bleeding. This can be given before or after conjunctival closure. A drop of local anaesthetic can be added.

Post Operative Management

Counselling

Parents can be told that their children return from the operating theatre hungry, confused and with sore eyes. Children will often sleep for an hour or so. Care needs to be exercised giving too much food quickly as the children may not be able to keep it down.

Normal activities are to be encouraged immediately although avoid swimming for 2–4 weeks.

No patch is required.

Medication

Use of post operative medication varies and may include a topical steroid, topical antibiotic or no drops.

Complications

Early discomfort should not be too severe and manageable with systemic paracetamol. Infection may occur in the periorbital tissues and endophthalmitis is rare [10]. Wound issues such as granuloma formation are also unusual.

Late under and over correction can occur leading to further surgery, as well as emergence of dissociated vertical deviation, inferior oblique overaction and manifest/latent nystagmus. Early surgery is thought to protect against these manifestations of poor binocular vision [11].

3 Acquired Esotropia in Childhood

3.1 Accommodative Esotropia

Introduction

The main purpose of surgery is to align eyes once refractive error and amblyopia is corrected. This main indication is to improve appearance. There may be some binocular development to gain in younger children, and binocular vision may be restored in children who had binocular vision prior to esotropia onset, for example following a sudden onset esotropia.

Once glasses have been prescribed, the angle of deviation at distance will be the main indication for surgery, and to guide the surgical dose. Care must be exercised to ensure that (a) the full hypermetropic prescription is as measured i.e. remove working distance only, and (b) the glasses are worn. Operating when these factors are not fulfilled may lead to recurrence and multiple unsuccessful procedures. Confirming parents understand that the surgery does not eliminate the need for glasses, nor the esotropia when glasses not worn.

History

The common presentation is of a young child whose parents, grandparents, or other care givers notice one eye turning in, intermittently, when tired. The frequency, length of time before presentation, and age of onset are highly variable. There is commonly a family history in first- or second-degree relatives, which may be a sensitive issue.

Prior Surgery

Not present.

Examination

Visual acuity recording and refraction are key features. The decision as to what initial glasses prescription to give is based on a cycloplegic refraction. Debate exists about the ideal drug or drugs to give for cycloplegia, and the length of time between administration and measurement. Commonly cyclopentolate 1% is administered with proxymetacaine anaesthetic first to reduce discomfort and enhance absorption. A delay of 30 min is recommended before retinoscopy. If there is a suggestion that cycloplegia is incomplete it is always worth repeating retinoscopy after a longer time period or consider an atropine refraction. In the presence of hypermetropia, the angle of deviation without optical prescription is of little relevance. The angle of deviation, measured at distance, with the full optical prescription with an alternating prism cover test, and following a period of adaption, is the most relevant to surgical planning.

Non Surgical Treatment

The "full" cycloplegic refraction is prescribed, meaning the lens power that neutralises the retinoscopic reflex minus working distance only. Full time wear is advised. A conversation about glasses fitting is essential, as poorly fitting frames will either not be worn or will be ineffective if the child is looking over the top. As children are small and look up frequently, the frames should be large enough to allow up gaze through the lenses.

There is no consensus as to what constitutes a significant hypermetropic prescription. There may be situations where as little as +1.00 dioptres are worth a trial, particularly if astigmatism and or anisometropia present.

Amblyopia treatment is completed if indicated before surgical intervention, either with an acceptable outcome (definition one line difference) or an acceptance that all avenues have been tried and abandoned (Fig. 2).

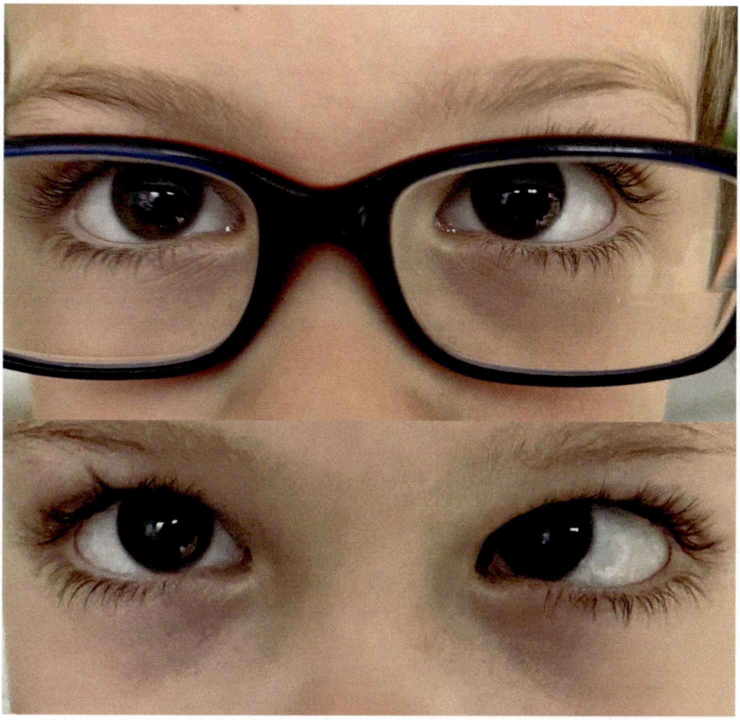

Fig. 2 Photograph of child showing large angle esotropia without glasses, and straight eyes with glasses

Surgical Aim/Planning

Timing of surgical correction is fluid. The aim is alignment or slight under correction and can be modified if binocular vision is expected.

Consideration of unilateral or bilateral surgery will be dictated by surgeon preference, age, and amblyopia. The surgical angle will usually require two muscle surgery. If there is a surgeon preference for bilateral medial rectus recession, then bilateral surgery may come as a surprise to parents and or child, as they see only one eye being the problem.

Predictability, reproducibility, reversibility, and post-operative course can be used as justification for bilateral medial rectus recession. However, if the child is beyond the age of amblyopia treatment and has an amblyopic eye with poor vision, then this justification may be outweighed by the small but real risk of damage to the operated eye if a complication were to arise, so unilateral recess resect on the strabismic eye may be preferred.

Some patients have a larger angle at near fixation, than distance fixation, in their full correction. If there is no binocular vision, aim for the distance angle and accept an under correction at near. (For those with binocular vision at distance and a near angle see high AC/A convergence excess esotropia.)

Prism Adaption

If there is potential for binocular vision, cases may be amenable to prism adaption. Temporary prisms are placed, equal to the surgical angle, over the distance correction and the binocular status is tested. If the angle grows and stabilises with binocular vision established, operate for the larger angle. If there is no binocular status established, or the angle just continues to grow above 50 prism diopters, operate on the initial angle [12].

Dosage

Dosage tables are available in literature [13, 14] and discussed in Sect. 5. Any surgeon should audit their own results and adjust accordingly.

Adjustable

Usually not relevant.

Patient/Parent Counselling

The parents need to be educated about the aim of surgery, to promote or restore binocular vision if relevant, the lack of any urgency (unless binocular vision probable), the absence of any upper age for surgery. Surgical complications need to be discussed, including the rate of exotropic drift [10, 15].

Surgical Technique

Forced Duction

Usually normal, although a tight medical rectus may be encountered in the strabismic eye. Adjusting the surgical dose is rarely needed.

Inspection

Normal conjunctiva and muscle anatomy.

Conjunctival Incision

Fornix or limbal incisions are commonly used.

Muscle Surgery

No particular issues should be encountered. As for infantile esotropia—direct attachment of the recessed muscle to the sclera may reduce long term exotropia drift or the development of a "stretched scar".

Adjustable

Not appropriate.

Local Anaesthesia

A small bolus of 1% lignocaine can be made in the tenons capsule around the operated muscles. This can be delivered using a lacrimal cannula avoiding the risk of causing bleeding. This can be given before or after conjunctival closure. A drop of local anaesthetic may also be used.

Closure

Conjunctival closure can be with 8/0 vicryl or in the case of fornix incisions, left alone. This is followed by a drop of broad spectrum antibiotic.

Post Operative Management

Counselling

Parents can be told that their children return from the operating theatre hungry, confused and with sore eyes. After initial return children will often sleep for an hour or so. Care needs to be exercised giving too much food quickly as the children may not be able to keep it down.

Normal activities are to be encouraged immediately although avoid swimming for 2–4 weeks.

No patch is required.

Medication

Use of post operative medication varies and may include a topical steroid, topical antibiotic or no drops as a routine.

Complications

The most common complication of accommodative esotropia is long term consecutive exotropia [15]. It is difficult to know what the lifetime risk might be, but a reasonable reference is 20%. Aiming for an undercorrection and secure medial rectus attachments are attempts to reduce this complication.

3.2 Sudden Onset Esotropia

Introduction

Sudden onset esotropia may present as an emergency or via routine channels. The assumption is that binocular vision was present prior to the sudden change. This may or may not be the case and may be difficult to elucidate.

History

A child age suddenly develops a large constant esotropia, or in some cases, esotropia may be intermittent. The initial presentation may occur at the time of an illness. Double vision is reported by older children.

Prior Surgery

Not relevant.

Examination

Visual acuity recording and refraction are key features. Acuity is usually equal and normal. If the acuity is unequal a thorough search should be made to exclude a structural cause of the reduced vision. Abduction is normal. Cycloplegic refraction is important and if there is a suggestion that cycloplegia is incomplete it is always worth repeating early, and or consider an atropine refraction.

Investigations

If there is no significant hypermetropia on cycloplegic refraction, there is concern that a sudden esotropia may be secondary to intracranial pathology. Demonstration of full abduction (to exclude sixth nerve paresis) and normal optic discs is helpful. However, if concern exists consideration of cranial imaging or referring for a paediatric opinion may be reasonable.

Non Surgical Treatment

The "full" cycloplegic refraction is given as per accommodative esotropia.

Aim/Planning

If alignment and binocular vision is not restored with glasses (usually due to insignificant amounts), the surgical intervention can be considered urgently.

The aim is to restore alignment as soon as possible to regain binocular vision. Botulinum toxin can be administered to the one or both medial recti. This would require a general anaesthetic in children [16]. However this may require multiple injections and so multiple general anaesthetics. If alignment is restored with toxin, and the esotropia recurs, surgical alignment is recommended as opposed to repeat toxin.

Consideration of unilateral or bilateral surgery as per accommodative esotropia [17].

Prism Adaption

Some cases may be amenable to prism adaption. The surgical angle is placed in temporary prisms and the binocular status is tested. If the angle grows and stabilises with binocular vision established, operate for the larger angle. If no binocular status is established or the angle grows to above 50 prism dioptres, operate on the initial angle [18].

Dosage

Dosage tables are available.

Adjustable

Usually not relevant.

Patient/Parent Counselling

As per accommodative esotropia.

Surgical Technique

As per accommodative esotropia.

Complications

The complication profile is greatly influenced by the presence of binocular vision. If the esotropia developed because of loss of control of an esophoria, and binocular vision is restored, the outcome should (in theory) be stable long term.

In some children re-alignment surgery may not be followed by the restoration of binocular vision. In these children the long term exotropic drift may be present as per accommodative esotropia.

3.3 *High AC/A, Convergence Excess Esotropia*

Introduction

The intention here is to describe treatment for those patients with binocular vision at distance (including a microtropia) using their hypermetropic correction if required. The indication for surgery in this group, is restoring comfortable binocular vision at near without the use of bifocal glasses [19].

Once refraction is prescribed many children will obtain binocular vision at distance and near (termed fully accommodative esotropia). In a proportion of children this state is complicated by an esotropia at near caused by increased accommodative driven convergence (high accommodative convergence per accommodation or AC/A). These children therefore break down to a manifest esotropia at near when concentrating on small detail. This may be developmental, i.e. they were initially fully accommodative and controlled, then developed the esodeviation at near over time.

History

The common presentation is of a young child whose parents notice one eye turning in, intermittently, commonly when tired as per accommodative esotropia, or noticing double vision at near having previously adapted well to hypermetropic glasses.

Prior Surgery

Not relevant.

Examination

Visual acuity recording and refraction are key features. The decision as to what initial glasses prescription to give is based on a cycloplegic refraction. If there is a suggestion that cycloplegia is incomplete it is always worth repeating early, and or consider an atropine refraction. Assessing AC/A is more accurate with minus lenses at distance to eliminate proximal convergence. The gradient method is ideal if this can be completed. Identification of the least possible additional lens required to establish binocular vision at near guides the power of the bifocal.

Non Surgical Treatment

The "full" cycloplegic refraction is given as per accommodative esotropia. Full time wear is advised. If a high AC/A is found, then bifocal glasses are recommended. This has a dual effect of allowing binocular vision to be re-established at near, and also allows whatever hypermetropic correction to be given at distance, no matter how small. Therefore, even small distance prescriptions should be given because the primary purpose of the glasses is for the bifocal. A split pupil bifocal is recommended. Prescribing these may require communication with the dispensing optometrist and a large "D seg" is preferred over an executive bifocal as the glasses are lighter (and cheaper).

A period of time may be needed for binocular vision to become re-established. If this fails to take place, and the child does not voluntarily raise their head to view a near target and so use the bifocal, the use of a bifocal can be abandoned, and the child managed as per accommodative esotropia with a near distance disparity.

Aim/Planning

As binocular vision is achieved by the bifocal the purpose of surgery is to eliminate the need for that bifocal. If bifocal glasses are an acceptable treatment, continued use is an option, and or conversion to a variable focus spectacle with the varifocal corridor set higher than would be ordered for an adult presbyope [20]. However, surgery may be more effective in restoring binocular function [21].

The surgical angle is the near angle without the bifocal (or through the distance segment) looking at an accommodative target [22]. This will usually require two muscle surgery. Bilateral medial rectus recession is often preferred.

Some authors have advocated a "Scott" modification (combined recession-resection) to try and reduce the risk of an exotropia drift [23]. Others have suggested posterior fixation sutures on the medial recti, slanted recession, augmented recession, and pulley surgery [24–26].

Dosage

The dose is based on the angle at near viewed through the distance prescription.

Adjustable

Usually not relevant.

Patient/Parent Counselling

As per accommodative esotropia

Surgical technique

As per accommodative esotropia with consideration of Scott and/or posterior fixation.

Complications

The most common complication of bilateral medial rectus recession is long term consecutive exotropia. Binocular vision should protect against this.

4 Sensory Esotropia

Introduction

In children a poorly sighted eye often becomes esotropic, opposite to the sensory exotropia seen in adults. Management to improve sight will take precedence. However, circumstances may dictate that the sight will remain poor (for example a unilateral optic nerve hypoplasia).

The aims of management are to obtain good appearance for the longest possible time.

History

The common presentation is of a young child whose parents notice one eye turning in.

There may be history of trauma.

Prior Surgery

Prior trauma or glaucoma surgery may have disturbed the conjunctiva and or muscles.

Examination

Visual acuity recording and refraction remain key features. The angle of deviation may require a prism reflection test.

Non Surgical Treatment

Any prescription of hypermetropia to the seeing eye may be considered. As per accommodative esotropia, the most powerful glasses that can be prescribed plus full time wear is advised. A conversation about glasses fitting is essential, particularly if the seeing eye does not require a prescription to see well. A hypermetropic prescription of the seeing eye will reduce the accommodative drive and help reduce any esotropic drift of the non seeing eye. Glasses have the secondary benefit of offering protection to any injury of the seeing eye. Counselling about protective frames and lenses is important. The parents and child to avoid environments where an eye injury may occur.

The lens to the non seeing eye will depend on any residual vision, a balance lens may be the most sensible if the acuity is very poor.

Surgical Aim/Planning

In adults there is a strong association with poorly sighted eyes drifting to exotropia. For this reason, consider of toxin as opposed to surgery to hold the eye in a cosmetically acceptable position in childhood. Recurrent injections may be required and if frequent, surgical alignment considered.

Unilateral surgery is advised due to the remote risk of damage to the eye during strabismus surgery.

5 Residual Esotropia

Introduction

This describes children who have already had one procedure for an esotropia and present with a residual or recurrent esotropia. The presentation can be early or late.

The aims of management are to obtain good appearance for the longest possible time.

Prior Surgery

By definition previous surgery will have been performed. This may have been bilateral medial rectus recession, or a unilateral recess resect—usually on the poorer acuity eye or amblyopic eye.

Examination

Visual acuity recording and refraction remain key features. Measure the distance angle with glasses to assess surgical dose.

Non Surgical Treatment

As per accommodative esotropia, the most powerful hypermetropic glasses that can be prescribed plus full time wear is advised. Ensure that the glasses are worn and fit well. If applicable it may be worth looking for a glasses mark on the temple during summer months. If there is any doubt that glasses are not being worn it is worth delaying further surgery or planning toxin.

Surgical Aim/Planning

This will really depend on what prior surgery has been performed.

If the initial surgery was a bilateral medial rectus operation, then a bilateral lateral rectus resection is the procedure of choice. Beware tables that state dosages for bilateral lateral rectus resection as a first operation. The following table is designed for bilateral lateral rectus as a second procedure following bilateral medial rectus recession (Table 1).

If the first operation was a unilateral recess resect, the next surgery could be a recess resect on the better seeing eye. This may be difficult to justify if the child

Table 1 Surgical dosage of symmetrical LR resection in each eye based on amount of residual esotropia [28]

Esotropia (in prism dioptres)	LR resection (in mm)
25	5.0
30	5.5
35	6.0
40	6.5
45	7.0
50	7.5
≥ 55	8.0

is beyond amblyopia treatment age and or the parents/child's wishes are for the strabismic eye to be operated.

In this situation, the surgical options may be dictated by the location of the previously operated medial rectus. If this is at or beyond 10 mm from the limbus, further recession may give an unacceptable risk of exotropia either immediately or over the next few years.

Options include toxin to the medial rectus and a re-resection of the lateral rectus, or a central tenotomy of the medial rectus with a re-resection of the lateral rectus, or lateral rectus resection alone.

References

1. Bhate M, Flaherty M, Martin FJ. Timing of surgery in essential infantile esotropia—what more do we know since the turn of the century? Indian J Ophthalmol. 2022;70(2):386–95.
2. Issaho DC, de Souza Carvalho FR, Tabuse MKU, Carrijo-Carvalho LC, de Freitas D. The use of botulinum toxin to treat infantile esotropia: a systematic review with meta-analysis. Invest Ophthalmol Vis Sci. 2017;58(12):5468–76
3. de Alba Campomanes AG, Binenbaum G, Eguiarte GC. Comparison of botulinum toxin with surgery as primary treatment for infantile esotropia. J AAPOS. 2010;14:111–6.
4. Mehner L, Ng SM, Singh J. Interventions for infantile esotropia. Cochrane Database Syst Rev. 2023;1(1).
5. Minkoff OV, Donahue SP. Three-muscle surgery for infantile esotropia in children younger than age 2 years. J Pediatr Ophthalmol Strabismus. 2005;42(3):144–8.
6. Wan MJ, Chiu H, Shah AS, Hunter DG. Long-term surgical outcomes for large-angle infantile esotropia. Am J Ophthalmol. 2018;189:155–9.
7. Stager DR, Weakley DR, Everett M, Birch EE (1994) Delayed consecutive exotropia following 7-millimeter bilateral medial rectus recession for congenital esotropia. J Pediatr Ophthalmol Strabismus 31(3):147–150. https://doi.org/10.3928/0191-3913-19940501-04
8. Harrison A, Allen L, O'Connor A. Strabismus surgery for esotropia, down syndrome and developmental delay; is an altered surgical dose required? A literature review. Br Ir Orthopt J. 2020;16(1):4–12.
9. Chung AKK, Rehman SU, Bradbury JA. Comparison of modified anchored "hang-back technique (HBT)" with conventional HBT in bimedial rectus recession. JPOS. 2005;9(3):234–9.
10. Bradbury JA, Taylor RH. Severe complications of strabismus surgery. J AAPOS. 2013;17:59–63.

11. Arslan U, Atilla H, Erkam N. Dissociated vertical deviation and its relationship with time and type of surgery in infantile esotropia. Br J Ophthalmol. 2010;94(6):740–2.
12. Efficacy of prism adaptation in the surgical management of acquired esotropia. Arch Ophthalmol. 1990;108(9):1248–56.
13. Parks MM. Atlas of strabismus surgery. Philadelphia: Harper and Row; 1983.
14. https://www.eyedocs.co.uk/ophthalmology-articles/neuro-ophthalmology/714-squint-tables.html
15. Ganesh A, Pirouznia S, Ganguly SS, Fagerholm P, Lithander J. Consecutive exotropia after surgical treatment of childhood esotropia: a 40-year follow-up study. Acta Ophthalmol. 2011;89(7):691–5.
16. Shi M, Zhou Y, Qin A, et al. Treatment of acute acquired concomitant esotropia. BMC Ophthalmol. 2021;21:9.
17. Clark AC, Nelson LB, Simon JW, et al. Acute acquired comitant esotropia. Br J Ophthalmol. 1989;73:636–8.
18. Prism adaption trial again: efficacy of prism adaptation in the surgical management of acquired esotropia. Prism Adaptation Study Research Group. Arch Ophthalmol 1990;108(9):1248–56.
19. Vivian A, Lyons C, Burke J. Controversy in the management of convergence excess esotrpia. BJO. 2002;86(8):923–9.
20. Akbari MR, Heirani M, Kundart J, Christian L, Khorrami-Nejad M, Masoomian B. Application of bifocal and progressive addition lenses in the management of accommodative esotropia: a comprehensive review of current practices. Surv Ophthalmol. 2022;67(5):1506–15.
21. Arnoldi KA, Tychsen L. Surgery for esotropia with a high accommodative convergence/accommodation ratio: effects on accommodative vergence and binocularity. Ophthalmic Surg Lasers. 1996;27(5):342–8.
22. Kushner BJ. Fifteen-year outcome of surgery for the near angle in patients with accommodative esotropia and a high accommodative convergence to accommodation ratio. Arch Ophthalmol. 2001;119(8):1150–3.
23. Somer D, Cinar FG, Oral B, Ornek F. Combined recession and resection surgery in the management of convergence excess esotropia with different levels of AC/A ratio. J AAPOS. 2017;21(1).
24. Ellis GS Jr, Pritchard CH, Baham L, Babiuch A. Medial rectus surgery for convergence excess esotropia with an accommodative component: a comparison of augmented recession, slanted recession, and recession with posterior fixation. Am Orthopt J. 2012;62:50–60.
25. Khalifa YM. Augmented medial rectus recession, medial rectus recession plus faden, and slanted medial rectus recession for convergence excess esotropia. Eur J Ophthalmol. 2011;21(2):119–24.
26. Mitchell L, Kowal L. Medial rectus muscle pulley posterior fixation sutures in accommodative and partially accommodative esotropia with convergence excess. J AAPOS. 2012;16(2):125–30.
27. Inal A, Ocak OB, Aygit ED, Celik S, OzturkKarabulut G, Inal B, Taskapili M, Gokyigit B. Medial rectus bridge faden operations in accommodative and partially accommodative esotropia with convergence excess. J Pediatr Ophthalmol Strabismus. 2017;54(6):369–74.
28. Nabie R, Manouchehri V, Meydan SR. Outcomes of bilateral lateral rectus resection in residual esotropia following bilateral medial rectus recession. J Curr Ophthalmol. 2022;34(2):247–50.
29. Magli A, Rombato L, Matarazzo F, Carelli R (2016) Infantile Esotropia: risk factors associated with reoperation. Clin Ophthalmol 10:2079–2083. https://doi.org/10.2147/OPTH.S116103
30. Wan MJ, Chiu H, Shah AS, Hunter DG (2018) Long-term Surgical Outcomes for Large-angle Infantile Esotropia. Am J Ophthalmol 189:155–159. https://doi.org/10.1016/j.ajo.2017.11.006. Epub 2018 Feb 19.

Esotropia in Adults

James R. C. Miller and Saurabh Jain

Abstract Adult-onset esotropia is commonly encountered in the context of lateral rectus weakness or thyroid eye disease, however there are numerous causes unrelated to either cranial nerve palsies or systemic pathology. These conditions are diverse but may be associated with myopic refractive errors or age-related tissue changes. This chapter will consider three significant causes of adult-onset esotropia: myopic esotropia, muscle heterotopy (heavy eye syndrome) and age-related esotropia (sagging eye syndrome). In each case the typical patient population, pathogenesis and management strategy will be discussed. A high index of suspicion should be maintained when assessing a new patient with adult-onset esotropia in order to ensure that more sinister underlying pathology is not missed.

Keywords Myopic esotropia · Muscle heterotopy · Heavy eye · Age related esotropia · Sagging eye

1 Introduction

Adults with esotropia greater at distance have a different underlying mechanism than children. New onset esodeviation in the adult patient carries a broad differential diagnosis, including (but not limited to) lateral rectus palsy, thyroid eye disease and myasthenia gravis. Given the potentially significant systemic implications of these conditions, a thorough assessment of any new patient presenting with an adult-onset esotropia is essential to exclude life or sight threatening pathology. Once this has been achieved, there are a number of increasingly recognised strabismic conditions which may be responsible. This chapter will address three of the most common causes:

- Myopic esotropia

J. R. C. Miller
University College London, London, UK

S. Jain (✉)
Royal Free Hospital, London, UK
e-mail: Saurabh.jain@nhs.net

S. Jain (ed.), *Surgical Management of Strabismus*,
https://doi.org/10.1007/978-3-031-80633-9_6

- Muscle heterotopy (heavy eye syndrome)
- Age-related esotropia (sagging eye syndrome).

The association of both myopic esotropia and muscle heterotopy with myopia is likely to explain the increasing prevalence of these conditions in the clinic [1, 2]. In contrast, age-related esotropia has no association with myopia but is thought to be due to degenerative changes in the connective tissue pulleys of the extraocular muscles. These conditions may respond very differently to specific surgical techniques, so accurate identification is essential for management planning.

2 Myopic Esotropia

Myopic esotropia is becoming an increasingly common condition in the adult strabismus clinic, and generally affects patients with low to moderate degrees of myopia [3].

2.1 Presentation

Presentation is typically with gradually progressive adult-onset of diplopia that is worse for distance vision. Motility is usually preserved, although some patients may demonstrate a mild limitation of abduction. The deviation is comitant and does not have any significant accommodative element. The effect on the near angle is variable and may range from orthotropia to worsening esophoria as the condition progresses.

2.2 Aetiology

The underlying cause of myopic esotropia remains unclear, however it has been suggested to be due to an imbalance between convergent and divergent muscle tone exacerbated by excessive near work. Guyton has proposed that tight adduction from near-target convergence leads to a shortening of the medial rectus muscle and reduced ability to maintain orthographic position at distance [4]. This is consistent with recent reports of increasing prevalence associated with factors such as home working and increased screen use [5], with two thirds of respondents in a large study reporting more than four hours of laptop or smartphone use per day at the time of symptom onset. Therefore, it is hypothesized that the esotropia in this cohort is due to the weakening of the lateral rectus muscle from prolonged near work, resulting in a slow progressive esodeviation that manifests initially at distance. However, further studies are required before this can be definitively confirmed. Additional neurological findings are typically absent in myopic esotropia, and their presence should prompt a careful reconsideration of the diagnosis. Although patients are often very symptomatic of diplopia in the distance, maintenance of near fusion will often allow a degree of binocularity to be preserved.

2.3 *Management*

Patients with myopic esotropia generally respond very well to surgical correction with bilateral medial rectus recessions, although there is a small risk of subsequent recurrence. Thorough pre-operative workup is essential to determine the full size of the deviation, and disruption of fusion with either prism adaptation or prolonged patching is recommended to unmask any residual angle. An increased surgical dose when performing horizontal recess-resect surgery is also often required (i.e. > 1 mm per 3 dioptres), with the patient's fusion range allowing them to control any subsequent tendency towards exodeviation. One report suggests an increase in surgical dose of 33% [5], although some authorities may increase their correction even more. The same publication has also suggested that a prolonged time between onset of diplopia and surgical correction is associated with reduced fusional reserve, and it may be prudent to plan surgery accordingly. As always, less invasive measures such as prisms or botulinum toxin injections to the medial rectus muscle may be more appropriate options for patients with smaller deviations and those who are not fit for or do not wish to undergo strabismus surgery.

3 Muscle Heterotopy

In contrast to the moderate refractive errors often seen in myopic esotropia, muscle heterotopy (also known as heavy eye syndrome or strabismus fixus) is associated with much higher degrees of myopia.

3.1 *Aetiology*

Studies of patient populations with muscle heterotopy have commonly found axial lengths in excess of 30 mm [6], and it is thought to be this characteristic that drives the pathogenesis of the condition. The underlying abnormality in muscle heterotopy is herniation of the globe through the surrounding muscle cone, with subsequent restriction of extraocular movements [7]. High myopia is associated with superotemporal dislocation of the posterior portion of the elongated globe from the muscle cone due to increased axial length, which causes inferior displacement of the LR leading to limitation of abduction and nasal displacement of the superior rectus (SR) leading to a limitation of elevation. The inferior displacement of LR leads to weakening of its abducting force and converts it into a depressor whereas nasalization of the SR weakens its elevating force and converts it into an adductor thereby leading to the eye fixed in an esotropic and hypotropic position. Hence, the patient develops a progressive esotropia and hypotropia [8].

3.2 Presentation

These positional changes cause the superior rectus to act as an adductor, and the lateral rectus to act as a depressor. The eye consequently develops a progressive incomitant esotropia and hypotropia with restriction of abduction and elevation (positive forced duction testing is often encountered). This limitation of extraocular movement is in contrast to the myopic esotropia discussed above, where motility is usually preserved. Diplopia is common although may be absent if one eye has been affecting by co-existing pathology such as myopic maculopathy or retinal detachment. Compensatory chin-up head posturing may be adopted as a result of the large angle deviation. The prevalence of this condition likely correlates with the degree of myopia, with patients with greater extremes of axial length being at increased risk.

3.3 Investigation

The recent use of high-resolution orbital imaging has greatly helped to clarify the aetiology of muscle heterotopy, particularly with regard to positioning of the globe and the resulting muscle sequelae. Orbital MRI has consistently demonstrated prolapse of the globe through the superotemporal muscle cone, alongside an increased angle formed between the superior rectus, the globe and lateral rectus as a result of muscle displacement [6]. This has been referred to as the angle of dislocation and may approach or even exceed 180° in some cases. Degenerative changes in the intermuscular septum between these two muscles have also been noted, having some overlap with the changes seen in age-related esotropia (discussed below). Indeed, investigation with MRI may be considered where the clinical diagnosis is in doubt and radiological confirmation of globe herniation is desired.

3.4 Management

Due to the large-angle deviation commonly seen in muscle heterotopy, there is generally limited benefit from conservative measures such as prisms. Treatment is primarily surgical, and while recess-resect techniques may be employed if the abduction deficit is not too severe, the optimal management strategies appear to be aimed at restoring the normal anatomy of the extraocular muscle cone. This allows the superior and lateral recti to regain their normal function and orientation, and relieves the often significant restrictions of abduction and elevation caused by the prolapsing globe.

The most common surgical technique is the Yokoyama procedure, which utilises a loop myopexy to connect the superior and lateral rectus muscles [9]. Sutures are commonly passed through the muscle bellies 15 mm posterior to their insertions, thereby reapproximating the superotemporal muscle cone. This operation has the significant advantage of not requiring any scleral suture passes, which are potentially hazardous in the thin sclera of highly myopic eyes. However, a muscle 'cheese-wiring' effect may occur if the sutures are not passed appropriately; the risk of this occurring may be reduced by the surgical assistant holding the muscles close together at the time the sutures are passed. The Yokoyama procedure has frequently been combined with an additional recession of the ipsilateral medial rectus muscle; however studies have suggested that this may not be required in order to achieve a satisfactory outcome [10, 11]. Where significant horizontal strabismus remains after initial surgical correction, a contralateral recess-resect procedure may be considered.

A novel modification of loop myopexy was proposed by Kekunnaya et al. using a 240 silicone band that is passed through a scleral tunnel and a sleeve to unite the muscles without using anchoring sutures on the sclera [12]. The authors' loop myopexy alone effectively corrects approximately 40 PD of esotropia and can be combined with MR recession in cases of tight MR muscle. This procedure eliminates the risk of anterior segment ischemia and has the advantage of being potentially reversible compared to suture loop myopexy. However, there can be a mild risk of foreign body granuloma and extrusion of the silicone sleeve.

Alternative surgical options for muscle heterotopy include the Yamada procedure, whereby the superior and lateral recti are split in half and the adjacent portions are sutured to a common point along the superotemporal sclera [13].

Myopic eyes are anatomically predisposed to the risk of scleral penetration and perforation due to the thin sclera, which is a consequence of axial elongation of the globe. In addition, high myopes can have pathological changes such as staphyloma, which can further increase the risk. The incidence of inadvertent scleral perforation following strabismus surgery according to recent reports is approximately 0.4% [14]. Keeping the spatulated needle tip under constant view while passing the scleral bite is imperative to avoid scleral perforation. In the event of scleral perforation, a prompt dilated fundus examination should be performed to confirm/rule out choroidal or retinal entry, and adequate retinal ablation with laser or cryotherapy should be considered if indicated.

Regardless of the technique selected, the common goal is to reform the extraocular muscle cone and reverse prolapse of the myopic globe (Fig. 1).

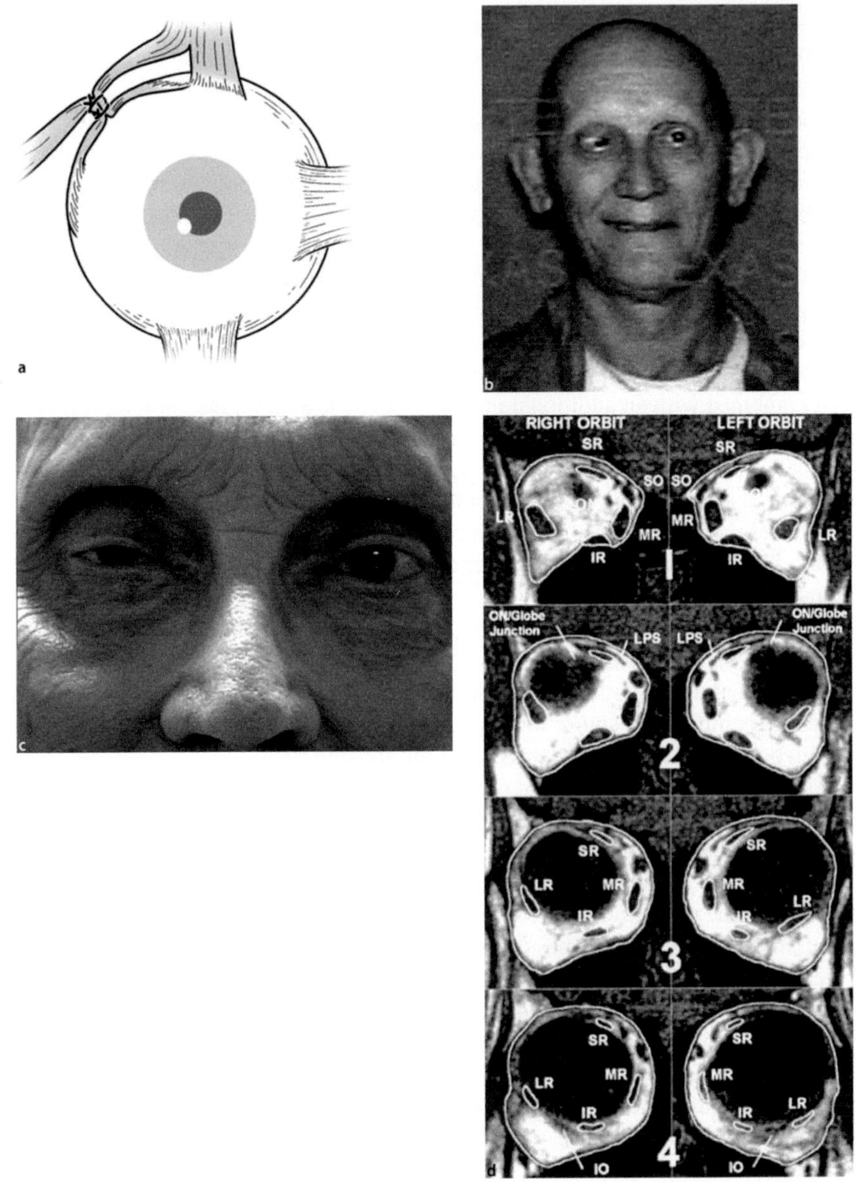

Fig. 1 Legend as above- from strabismus surgery and its complications, Springer 2007. David Coats, Scott Olitsky-rights obtained

4 Age-Related Esotropia

Age-related esotropia is a relatively recently described condition, that may also be referred to as sagging eye syndrome or divergence insufficiency esotropia (DIET). Divergence insufficiency esotropia is most commonly defined as an acquired comitant esotropia that is at least 10^{Δ} larger at distance than at near [15]. While there is some overlap with the features encountered in muscle heterotopy, the aetiology is distinct. Notably, age-related esotropia has no association with myopia, and may affect patients of any axial length.

4.1 Aetiology

Initially, divergence weakness or paralysis was considered to be the underlying cause of this acquired distance esotropia. Recently, the term "divergence insufficiency" has been challenged, since alternate aetiologies have been introduced that do not necessarily imply insufficient divergence amplitudes as the cause of this disease-state. Also, divergence amplitudes in older patients tend to be normal and attention shifted to the medial recti as the possible culprits. Both limited relaxation of the medial rectus muscles during divergence and the high accommodative vergence to accommodation ratio may lead to secondary contracture of the medial rectus muscles. Supporting clinical evidence is the observation that bilateral medial rectus recession successfully corrects DI pattern esotropia in adults [16, 17].

With the advent of functional MRI, there has been a change in thinking around the condition and the primary cause of age-related esotropia is now thought to be degenerative change in the connective tissue band between the superior and lateral rectus muscles [18]. This band normally provides vertical support for the lateral rectus, allowing it to maintain its appropriate vector of action. Degeneration of the connective septum causes the lateral rectus muscle to sag, thereby reducing its action as an abductor. This inferior displacement is comparable to that seen in muscle heterotopy, and again causes an increased angle of dislocation between the superior and lateral rectus muscles. Imaging studies have suggested that this change is less severe than that seen in muscle heterotopy [19], which is consistent with the absence of associated medial displacement of the superior rectus in age-related esotropia. It should be noted that the co-existence of esotropia and high myopia does not guarantee that a patient has muscle heterotopy, as myopic eyes are also prone to the degenerative changes that lead to age-related esotropia. Vertical deviations may also be seen where the lateral recti are affected asymmetrically between the two eyes.

4.2 Presentation

The typical presentation is in older individuals, as a gradual or subacute onset of horizontal double vision (diplopia). Initially, most patients experience intermittent horizontal binocular diplopia at long distances, such as while attending the theatre or driving. Over several months, this diplopia becomes more persistent and is noticed during activities like driving, watching television, and other situations involving long-distance vision. Patients generally report no diplopia at close range. The deviation at a distance usually falls within the range of 10–20Δ, and patients often have no deviation (orthotropic) or a controlled inward deviation (esophoria) at near distances. The esotropia at a distance is horizontally consistent and may be associated with either normal or reduced divergence amplitudes. In contrast to muscle heterotopy, there is no significant restriction of abduction or prolapse of the globe through the extraocular muscle cone. The senescent nature of this condition means it often co-exists with other adnexal findings such as ptosis and a deep upper lid sulcus [18]. The rest of the neurological examination should be normal, with no signs of cranial nerve impairments or difficulties in eye abduction. It is crucial to exclude a neurological cause of esotropia, as unilateral and bilateral abducens nerve palsies can present similarly. The presence of lateral incomitance or other cranial nerve issues should lead to further neurological evaluation [15, 20].

As may be expected, its frequency among all causes of esotropia increases with the age of the population studied; one study of 945 patients with diplopia found a proportion of 4.7% in patients under the age of 50, that increased to 60.9% in patient over 90 [21]. Care should be taken to avoid confusion with a lateral rectus palsy, which also notably presents with esodeviation worse for distance, and has a high prevalence among a patient population at increased risk of microvascular complications.

4.3 Management

Management of age-related esotropia is dependent on the size of the deviation and its symptomatic effect on the patient. If the angle encountered is small, it may respond well to conservative treatment with prisms. Where surgery is required to correct horizontal deviations either a medial rectus recession and/or lateral rectus resection is used, with either one or two muscles being selected depending on the size of the deviation. Both these have their own proponents but a recent study by Demer and colleagues concluded that medial rectus recession is as effective as lateral rectus resection in this population of patients [22]. However, they did note larger amounts of recession were required in this population, and suggested that double the distance angle of esotropia should be used as the surgical target. Interestingly, a larger preoperative distance-near incomitance was associated with greater reduction in the incomitance irrespective of which muscles underwent surgery [23].

Co-existing vertical misalignment may also need to be addressed, for example with inferior rectus tenotomy [24]. Surgical intervention is generally effective however there may be recurrence post-operatively should progressive degeneration of the intermuscular band occur [25].

5 Conclusion

Adult-onset esotropia comprises a broad range of conditions beyond frequently considered entities such as lateral rectus palsy and ocular myasthenia. While there are strong associations with myopia, they may affect patients of any axial length and careful characterisation of a newly presenting patient is required to reach an accurate diagnosis. This is vital for effective management planning, as conditions such as muscle heterotopy may not respond well to conventional recess-resect surgery. Patients with adult-onset esotropia generally respond well to treatment, although factors such as time from the onset of diplopia to surgical correction may affect the prognosis for binocular vision. As already stated, a full systemic workup should be considered if there is any doubt regarding the underlying cause of a new onset esodeviation.

References

1. Dahlmann-Noor A, Jaselsky A, Whiting C, Kana Y, Da Cruz L. Increasing prevalence of myopia in patients undergoing retinal detachment repair: an 11-year service evaluation. Eye (Lond). 2024;38(7):1231–2.
2. McCullough SJ, O'Donoghue L, Saunders KJ. Six year refractive change among white children and young adults: evidence for significant increase in myopia among white UK children. PLoS ONE. 2016;11(1):e0146332.
3. Webb H, Lee J. Acquired distance esotropia associated with myopia. Strabismus. 2004;12(3):149–55.
4. Guyton DL. The 10th Bielschowsky lecture. Changes in strabismus over time: the roles of vergence tonus and muscle length adaptation. Binocul Vis Strabismus Q. 2006;21:81–92.
5. Roda M, Di Geronimo N, Valsecchi N, Gardini L, Fresina M, Vagge A, et al. Epidemiology, clinical features, and surgical outcomes of acute acquired concomitant esotropia associated with myopia. PLoS ONE. 2023;18(5):e0280968.
6. Maiolo C, Fresina M, Campos EC. Role of magnetic resonance imaging in heavy eye syndrome. Eye (Lond). 2017;31(8):1163–7.
7. Hennein L, Robbins SL. Heavy eye syndrome: myopia-induced strabismus. Surv Ophthalmol. 2021;66(1):138–144.
8. Kekunnaya R, Chandrasekharan A, Sachdeva V. Management of strabismus in myopes. Middle East Afr J Ophthalmol. 2015;22(3):298–306.
9. Yamaguchi M, Yokoyama T, Shiraki K. Surgical procedure for correcting globe dislocation in highly myopic strabismus. Am J Ophthalmol. 2010;149(2):341-346.e2.
10. Wabbels B, Fricke J, Schittkowski M, Graf M, Lorenz B, Bau V, et al. Yokoyama procedure for esotropia associated with high myopia: real-world data from a large-scale multicentre analysis. Acta Ophthalmol. 2021;99(8):e1340–7.

11. Bansal S, Marsh IB. Unaugmented muscle union surgery for heavy eye syndrome without combined medial rectus recession. J Pediatr Ophthalmol Strabismus. 2016;53(1):40–3.
12. Shenoy BH, Sachdeva V, Kekunnaya R. Silicone band loop myopexy in the treatment of myopic strabismus fixus: surgical outcome of a novel modification. Br J Ophthalmol. 2015;99:36–40.
13. Godeiro KD, Kirsch D, Tabuse MK, Cronemberger M. Yamada's surgery for treatment of myopic strabismus fixus. Int Ophthalmol. 2009;29(4):305–8.
14. Dang Y, Racu C, Isenberg SJ. Scleral penetrations and perforations in strabismus surgery and associated risk factors. J AAPOS. 2004;8:325–31.
15. Divergence PS, Esotropia I. Surgical treatment. Am Orthopt J. 2015;65:35–9.
16. Bothun ED, Archer SM. Bilateral medial rectus muscle recession for divergence insufficiency pattern esotropia. J AAPOS. 2005;9(1):3–615729272.
17. Herlihy EP, Phillips JO, Weiss AH. Esotropia greater at distance: children vs adults. JAMA Ophthalmol. 2013;131(3):370–5.
18. J Chaudhuri Z, Demer JL. Sagging eye syndrome: connective tissue involution as a cause of horizontal and vertical strabismus in older patients. JAMA Ophthalmol. 2013;131(5):619–25.
19. Tan RJD, Demer JL. Heavy eye syndrome versus sagging eye syndrome in high myopia. J AAPOS. 2015;19(6):500–6.
20. Godts D, Mathysen DG. Distance esotropia in the elderly. Br J Ophthalmol. 2013;97:1415–9.
21. Goseki T, Suh SY, Robbins L, Pineles SL, Velez FG, Demer JL. Prevalence of sagging eye syndrome in adults with binocular diplopia. Am J Ophthalmol. 2020;209:55–61.
22. Chaudhuri Z, Demer JL. Medial rectus recession is as effective as lateral rectus resection in divergence paralysis esotropia. Arch Ophthalmol. 2012;130:1280–4.
23. Archer SM. The effect of medial versus lateral rectus muscle surgery on distance-near incomitance. J AAPOS. 2009;13:20–6.
24. Chaudhuri Z, Demer JL. Graded vertical rectus tenotomy for small angle cyclovertical strabismus in sagging eye syndrome. Br J Ophthalmol. 2016;100(5):648–51.
25. Chaudhuri Z, Demer JL. Long-term surgical outcomes in the sagging eye syndrome. Strabismus. 2018;26(1):6–10.

Alphabet Pattern Strabismus

Alasdair Kennedy

Abstract This chapter defines the various alphabet patterns and their aetiologies. Practical steps in their assessment are offered as well as a structured approach to planning surgery. Oblique muscle over- or under-action should be addressed first prior to moving onto horizontal muscle transpositions. It is important to consider other causes of alphabet patterns which require a different management such as in Duane or Brown syndrome. Other rarer patterns are discussed as well as complications of alphabet pattern surgery.

Keywords Alphabet-pattern · V-pattern · A-pattern · Y-pattern · λ-pattern · Arrow-pattern · X-pattern · Diamond-pattern · Oblique muscle dysfunction · Horizontal muscle transposition

1 Introduction

- Alphabet patterns are a form of horizontal strabismus which are incomitant in the vertical plane.
- The deviation in primary position, upgaze and downgaze varies.
- The most common patterns are "V" and "A"
- Other patterns, such as "Y", "↓" (arrow) and "λ" are variations of these.
- "X" and "⬩" (diamond) patterns are a separate and rare entity.
- Once the aetiology of the pattern has been appropriately investigated, then surgery can be planned.
- If the pattern is not clinically significant, the surgeon can ignore it and address the deviation in primary position as normal.
- If the pattern is significant, the orthoptic examination will indicate which surgical technique is required.

A. Kennedy (✉)
Moorfields Eye Hospital, London, UK
e-mail: alasdairkennedy@nhs.net

S. Jain (ed.), *Surgical Management of Strabismus*,
https://doi.org/10.1007/978-3-031-80633-9_7

- This chapter provides the reader with definitions of the various types of alphabet patterns and practical steps in their assessment and management.

2 Definitions

V-pattern strabismus

(1) **V-pattern exotropia**: this is the most common type of pattern strabismus where the deviation is more in upgaze than downgaze (Fig. 1)
(2) **V-pattern esotropia**: here the deviation is more in downgaze than upgaze (Fig. 1)
(3) **Y-pattern exotropia**: this is a variation of V-pattern where the deviation in primary position and downgaze are stable but the divergence is greater in upgaze (Fig. 2)
(4) **↓-pattern esotropia**: another variant, in this pattern primary gaze and upgaze are stable but the eyes converge more in downgaze.

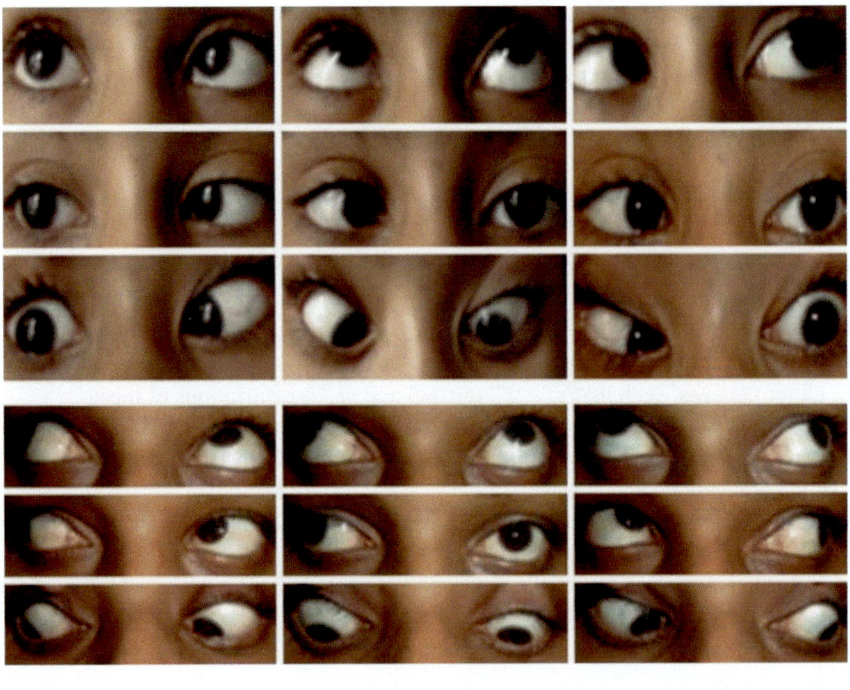

Fig. 1 V-pattern esotropia and exotropia (from Strabismus, S Agrawal 2019, Springer—Rights obtained)

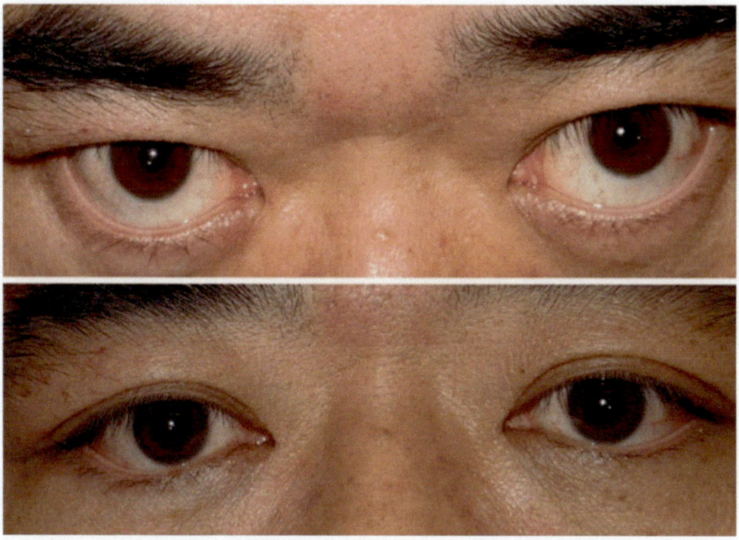

Fig. 2 Y-pattern exotropia. From simplifying strabismus: a practical approach to diagnosis and management, 2nd edition, 2024. Springer—Rights obtained

A-pattern strabismus

(1) **A-pattern esotropia**: in this pattern, the esotropia measures less in downgaze than upgaze (Fig. 3)
(2) **A-pattern exotropia**: here, the deviation increases from upgaze to down gaze (Fig. 3)
(3) **λ-pattern exotropia**: a variation of A-pattern exotropia, the deviation is stable in upgaze and primary position but the divergence is greater in downgaze.

3 Aetiology

Conventional alphabet patterns

- The most common alphabet patterns are A- and V-patterns
- Oblique muscle over- or under-action is the most popular aetiological theory [1, 2]
- The pattern may either be due to the primary torsion or the tertiary abducting action of these muscles [1, 2]
- Vertical rectus muscle over- or under-action may also be a significant cause of a pattern
- In the absence of oblique muscle or vertical rectus involvement, there may be no apparent cause for the alphabet pattern

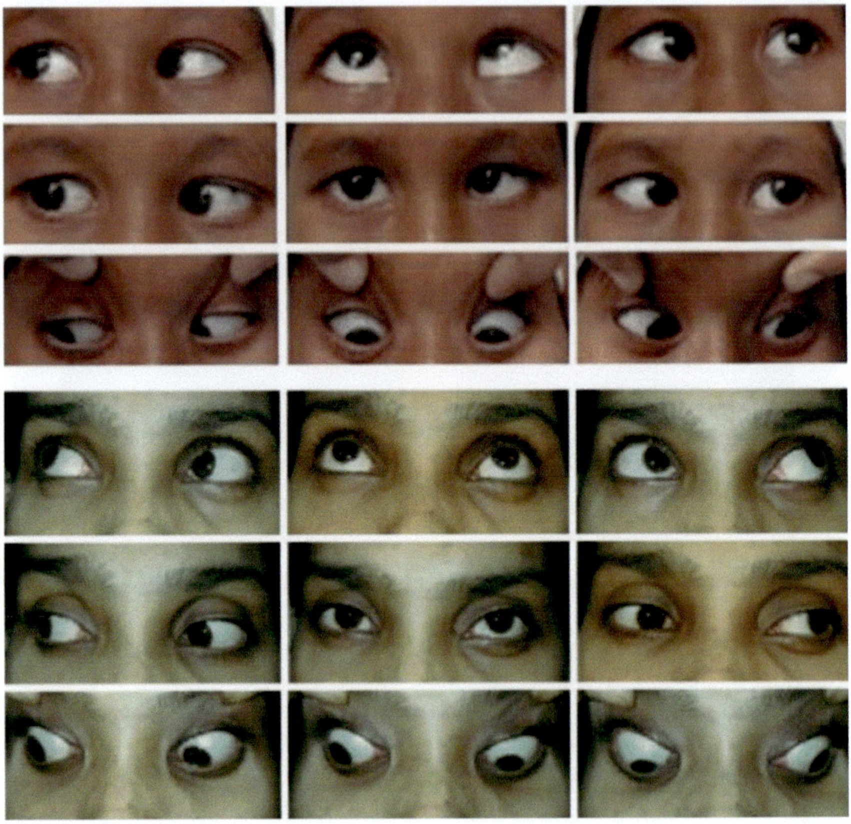

Fig. 3 A-pattern esotropia (upper) and exotropia (lower)-(from Strabismus, S Agrawal 2019, Springer—Rights obtained)

- Other theories include:
  - Horizontal muscle over- and under-action: the medial rectus is more active in downgaze and the lateral rectus in upgaze [3]—this has been disproved by electromyographic studies.
  - Primary under-action of the superior or inferior oblique muscles causing fixation duress and over-action of the yoke oblique muscle [4]—further evidence is however required to prove this.
  - Heterotopia of extraocular muscle pulleys: MRI studies have shown that pulley heterotopia (small displacements) can cause vertical gaze incomitance and therefore alphabet patterns [5].

  - Theory of saggitalisation of oblique muscles: abnormal saggitalisation of the inferior oblique muscle causes incylorotation and a resultant compensatory over-action of the inferior oblique thus eliminating the torsion [6]—this theory is unlikely as patients with conventional V-patterns tend to have excyclorotation.

Aetiology of conventional alphabet patterns

- The cause of the over- or under- action must be considered and, if appropriate, investigated first prior to undertaking surgical intervention
- Oblique muscles:
  - Inferior oblique over-action: can be isolated but also frequently seen in congenital horizontal strabismus and as part of the muscle sequelae seen in 4th nerve palsy.
  - Inferior oblique under-action is rare and can be congenital or acquired (e.g. trauma, vascular lesions or myasthenia gravis) [7]
  - Superior oblique over-action: rare and can be isolated or associated with brain lesions such as Chiari malformations or hydrocephalus [8]
  - Superior oblique under-action: can be caused by a congenital or acquired 4th nerve palsy (see Chap. 9).
- Vertical muscles:
  - Under- and over-actions may be idiopathic or forming part of muscle sequelae but other causes such as myasthenia gravis, neurological conditions, compressive lesions, thyroid eye disease and trauma must be excluded.
- Orbital structure anomalies: alphabet patterns are frequently seen in craniofacial syndromes such as Crouzon syndrome where the globe is excylotorotated or in hydrocephalus (Fig. 4). [9] Similarly, patients with up-slanting palpebral fissures can present with an A-pattern esotropia, and patients with down-slanting fissures with a V-pattern exotropia (Fig. 5).

Other causes of alphabet patterns

There are some important diagnoses to exclude which may mimic conventional alphabet patterns. See Chap. 12 for the management of these conditions:

- Brown syndrome: the abnormal superior oblique seen in Brown syndrome can be difficult to differentiate from an inferior oblique weakness. However, in Brown syndrome, there may be a Y-pattern exotropia whereas in inferior oblique under-action, it is more common to see an A-pattern secondary to the unopposed action of the superior oblique.
- Duane syndrome and other Congenital Cranial Dysinnervation Syndromes: abnormal movements can be seen in these conditions which may cause A- or V-patterns or any of their variants.

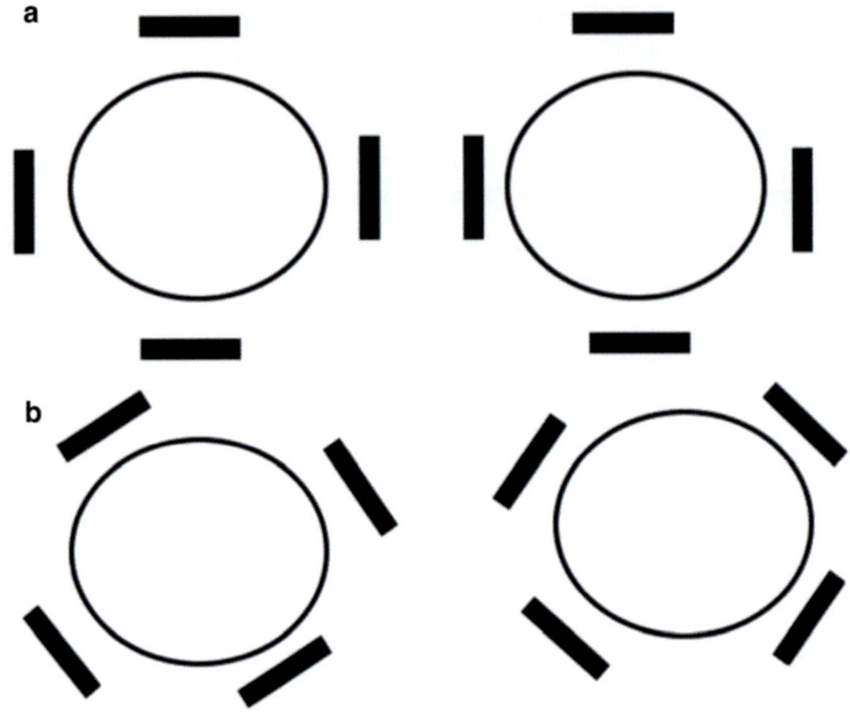

Fig. 4 a Normal arrangement of rectus muscles around the globe. b Abnormal recuts muscle arrangement seen in Crouzon syndrome. The medial rectus is supero-placed leading to increased elevation following adduction and a V-pattern exotropia. From simplifying strabismus: a practical approach to diagnosis and management, 2nd edition, 2024. Springer—Rights obtained

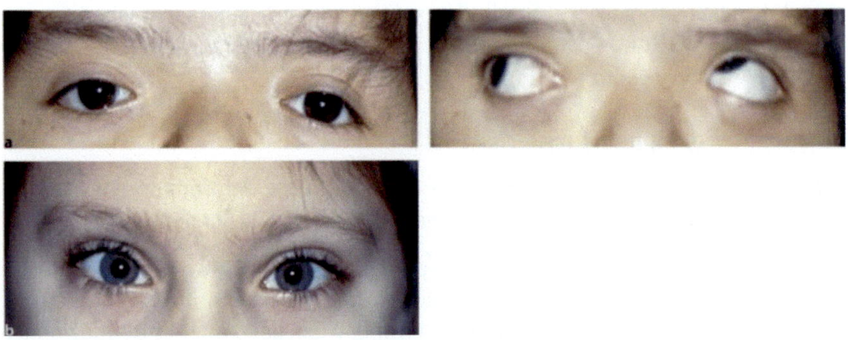

Fig. 5 V-pattern in patient with down-slanting palpebral fissures b: A-pattern in patient with up-slanting palpebral fissures

- Restrictive causes: thyroid eye disease or trauma can cause restrictive patterns which may mimic conventional alphabet patterns.
- Myasthenia gravis can mimic almost any form of strabismus and should always be considered.

4 Assessment of Alphabet Patterns

A careful orthoptic assessment is key to the successful management of a patient with an alphabet pattern strabismus. Below is a structured approach to such patients.

(1) **What is the primary horizontal deviation**?

This is the first step in defining the alphabet pattern. The deviation will either be predominantly an esotropia or exotropia in either primary, up-gaze and/or down-gaze.

(2) **What is the type of alphabet pattern?**

- Using the classification above, the pattern deviation can be defined.
- Orthoptic measurements should be in full optical correction and include prism cover tests in primary position, 20–25° in up-gaze and down-gaze using an accommodative target at 6 m to remove the near reflex.

(3) **Is the pattern significant?**

Once the pattern has been defined, the next step is to establish if the deviation is significant.

- V-pattern strabismus and variations: by convention, these patterns are deemed clinically significant if the deviation measures more than **15 prism dioptres** (PD) between upgaze and downgaze as some V pattern is physiological due to the convergence in accommodation.
- A-pattern strabismus and variations: by convention, these patterns are deemed clinically significant if the deviation measures more than **10 prism dioptres** (PD) between upgaze and downgaze

(4) **Is surgery indicated?**

- A patient with a symptomatic alphabet pattern will benefit from surgery.
- Common indications include a large deviation in primary position or diplopia on down gaze which may become more obvious at the onset of presbyopia when down-gaze is required for the use of bifocals
- Patients may also be aware of the cosmetic and visual disturbances caused by over-actions in up- or down-gaze
- By convention, the surgeon may be able to ignore an alphabet pattern if it is not significant. However, there may be exceptions, for example:
  - the deviation does not meet the significance criteria, but the patient may still benefit from surgery to collapse the pattern; for example, if there is a risk of postoperative overcorrection in downgaze of a V-pattern exotropia

– the opposite may also be true. A patient may have a significant Y-pattern exotropia but may not be particularly symptomatic. In such cases, it may be wise to not operate on these patients to avoid overcorrection and diplopia in primary position.

5 Planning Surgery

Once an alphabet pattern has been identified and surgical intervention is deemed beneficial, a structured approach is required when planning surgery. The aim of surgery is to both address the primary horizontal deviation and collapse the pattern:

(1) **Rule out the oblique muscle overaction first**

- When faced with an alphabet pattern strabismus, the first aetiology to consider is the under or over-action of either the superior or inferior oblique muscles.
- If these over- or under-actions are large (a guide is + 2 over-action or more), they could be addressed before considering surgery to the rectus muscles – in such cases, oblique muscle surgery alone may be sufficient in addressing both the pattern and the horizontal deviation.
- A careful assessment of ocular motility in the nine positions of gaze will establish if there are any significant over- or under-actions of the oblique muscles:

  – Inferior oblique over-action/Superior oblique under-action:

    Confirmed on ocular motility testing where an up-drift is seen in adduction
    Superior oblique under-action tends to be worse in adduction combined with depression
    Inferior oblique over-action tends to be worse in adduction with elevation
    Can cause a V-pattern exotropia, esotropia or Y-pattern
    An $\downarrow$-pattern esotropia may be seen in bilateral superior oblique weakness

  – Superior oblique over-action/Inferior oblique under-action:

    Confirmed on ocular motility testing where a down-drift is seen in adduction
    Can be the principal cause of a A-pattern exotropia or esotropia
    Bilateral cases may result in a λ-pattern exotropia
    Inferior oblique under-action is very rare and usually presents with an A-pattern combined with ipsilateral hypotropia

(2) **Rule out vertical rectus muscles next**

- Inferior or superior rectus under- or over-action should be considered next if there is no significant oblique muscle involvement
- Once again, careful assessment of ocular motility is required
- Both muscles are adductors and will only influence the deviation in their field of action potentially causing an alphabet pattern
  - Inferior rectus weakness is most commonly described. The under-action results in weakened adduction in down-gaze and a possible A-pattern
  - Similarly, superior rectus over-action may cause increased adduction in up-gaze and an A-pattern
  - In bilateral inferior rectus weakness, a λ-pattern exotropia may be observed
  - Inferior rectus over-action and superior rectus under-action may result in V-patterns.

(3) **That leaves the horizontal rectus muscles**

- If the oblique muscles, vertical muscles and other causes or mimics of conventional alphabet patterns have been ruled out, it is reasonable to proceed with horizontal rectus muscle surgery

6 Surgical Approach to Alphabet Patterns

- **Oblique muscle surgery**
- General considerations
  - In cases of large alphabet pattern strabismus caused by oblique muscle over- or under-action, it is reasonable to operate on these muscles first
  - Residual horizontal deviations can then be addressed at a later date to avoid over-correction
  - In mild to moderate patterns, oblique muscle surgery may be combined with conventional horizontal rectus surgery
  - Care must be taken to assess patients for torsion. Oblique surgery will address excessive abduction in upgaze for V-patterns and in down-gaze for A-patterns but will also influence torsion depending on the surgical technique used
  - In unilateral cases, only the over- or under-acting muscle should be addressed
  - In symmetrical bilateral cases, symmetrical surgery should be performed to prevent a secondary vertical deviation or other unexpected results.
  - In asymmetric bilateral cases, asymmetric surgery can be performed.
- Inferior oblique over-action (V- or Y-pattern)
  - Can be addressed with any technique listed in Chap. 3
  - If there is a vertical deviation in primary gaze or one inferior oblique is over-acting more than the other, asymmetric surgery can be performed

  - Anteriorisation is a more powerful operation than other weakening techniques and can therefore be used on the more over-acting side or on the hypertropic eye combined with an inferior oblique recession, myectomy or myotomy on the contralateral eye
  - It is generally agreed that bilateral inferior oblique surgery can correct between 15 to 20 PD of exotropia in up-gaze with minimal effect in primary position [10]

- Superior oblique under-action (V- or ↓-pattern)

  - Can be addressed with a superior oblique tuck as described in Chap. 3
  - ↓-pattern esotropia, as can be seen in bilateral under-action, should be treated with bilateral Superior Oblique tucks allowing for any asymmetry.

- Superior oblique over-action (A- or λ-pattern)

  - Various techniques have been described for superior oblique weakening
  - All techniques begin with identifying the superior oblique tendon as described in Chap. 3
  - Care must be taken to avoid cutting the vortex vein when cutting the tendon
  - Nasal tendon surgery is more impactful than temporal approaches and therefore can be used in larger A-patterns but may result in a higher incidence of complications, over-correction and V-patterns [11, 12]
  - Techniques can be divided into anterior fibre sparing or involving.
  - Anterior fibre sparing:

    There is an advantage to maintaining the anterior 10% of fibres because they are responsible for incyclorotation and the remaining posterior fibres for depression and abduction [13]. However, there may be a loss of function of the muscle and iatrogenic superior oblique paresis with these techniques [14]

    Superior oblique posterior tenotomy (Fig. 6)

    - The superior oblique tendon is identified temporally
    - The posterior 4/5th of the tendon close to the insertion are cut tangentially to the globe

    Superior oblique posterior tenectomy [12] (Fig. 7)

    - The superior oblique tendon is identified temporally
    - The posterior 4/5th of the tendon close to the insertion are cut tangentially to the globe
    - The scissors are then rotated in the direction of the tendon fibres and a triangle of 12 mm in length [12] or a rectangle of 10 mm in length [15] is excised leaving behind the anterior 1/5th of the tendon

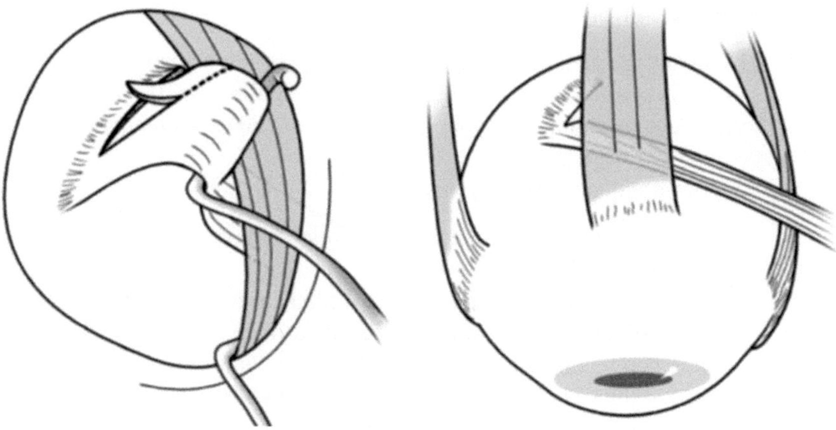

Fig. 6 Posterior tenotomy of the superior oblique—from Strabismus surgery and its complications. David K. Coats, Scott E. Olitsky, Springer 2007—rights obtained

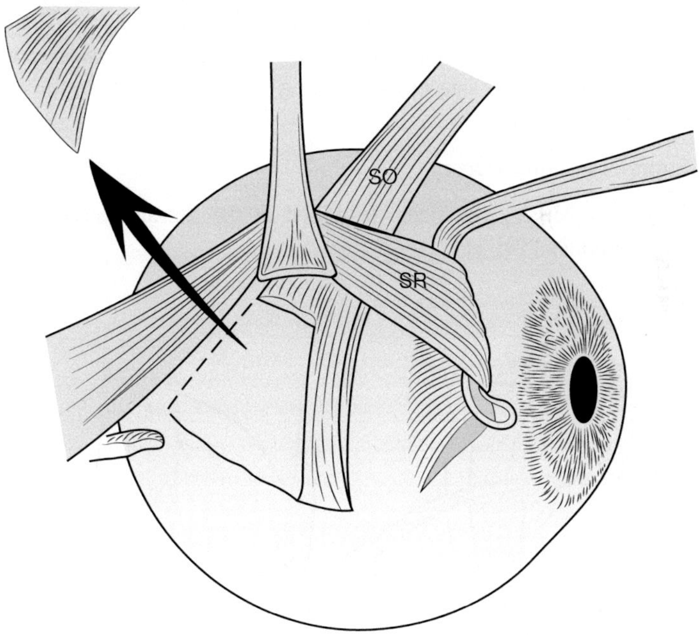

Fig. 7 Rectangular posterior tenectomy of the superior oblique- from Colour atlas of strabismus surgery 2015 Ken Wright. Springer- rights obtained

– Anterior fibre involving:

The advantage of surgery to the whole tendon is that graded and controlled surgery is possible with maintenance of muscle function. If there is significant incyclorotation, this may be preferable. These techniques are also potentially reversible.

Superior oblique recession [16] (Fig. 8):

- In this technique, the entire superior oblique muscle is recessed from its insertion
- Once the temporal superior oblique tendon has been identified, a double ended non-absorbable suture is inserted through it close to its insertion
- The tendon can then be disinserted and the suture passed through the sclera at the site of the insertion much like in a conventional recession
- The superior rectus can be manipulated to allow the superior oblique to pass beneath it or the tendon can be pulled nasally from the nasal side of the superior rectus
- Graded recession has been reported to give a 2PD reduction in A-pattern per mm recessed after an initial 8mm recession [17]
- Conversely, it has been reported that the amount of pattern corrected is correlated to the size of the initial A-pattern rather than the amount of recession [18]

Superior oblique spacer:

- Spacer surgery has been described in the literature. see Chap. 3 for techniques [19].

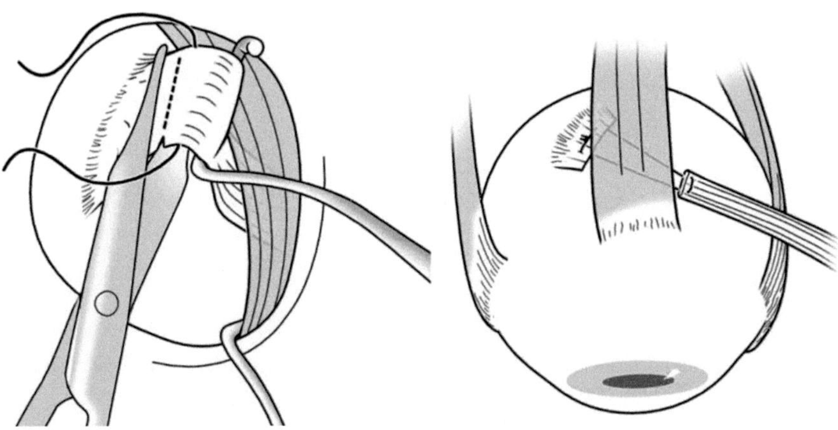

Fig. 8 Superior oblique recession. A double ended non-absorbable suture is inserted through the superior oblique tendon close to its insertion. The tendon is disinserted and the suture passed through the sclera at the site of the insertion. The superior oblique is passed beneath the superior rectus and pulled nasally—from Strabismus surgery and its complications. David K. Coats, Scott E. Olitsky, Springer 2007-rights obtained

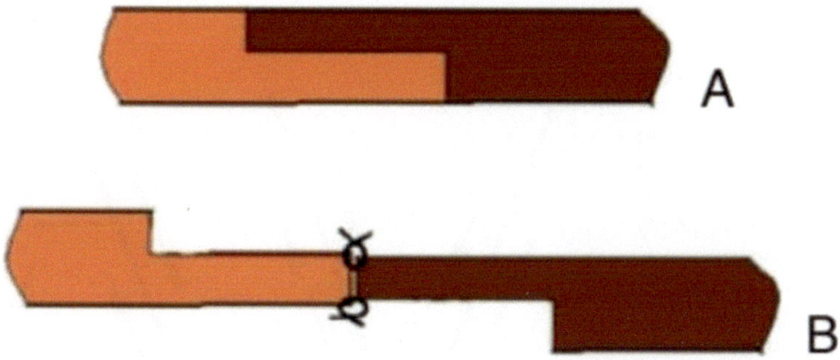

Fig. 9 Z-tendon lengthening of SO tendon—from Colour atlas of strabismus surgery 2015 Ken Wright. Springer-rights obtained

Z-tendon lengthening (Fig. 9):

- The superior oblique tendon is identified and hooked nasally
- The tendon is spread out with two hooks
- The tendon is split longitudinally in the middle with scissors and extended to around 8mm bluntly with one of the hooks
- 1 non-absorbable suture is passed twice through the temporal slit as far temporally as possible and tied off and another twice through the nasal split as far nasally as possible and tied off
- The posterior tendon is cut temporal to its suture and the anterior tendon cut nasal to its suture
- The two ends are apposed by passing the nasal suture through the posterior split and vice versa
- This produces a controlled lengthening of the tendon

- Inferior oblique under-action (A-pattern)
  - A forced duction test at the start of surgery should be performed to differentiate this condition from a Brown syndrome
  - There is no reported effective tightening or other similar procedure for the inferior oblique
  - Ipsilateral superior oblique weakening, as described above, or contralateral superior rectus recession can be effective [7]

- **Horizontal rectus muscle surgery**
- Vertical transposition
  - Horizontal rectus muscle vertical transposition is indicated in cases where over-action of the oblique muscles is absent or insignificant and other causes of alphabet patterns have been ruled out
  - No modification is required to the usual surgical dose calculation for the horizontal deviation—the dosage is based on the largest deviation within the pattern

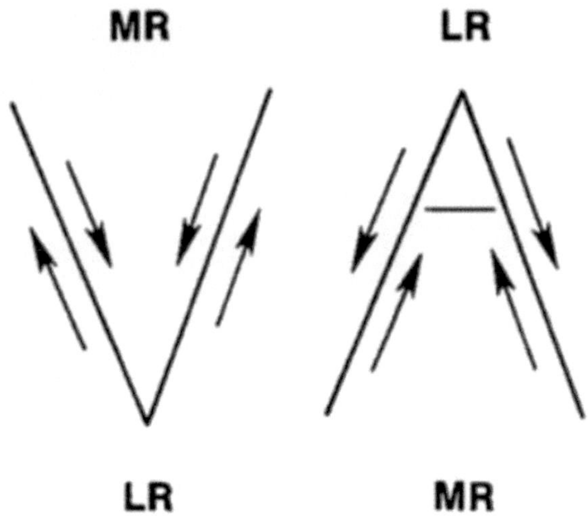

Fig. 10 This diagram demonstrates the "MALE" mnemonic with the medial recti transposed to the apex of the pattern, superiorly in A-patterns and inferiorly in V-patterns. The lateral recti are transposed to the empty space of the pattern, superiorly in V-patterns and inferiorly in A-patterns—from Colour atlas of strabismus surgery 2015 Ken Wright. Springer-rights obtained

- When a horizontal muscle is transposed, its primary action is weakened in the field of gaze which it has been moved to and enhanced in the opposite field
- For example, if the lateral rectus is transposed superiorly, it is a weaker abductor in up-gaze and a stronger abductor in down-gaze
- The useful mnemonic "MALE" helps guide the surgeon as to which direction to transpose and stands for **M**edial to **A**pex and **L**ateral to **E**mpty space of the pattern (Fig. 10)

  Medial recti should therefore be transposed inferiorly in V-patterns and superiorly in A-patterns
  Lateral recti should be transposed superiorly in V-patterns and inferiorly in A-patterns

- The operated muscle should be transposed respecting the spiral of Tillaux. Dosage calculations can be made by measuring radially from the limbus to prevent any over- or under-estimation (Figs. 11 and 12).
- Half a muscle width will address up to 15 PD of the alphabet pattern and a full muscle at least 20 PD.
- Symmetric bilateral surgery should be carried out where possible to avoid iatrogenic vertical deviations or torsion which can occur after unilateral recess/resect surgery [20].

  For example, bilateral lateral rectus with superior vertical transposition in a V-pattern

- If unilateral surgery is required, no more than a half-tendon width transposition is preferable to avoid a new iatrogenic deviation.
- If the alphabet pattern measures 25 PD or more, care must be taken to ensure oblique muscle dysfunction is not present as this is usually the cause.

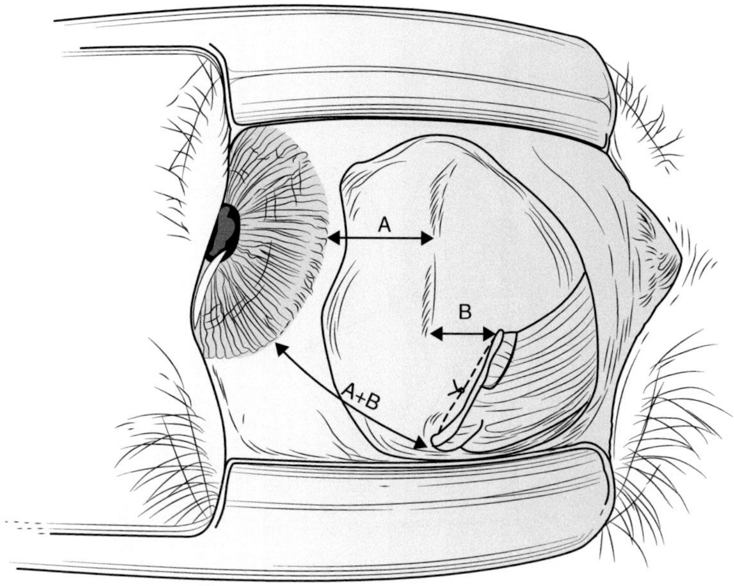

Fig. 11 In an inferior full or half tendon width recession, it is easier to start by recession the superior pole. In a full tendon width recession, the superior pole of the muscle is aligned with the inferior pole of the insertion and recessed adding the distance from the limbus to the insertion (A) with the planned amount of recession (B). The recession for the inferior pole of the muscle is then measured radially from the limbus (A + B) ensuring the poles of the muscle are appropriately spread. The converse is true for a superior transposition. In a half tendon width inferior or superior recession, the principles are the same but the superior or inferior pole are recessed through the mid-point of the insertion respectively—from Colour atlas of strabismus surgery 2015 Ken Wright. Springer-rights obtained

- Insertion slanting

    Slanting the superior or inferior pole of the muscle involves recessing one pole more than the other
    In theory, it simulates vertical transposition whilst avoiding inducing unwanted torsion
    However, there are two contradictory theories

    Biomechanical [21]:

    In downgaze, the superior border of the muscle is tighter
    In upgaze, the inferior border is tighter
    According to this theory, the following rules would apply to collapse an alphabet pattern:

    V-pattern esotropia: greater recession of superior pole of medial rectus
    A-pattern esotropia: greater recession of inferior pole of medial rectus
    V-pattern exotropia: greater recession of inferior pole of lateral rectus
    A-pattern exotropia: greater recession of superior pole of lateral rectus

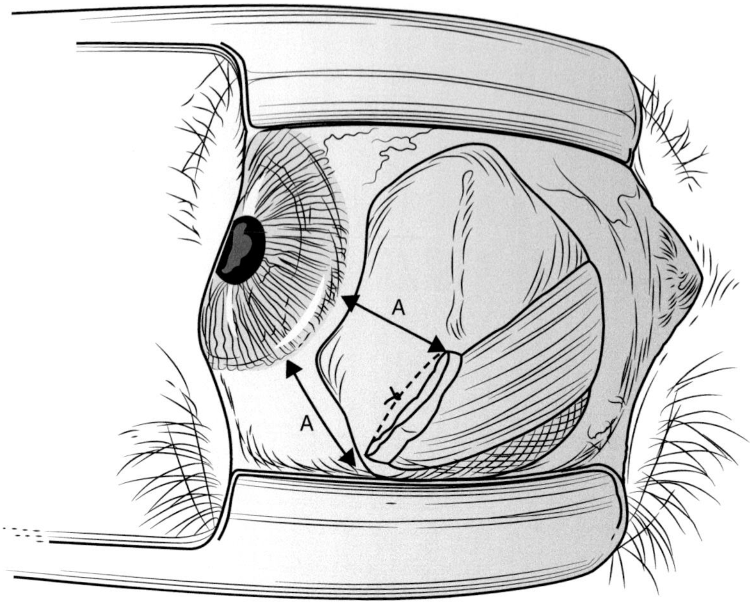

Fig. 12 In an inferior full or half muscle width resection, after resecting the required amount of muscle, it is easier to re-insert the superior pole of the muscle first through the inferior pole of the insertion. The same distance (A) from the limbus is then measured radially for the re-insertion of the inferior pole of the muscle making sure the muscle poles are appropriately spread. The converse is true for a superior transposition. In a half tendon width inferior or superior resection, the principles are the same but the superior or inferior pole are re-inserted through the mid-point of the insertion respectively—from Colour atlas of strabismus surgery 2015 Ken Wright. Springer-rights obtained

Segmental innervation [22]:

Increased contraction of inferior half of medial rectus in down-gaze and of superior half in up-gaze and vice-versa for the lateral rectus
According to this theory, the following would apply:

V-pattern esotropia: greater recession of inferior pole of medial rectus
A-pattern esotropia: greater recession of superior pole of medial rectus
V-pattern exotropia: greater recession of superior pole of lateral rectus
A-pattern exotropia: greater recession of inferior pole of lateral rectus

These contradictory theories imply that either slanted recessions do not work, or the evidence is inadequate. The positive results reported on both sides of the argument suggest that the accompanying recession or resections may be responsible for the surgical effect [23]

Surgical dosage: in both techniques, the surgical dosage is based on the largest and smallest deviations of the pattern.

The dosage pole requiring more recession is based on the largest deviation. The dosage pole requiring the least recession is based on the smallest deviation.

- Horizontal muscle pulley surgery
  - If heterotopia of extraocular muscle pulleys is suspected, then pulley surgery can be considered [24]
- **Vertical muscle transposition**
  - Horizontal transposition of a vertical rectus muscle by 7mm can be combined with horizontal rectus muscle recession [25, 26]
  - This creates a force vector in the direction of transposition.

    V-esotropia: Bilateral inferior rectus transposition temporally with medial rectus recessions
    V-exotropia: Bilateral superior rectus transposition nasally with lateral rectus recessions
    A-esotropia: Bilateral superior rectus transposition temporally with medial rectus recessions
    A-exotropia: Bilateral inferior rectus transposition nasally with lateral rectus recessions

  - This technique is unpopular as it sometimes requires surgery to an extra rectus muscle thus limiting further operations due to risk of anterior segment ischaemia

7 Other Alphabet Patterns

- X- and ◆- pattern strabismus have a different aetiology to conventional patterns and are thus treated differently
- Both patterns are rare and therefore there is limited evidence to support either their aetiological theories or the best surgical intervention
- **X-pattern exotropia**:
  - increased divergence in up-gaze and down-gaze
  - Several aetiological theories exist

    Tight lateral recti [27]: may arise from longstanding exotropia or from bilateral Type 2 Duane Retraction Syndrome
    Over-action of all four oblique muscles [28]
    Slip of all four oblique muscles to polar cap [29]

Mixed horizontal and oblique muscle dysfunction [30]

- Regardless of the possible theory, conventional horizontal muscle surgery appears to be an effective operation [31]

- **◆-pattern strabismus**: increased convergence in up-gaze and down-gaze
  - Even less well described, may be caused by tight medial recti.
  - Surgery on the medial recti may be beneficial.

8 Complications of Alphabet Pattern Surgery

- Each of the surgical techniques described above carries the risk of over-correction either resulting in an iatrogenic pattern strabismus, torsion or a vertical deviation
- Where possible, and if required, the original surgery may have to be reversed.
- Some operations are harder to reverse than others and therefore care must be taken when electing a surgical technique.
- If over-correction is identified as a risk or the patient is binocular, then the least involved and more readily reversible surgery should be considered.
- Similarly, stepped surgery, for example addressing the oblique muscles first rather than operating on the oblique muscles and horizontal recti at the same time, may help prevent unexpected results.
- Common iatrogenic alphabet patterns and other complications
  - Inferior oblique surgery:

    May result in limited upgaze and a V- or Y-pattern.

    More likely after inferior oblique anteriorisation due to anti-elevation syndrome as described in Chap. 3.

    Many cases settle down, but exploration and recession of the inferior oblique and release of adhesions and scarring with amniotic membrane to aid conjunctival closure may be required. Failing this, and combined recession and resection on the contralateral superior rectus to match the up-gaze limitation may be required.

  - Superior oblique surgery

    Superior oblique weakening surgery may cause an overcorrection and an A-pattern

      Depending on the technique employed, revision of the superior oblique can be challenging.

      Ipsilateral inferior oblique weakening may be a safer option in the first instance.

The incylorotation and excyclorotation produced by superior oblique tucks and weakening procedures respectively can be anticipated by marking the eye prior to starting the surgery.
During tucks, if significant excyclorotation is noted, ipsilateral inferior oblique weakening surgery may be indicated. This can also be completed as a second stage procedure.
Asymmetric superior oblique surgery for an A-pattern can cause a vertical deviation. Care should be taken to ensure the surgery is symmetric.

– Horizontal muscle vertical transpositions

  Over-transposing the horizontal recti can rarely cause an overcorrection.
  Similarly, a vertical deviation or torsion may be induced.
  Bilateral symmetric recession surgery is reversible and therefore may be safer option than unilateral recess/resect procedures, especially if a full tendon width transposition is indicated.

– Inferior rectus surgery

  Over-vigorous inferior rectus recessions can cause an A-pattern
  This occurs due to weakening of the adducting power of the muscle
  Re-advancement may be required, particularly if there has been a reversal of height in downgaze.
  However, this may not be possible for example in a patient with thyroid eye disease
  If there has been no significant reversal of height, then ipsilateral superior oblique weakening may be considered (Fig. 13).

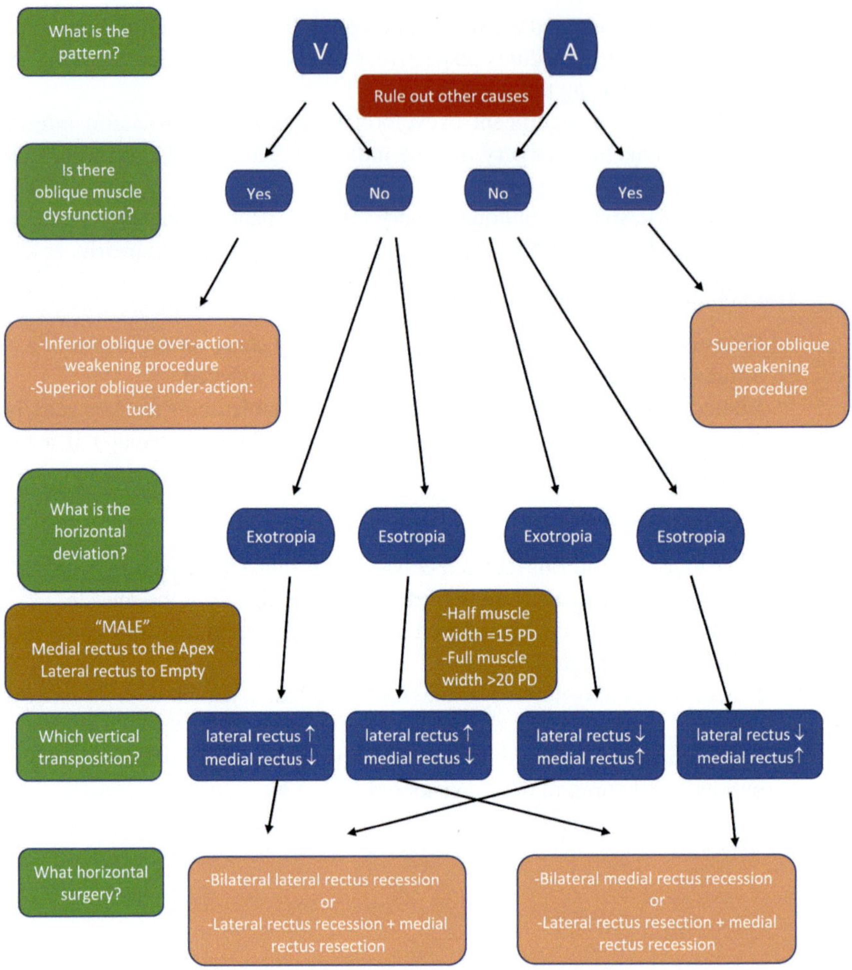

Fig. 13 Flowchart for decision making in alphabet pattern strabismus

References

1. Kushner B. The role of ocular torsion on the etiology of A and V patterns. J Pediatr Ophthalmol Strabismus. 1985;22:171–9. PMID: 4045645.
2. P, Knapp. Vertically incomitant horizontal strabismus: the so-called "A" and "V" syndromes. Trans Am Ophthalmol Soc. 1959;57:666–9.
3. Urist M. The etiology of the so-called "A" & "V" syndromes. Am J Ophthalmol 1958;46:835–44.
4. Brown H. Vertical deviations. Trans Am Acad Ophthalmol Otolaryngol. 1953;57:157–62. PMID: 13049450.
5. Clark RA, Miller JM, Rosenbaum AL, Demer JL. Heterotopic muscle pulleys or oblique muscle dysfunction. J AAPOS. 1998;2:17–25.

6. Gobin MH. Sagittalization of the oblique muscles as a possible cause for the 'A', 'V', and 'X' phenomena. Br J Ophthalmol. 1968;52:13–18.
7. Yan J-H, Wu XF. Diagnosis and surgical management of isolated inferior oblique palsy. Int J Ophthalmol. 2020;13:349–55. PMID: 32090047.
8. Brodsky MC, Donahue SP. Primary oblique muscle overaction the brain throws a wild pitch. Jama Ophthamol. 2001;119:1307–1314.
9. Miller M, Folk E. Strabismus associated with craniofacial anomalies. Am Orthopt J. 1975;25:27–37. PMID: 1200461.
10. Zhale R, Norouzi S, Sabbaghi H, Yaseri M, Abdi S, Faghihi M. The effect of inferior oblique muscle weakening on horizontal alignment. J Current Ophthalmol. 2019;13:298–304.
11. Buckley EG, Flynn JT. Superior oblique recession versus tenotomy: a comparison of surgical results. J Pediatr Ophthalmol Strabismus. 2013;20:112–7.
12. Julio Prieto-Diaz MD. Posterior tenectomy of the superior oblique. J Pediatr Ophthalmol Strabismus. 2013;16:321–323.
13. Sharma P, Saxena R, Venkateswara Rao B, Menon V. Effect of posterior tenectomy of the superior oblique on objective and subjective torsion in cases of superior oblique overaction. J Pediatr Ophthalmol Strabismus. 2005;42:284–9.
14. Kutschke PJ, Scott WE. Postoperative results in inferior oblique palsy. J Pediatr Ophthalmol Strabismus. 1996;33:72–78.
15. Heo H, Lee KH, Ahn JK, Kim DH, Park YG, Park SW. Effect of 10-mm superior oblique posterior tenectomy combined with frenulum dissection in a-pattern with superior oblique overaction. Am J Ophthalmol. Vol. 2009;148:794–9.
16. Caldeira JA. Graduated recession of the superior oblique muscle. Br J Ophtalmol. 1975;59(10):553–9.
17. Romano P, Roholt P. Measured graduated recession of the superior oblique muscle. J Pediatr Ophthalmol Strabismus. 1983;20:134–140.
18. Drummond GT, Pearce WG, Astle WF. Recession of the superior oblique tendon in A-pattern strabismus. Can J Ophthalmol. 1990;25:301–305.
19. Wright K. Superior oblique silicone expander for brown syndrome and superior oblique overaction. J Pediatr Ophthalmol Strabismus. 2013;28:101–107.
20. Sharma P, Halder M, Prakash P. Torsional changes in surgery for A-V phenomena. Indian J Ophthalmol. 1997;45:31–35.
21. van der Meulen-Schot HM, van der Meulen SB, Simonsz HJ. Caudal or cranial partial tenotomy of the horizontal rectus muscles in A and V pattern strabismus. Br J Ophthalmol. 2008;92:245–51.
22. Bietti GB. On a technical procedure (recession and fan-shaped oblique reinsertion of the horizontal rectus muscles) for correction of V or A exotropias of slight degree in concomitant strabismus. Boll Ocul. 1970;49:581–8.
23. Kushner BJ. Insertion slanting strabismus surgical procedures. Arch Ophthalmol. 2011;129:1620.
24. Clark RA, Miller JM, Demer JL. Location and stability of rectus muscle pulleys. Muscle paths as a function of gaze. Invest Ophthalmol Vis Sci. 1997;38:227–40.
25. Fink WH."A" and "V" syndromes. Am Orthopt J. 1959;9:105–10.
26. Miller JE. Vertical recti transplantation in the "A" and "V" syndromes. Arch Ophthalmol. 1960;61:689–700.
27. Wright KW. Alphabet patterns and oblique muscle dysfunctions. Pediatric Ophthalmol Strabismus. 2002:232–49.
28. Jampolsky A. Oblique muscle surgery of the A and V patterns. J Pediatr Ophthalmol. 1965;2:31–36.
29. de Decker W.Heterotropie. In: Kaufmann H, editor. Strabismus; 2004. p. 188–234. vol. 3.
30. von Noorden GK, Campos EC. A and V patterns. In: von Noorden GK, Campos EC, editors. Binocular vision and ocular motility: theory and management of strabismus. 2002. p. 396–413. vol. 6.
31. Brandner M, et al. Biomechanical analysis of X-pattern exotropia. 2011;152:0–142.

Surgical Management of Strabismus Third Nerve Palsy

Neha Yadav and Stephanie K. West

Abstract Management of third nerve palsy (oculomotor nerve palsy) requires a multifaceted approach tailored to the clinical presentation. The goal is to address the underlying cause, alleviate symptoms, and improve ocular alignment and function. The initial step in management is a thorough clinical evaluation to determine the etiology, which may include vascular, traumatic, neoplastic, inflammatory, or idiopathic origins. Neuroimaging and other diagnostic tests are often necessary to identify the underlying pathology. Non-surgical options like prisms and botulinum toxin have limited efficacy in complete palsies where occlusive patches can be used to manage diplopia. Surgical intervention aims to align the visual axis in the primary position, and patient expectations must be managed, as postoperative diplopia is common. Various surgical techniques, such as supramaximal recession and resection, split lateral rectus transposition, and globe fixation, are used based on the specific characteristics of the palsy. For partial palsies, surgical plans are tailored to optimise the affected eye's position and movement, often involving contralateral eye surgery to balance residual deficits. The management of superior and inferior division palsies and single muscle palsies involves specific strategies, including the use of botulinum toxin for sensory outcome assessment and a combination of recession and resection procedures. This chapter also discusses the technical details and potential complications of these surgical interventions, supported by case studies illustrating various management approaches.

Keywords Third nerve palsy · Supramaximal recession · Globe anchoring · Split lateral rectus transposition · Choroidal effusion · Scott's procedure · Vertical transposition.

N. Yadav · S. K. West (✉)
University Southampton NHS Foundation Trust, Southampton, UK
e-mail: Stephanie.West@uhs.nhs.uk

S. Jain (ed.), *Surgical Management of Strabismus*,
https://doi.org/10.1007/978-3-031-80633-9_8

1 Introduction

The management of third nerve palsies is challenging due to the involvement of four out of six extraocular muscles. In children, common causes of isolated third nerve palsies include congenital issues, trauma, and inflammation. In adults, vascular causes are more prevalent, such as those related to diabetes, hypertension, hypercholesterolemia, smoking, as well as conditions like migraines, aneurysms, and trauma [1].

In all acquired cases it is important to allow time for recovery and stability of the eye movements before considering surgical intervention.

2 Classification

Third nerve palsies can be broadly divided into two categories: Complete and Incomplete (partial).

Complete

- involves both upper and lower division affecting all extraocular muscles innervated by the third nerve.
- Pupil involvement may or may not be present.

Incomplete

This, also, may or may not involve the pupil.

- Superior division affecting superior rectus and levator muscles.
- Inferior division affecting medial and Inferior recti, Inferior oblique, iris sphincter and ciliary body.
- It is also possible to have single muscle involvement (Table 1).

Table 1 Classification of third nerve palsy

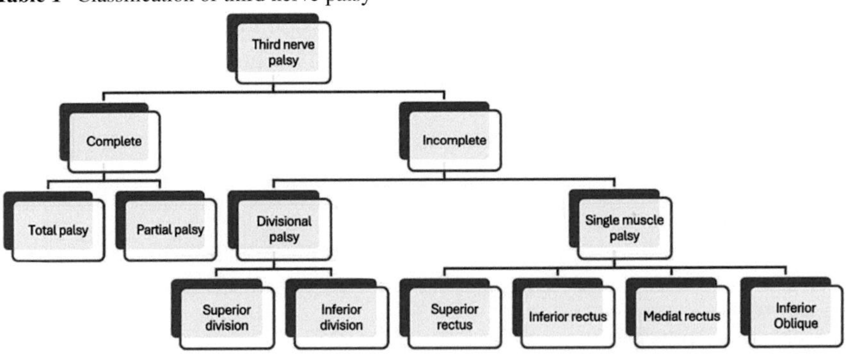

The aim of surgical intervention is to try and align the visual axis in primary position. It is important that patient expectations are appropriately managed. In binocular patients post operative diplopia should be expected and anticipated.

Ability to assess tolerance or acceptance of residual deviation is difficult as botulinum toxin is often not effective enough or the size of deviation prevents successful use of fresnel prisms.

The management of postoperative diplopia should be thoroughly discussed with the patient. This includes the potential need for eye occlusion (using a frosted lens or patch) if diplopia is intolerable after surgery [2]. Additionally, the possibility of using an occlusive contact lens should be evaluated preoperatively.

3 Management of Complete Third Nerve Palsy

The clinical features of a complete third nerve palsy include exotropia and hypotropia. Intorsion is also present although patients are not usually symptomatic. The sequalae of this includes overaction of the contralateral lateral and superior recti as well as the superior and inferior obliques.

There will be no diplopia nor abnormal head position if there is ptosis obscuring the visual axis however if only partial then contralateral lid retraction may be present.

It is important to look for signs of aberrant regeneration if there is a history of trauma or nerve compression which may include synergistic movement of either the lids or extraocular muscles with jaw movements, horizontal gaze-eyelid synkinesis, a pseudo von Graefe's sign (elevation or retraction of the upper eyelid when the eye is looking downwards and inwards.), adduction of the eye on attempted vertical movements with retraction of globe on attempted vertical movement and a pseudo Argyll-Robertson pupil (constricts to accommodation and has a slight response to light (miosis) as opposed to Argyll Robertson pupils were there is no response to a light stimulus). If there is ciliary body involvement there may be an accommodative deficit as well as a dilated pupil [3, 4].

3.1 Non-surgical Management

Non-surgical treatment options are limited. Prisms are unlikely to provide benefit in complete palsies since diplopia tends to reverse across different positions, but they may prove helpful in partial cases. Similarly, botulinum toxin can aid in assessing residual muscle function, such as that of the medial rectus, but is unlikely to substantially alter eye position in a complete palsy [5]. Significant ptosis can be advantageous in obscuring the second image; otherwise, alternative methods of occlusion may be necessary if the ability to ignore or suppress the second image is absent.

Photophobia from pupil dilation can be managed with tinted glasses, pilocarpine 1% or a painted miosed contact lens [6].

3.2 Surgical Management

The aim of successful surgery, for complete third nerve palsy, is good alignment in primary position which involves correcting both the exotropia and the hypotropia. To achieve this, and minimise the risk of exotropia recurrence, all eye movements and especially abduction need to be limited.

Options to achieve this include:

(1) Maximal recession of lateral rectus (12–16 mm) and resection of medial rectus (8–12 mm) can be done to correct the exotropia. This can be combined with supraplacement of the horizontal recti (modified Knapp's procedure) or superior oblique weakening (tenotomy or expander) to address the hypotropia. Additionally, traction sutures can be placed around the vertical recti, brought out through the upper and lower lids, and left in situ for six weeks [7–9].

(2) Superior oblique transposition to insertion of medial rectus combined with lateral rectus recession. This requires superior oblique function to be intact and acts to leash the eye limiting depression as well as abduction. Anecdotal evidence is that the outcome of this procedure lacks longevity and it has lost favour in current practice [7, 10–12].

(3) Split lateral rectus transposition. This is our preferred option for complete third nerve palsy, details of the procedure are outlined further on in this chapter [8, 13, 14].

(4) Globe fixation procedures. Non absorbable sutures or fascia lata can be used to fixate the globe, for example removing lateral rectus and suturing the medial rectus to the periosteum with or without muscle resection [8, 15–18] (Figs. 1, 2 and 3).

3.2.1 Split Lateral Rectus Transposition

Video 3.9: Split lateral rectus transposition to the medial rectus in third nerve palsy.

A recent global study deemed this procedure successful (within 15 PD of orthophoria) in 69% of cases and in 100% of those who had concurrent superior oblique tenotomy. The researchers found no link between success and factors such as the surgeon's experience, age at surgery, sex, history of strabismus surgery, aetiology, concurrent inferior oblique myectomy, or the use of adjustable or augmentation sutures. Technical difficulties were encountered in 30% of cases with a previous history of strabismus surgery. Additionally, the authors noted that postoperative alignment under general anaesthesia was a strong predictor of alignment after recovery. They recommend aiming for 10 PD BO esotropia during surgery [13].

Fig. 1 a and b: Fixation of the lateral rectus to the taeral orbital wall

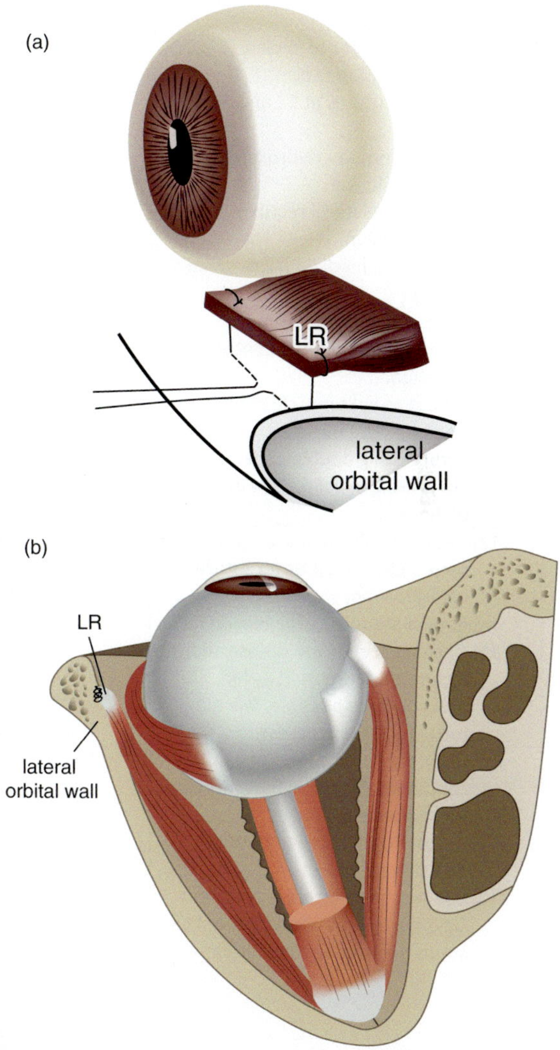

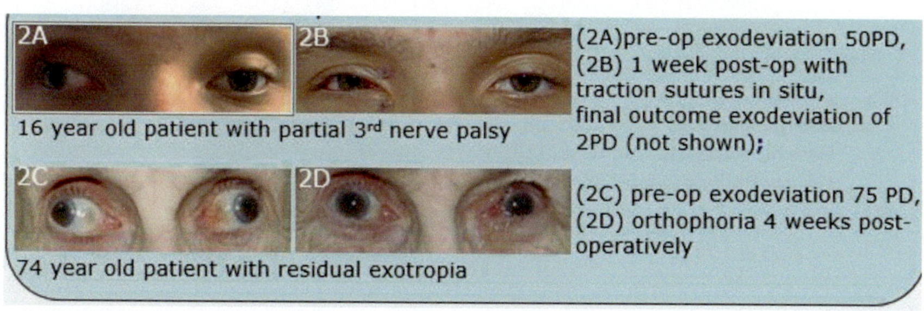

Fig. 2 Results of medial and lateral orbital fixation and traction sutures in two patients- courtesy Gill Adams

1) Full face drape 2) Vasoconstrictor of choice 3) Forced duction test. 4) Traction sutures at 12 and 6 o'clock 5) Protect cornea - Hydroxypropyl methylcellulose. 6) Expose the lateral rectus – limbal based incision. 7) Expose the medial rectus – limbal incision	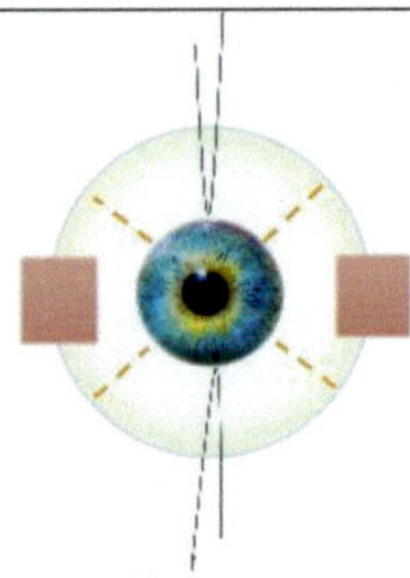
8) Hook and expose LR. 9) Measure and identify centre of insertion. 10) Dissect to split muscle in half. 11) Hook half the muscle 12) Suture using double ended 6.0 vicryl using usual recession technique	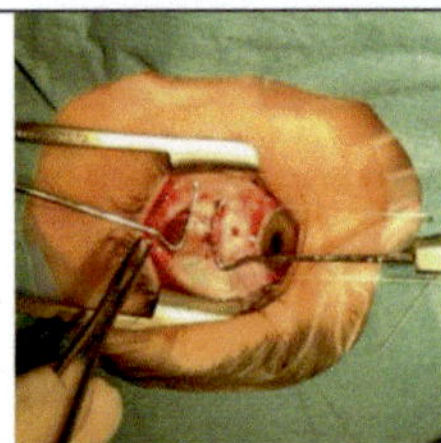
13) Disinsert half the muscle and secure loose sutures for future identification. 14) Repeat steps 9-11 for second half. 15) Once both ends are disinserted, ensure muscle is split as far posteriorly as possible, use a retractor to gain access	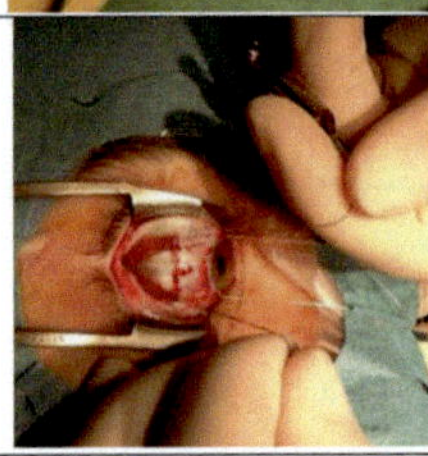
16) Hook the IO through same conjunctival incision using stevens tenotomy hook. 17) Expose IO and spread between two stevens hooks. 18) Use mosquito artery forceps or Gass hook to pass inferior split LR sutures posterior to anterior	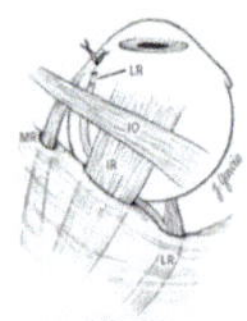 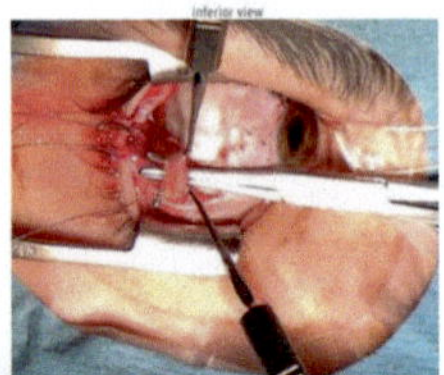
19) Hook the IR using existing incisions. 20) Use mosquito artery forceps or Gass hook to pass inferior split LR sutures under the inferior rectus	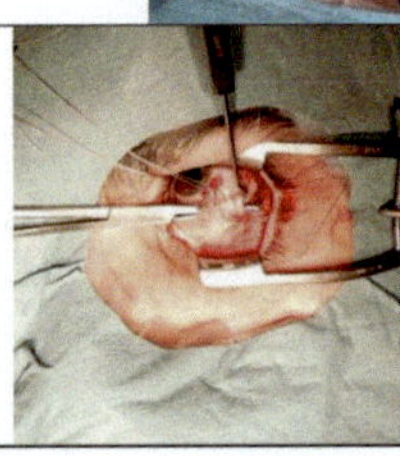

Fig. 3 Split lateral rectus transposition procedure, step by step. LR = lateral rectus, IO = inferior oblique, IR = inferior rectus, SR = superior rectus, SO = superior oblique

21) Hook the SR using existing incisions from the medial side. 22) Identify the SO tendon to ensure LR passes underneath	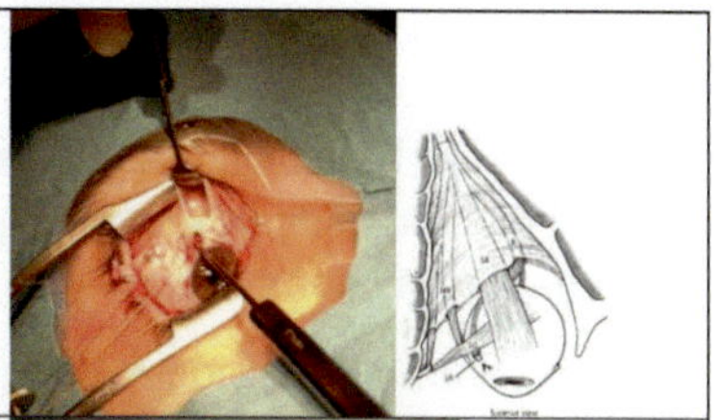
23) Use mosquito artery forceps or Gass hook to pass inferior split LR sutures under the superior rectus	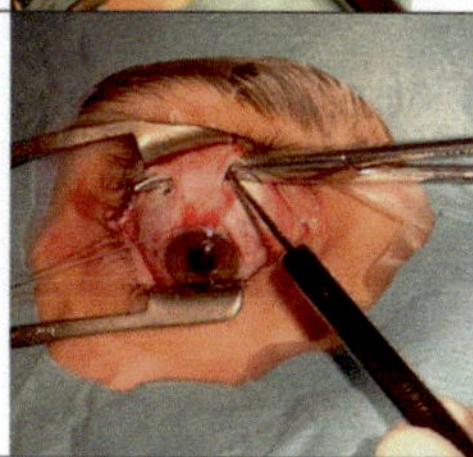
24) Suture LR adjacent to superior and inferior border of MR respectively using an adjustable suture e.g. bow. 25) Use light reflex on both eyes to adjust, aim for approx. 10ET	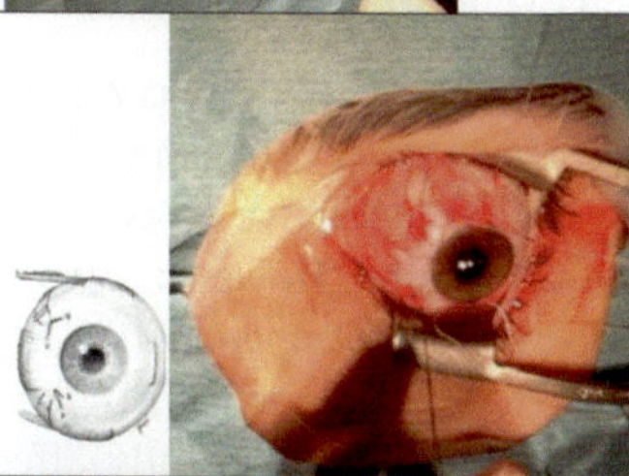
26) Reposition and suture the conjunctiva – 8.0 silk	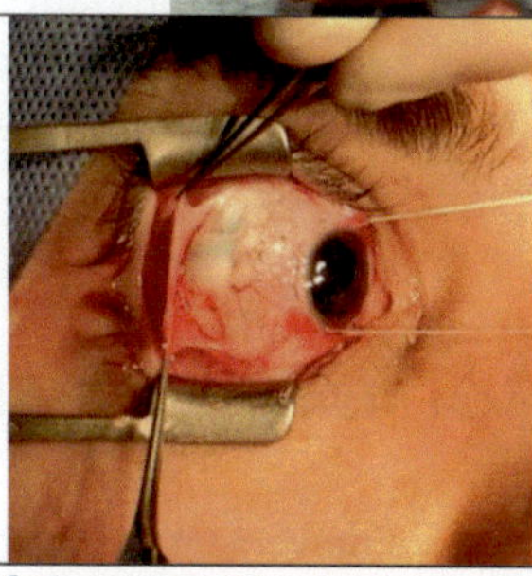

LR= lateral rectus, IO= inferior oblique, IR=inferior rectus, SR=superior rectus, SO= superior oblique

Fig. 3 (continued)

3.2.1.1 Variations

The steps involving the superior and inferior oblique can be simplified by performing superior oblique and Inferior oblique tenotomies. The procedure can be combined with a medial rectus resection. The use of fascia lata has been described, to extend the insertions of the lateral rectus [19].

3.2.1.2 Potential Pitfalls and Complications

This surgery can be technically challenging especially in cases that have had previous surgery. Potential complications include.
Vision threatening complications (11%) [13, 20]

- Serous choroidal effusions
- Central Serous Retinopathy
- Optic nerve compromise
- Anterior segment ischaemia.

Transient ocular hypertension

Intractable diplopia

Limited eye movements

The occurrence rate of these complications was not associated with age at the time of surgery, the interval between diagnosis and surgery, history of previous strabismus surgery, or intraoperative procedures such as superior oblique tenotomy and inferior oblique myectomy. However, complications were correlated with a higher degree of preoperative exotropia and the average placement of the split lateral rectus (LR) relative to the medial rectus (MR) insertion. Transpositions located more posteriorly on the globe may significantly affect the vortex veins. In contrast, transpositions where the split ends are closer to the MR muscle insertion (within 4.25 mm) may create an anterior arc of contact with the globe, thereby reducing the impact on posterior circulation [8, 13, 20–24].

4 Surgical Management of Partial Third Nerve Palsy

Less limitation of movement means that these patients have a better chance of getting a central area of binocular single vision.

The general principles are:

- Botulinum toxin can be used to investigate the potential sensory outcome.
- Surgical planning should aim to optimise the position and range of movement in the affected eye.
- The residual movement deficits can then be balanced by operating on overacting synergists in contralateral eye.

4.1 Surgical Management

This depends on if there is just a horizontal deviation or a vertical component as well.

Horizontal deviation only.

- Perform an adjustable lateral rectus recession and medial rectus resection on the affected eye. If there is any residual limitation of adduction in the affected eye, consider a lateral rectus recession on the contralateral eye or a Scott or Faden's procedure if the primary position is optimal [23, 24].

Horizontal and Vertical deviation

- Technically it is possible to combine vertical transposition of the horizontal muscles with recession or resection however the results are reported to be disappointing.
- The other option is to consider further surgery on contralateral unaffected eye to correct any residual deviation.

5 Incomplete Palsy

5.1 Superior Division

The superior division of the third nerve supplies motor innervation to the superior rectus and levator palpebrae superioris muscles. Additionally, sympathetic fibers travel alongside the superior branch to innervate the superior tarsal muscle. Acquired superior division palsies are frequently linked with aneurysms, underscoring the importance of excluding and effectively managing them as a priority.

5.1.1 Clinical Features

- The affected eye will be hypotropic with an element of pseudoptosis as well as a true ptosis.
- Superior rectus underaction is often partial, and eyelid retraction is typically present on the contralateral side when fixating with the affected eye.
- Binocular patients will adopt a head elevation posture.

5.1.2 Management

Conservative management may be appropriate in terms of prisms or sector occlusion of the upper part of their spectacles.

Strabismus surgery should be undertaken prior to their ptosis surgery.

- Incomitant vertical deviation
  - If the vertical deviation is incomitant with contralateral inferior oblique overaction, this should be weakened first.
- Concomitant deviation

- For concomitant deviation in downgaze and in the contralateral field of gaze measuring less than 15 prism dioptres in primary position perform a contralateral superior rectus recession.
- For more than 15 prism dioptres combine this with an ipsilateral inferior rectus recession.
- Alternative is to consider an ipsilateral inferior rectus recession/ superior rectus resection.

For marked Superior rectus palsies a forced duction test should be performed. If the inferior rectus is tight this should be recessed taking care to separate the lower lid retractors to avoid post operative lid changes.

If the force duction test is normal, then an ipsilateral Knapp's or vertical Nishida procedure should be performed. It is important to warn the patient that this may unmask an ipsilateral inferior rectus palsy and they may get diplopia in downgaze. Knapp procedures can be enhanced with posterior fixation sutures [25, 26].

If further surgery is required, this can be undertaken on the contralateral eye to reduce the overaction of the inferior oblique or superior rectus.

5.2 *Inferior Division*

This is a rare occurrence of medial rectus, inferior rectus, and inferior oblique palsy as well as sphincter pupillae and ciliary muscle involvement.

The clinical features include exotropia, hypertropia and intorsion with pupil dilation. There is overaction of the contralateral lateral rectus, superior rectus, and superior oblique. Accommodation is defective in the affected eye. Due to the incomitance and intorsion it is unlikely any field of binocular single vision can be achieved, and so no abnormal head posture is present and non-surgical management is ineffective.

5.2.1 Surgical Management

- Partial inferior division palsies- Lateral rectus can be recessed and medial rectus resected combined with inferoplacement of both insertions.
- Total inferior division palsies. Medial transposition of the lateral rectus and nasal tenotomy of the superior oblique have been described [27].

6 Single Muscle Palsies

6.1 Medial Rectus

Medial rectus palsies are often due to internuclear ophthalmoplegia, myasthenia gravis, or trauma. Patients typically exhibit a head turn towards the unaffected side if they can achieve binocular single vision. Management options include conservative approaches with prisms or surgical interventions such as lateral rectus recession combined with medial rectus resection. In cases of complete palsy, vertical rectus transposition with medial rectus resections (typically 5 mm to reduce slack) can be considered.

6.2 Inferior Rectus

Inferior rectus palsies may be congenital or acquired, linked to conditions like myasthenia gravis, skew deviations, or mechanical issues. Acquired isolated palsies could be due to a vascular event affecting the third nerve nuclei or a brainstem tumor.

Clinically, these cases present with hypertropia, occasionally accompanied by slight exotropia. An 'A' pattern may indicate bilateral involvement. Overaction of the contralateral superior rectus and secondary inhibition of the contralateral inferior oblique are common sequelae. Patients may adopt a downward head posture, with a tilt to the unaffected side due to hypertropia and torsion. The Bielschowsky head tilt test is unreliable in these cases.

6.2.1 Surgical Management

6.2.1.1 Ipsilateral Eye Surgery

Treatment options include inferior rectus resection or superior rectus recession on the affected eye, or an inverse Knapp procedure. If the primary position deviation is less than 5 prism diopters, there is a risk of reversal in both primary position and contralateral gaze, so a half tendon width transposition is recommended. It can take up to six months for binocular single vision improvement. If further surgery is needed, residual deficits can be addressed by weakening the overacting contralateral superior or inferior recti.

Table 2 Surgical management of inferior rectus palsy

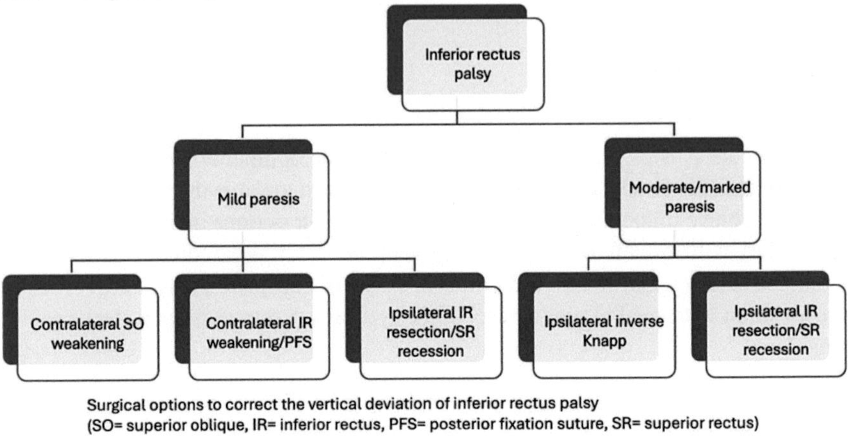

6.2.1.2 Contralateral Eye Surgery

Procedures may include superior oblique weakening through posterior tenotomy or spacer placement. Once concomitance has spread, recession of the contralateral inferior rectus with or without posterior fixation sutures can be performed. A posterior fixation suture or Scott procedure to the contralateral inferior rectus may be indicated if the patient has binocular single vision in the primary position (Table 2).

6.3 Superior Rectus Palsy

Typically bilateral and congenital, superior rectus palsies are often associated with a V-pattern exotropia (XT). Management recommendations align with those for superior division palsy.

7 Aberrant Regeneration

In cases of acquired compressive or traumatic palsy, checking for aberrant regeneration is crucial. Signs include eyelid elevation during attempted adduction. If surgery for exotropia is necessary, operating on the contralateral horizontal recti is advised, as this can improve ptosis and eyelid movements by increasing stimulation to the lateral rectus and medial rectus synergist [28].

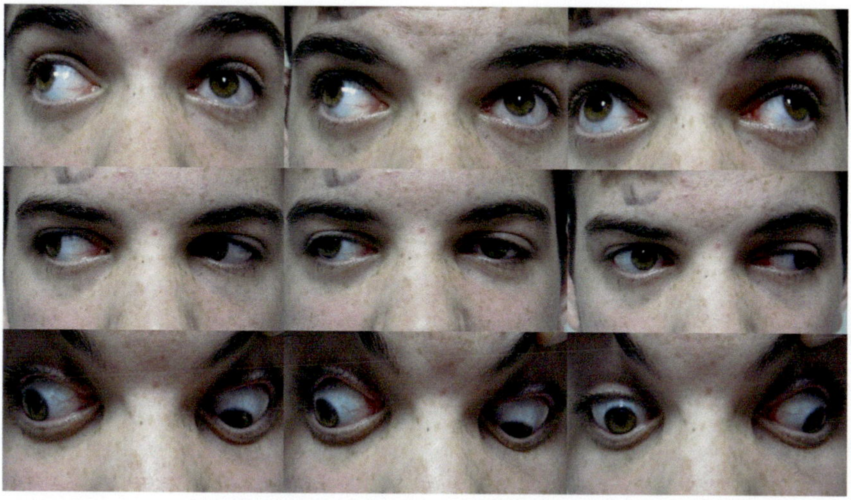

Fig. 4 9-year-old with right third nerve palsy preoperatively

8 Example Cases

8.1 Case 1

An 18-year-old represents with right third nerve palsy resulting from a midbrain pilocytic astrocytoma diagnosed at age 9. They are experiencing persistent diplopia and are managed with occlusion. Previous administration of botulinum toxin to the right lateral rectus reduced the exotropia but did not achieve fusion. Preoperatively, the patient had a 60 PD right exotropia and 8 PD right hypertropia, accompanied by deficits of − 3 in adduction and − 2 in depression and elevation (Figs. 4 and 5).

Split lateral rectus transposition was performed as described earlier in this chapter; 4 months later there was a stable residual deviation, fixing with his left eye, of 12 PD right exotropia and 6 PD right hypertropia. Patient was pleased with the cosmetic outcome but still troubled by diplopia which was managed with an occlusive contact lens (Fig. 6).

8.2 Case 2

A 59-year-old man represents with superior division third nerve palsy resulting from a road traffic accident 50 years ago. He previously underwent ipsilateral inferior rectus recession and contralateral superior rectus recession with adjustment ten years ago.

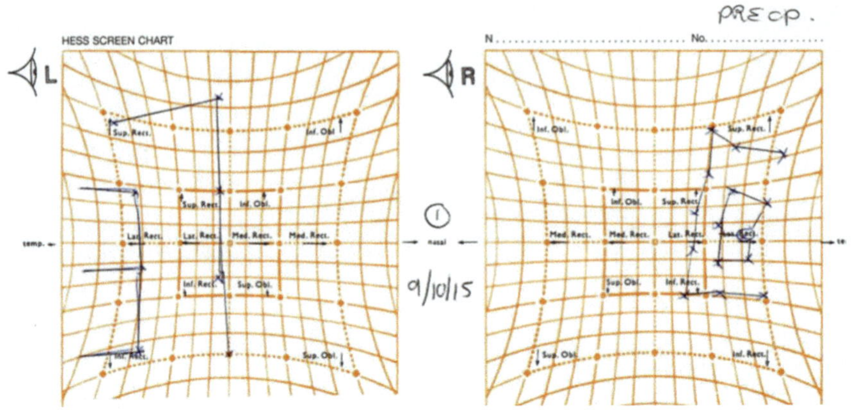

Fig. 5 Hess chart showing right third nerve palsy corresponding sequelae with contralateral overactions

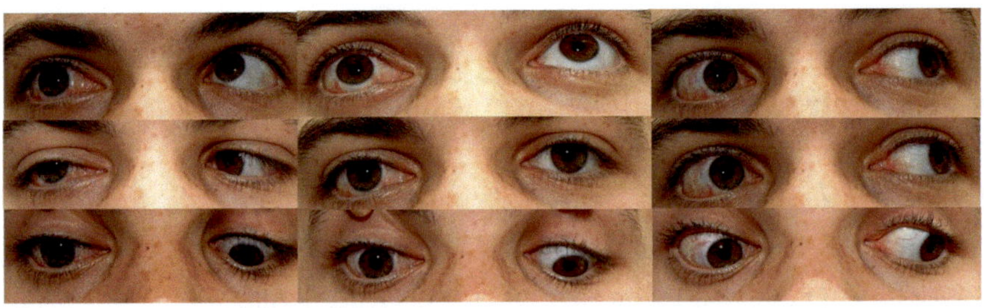

Fig. 6 Post operative eye movements for case 1

He now has 35 PD right hypotropia and right ptosis, accompanied by a limitation of elevation of – 5 and an adduction deficit of – 1 (Fig. 7).

Right Knapp procedure was performed with full tendon transposition of lateral and medial rectus muscles to the border of the superior rectus, augmented with 5.0 ethibond posterior fixation sutures 8 mm posterior to superior rectus insertion (Fig. 8).

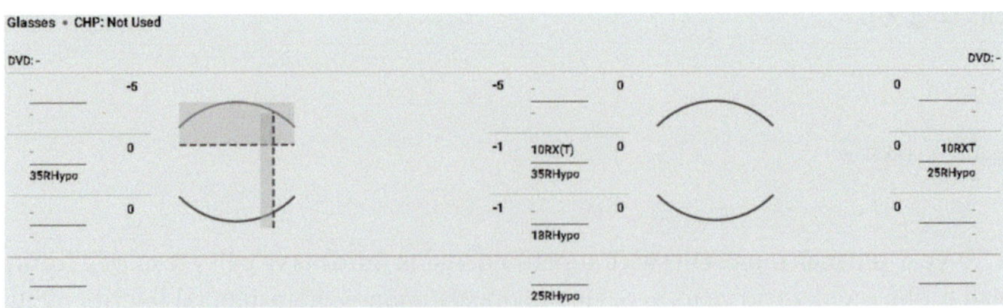

Fig. 7 Pre-operative orthoptic report for case 2

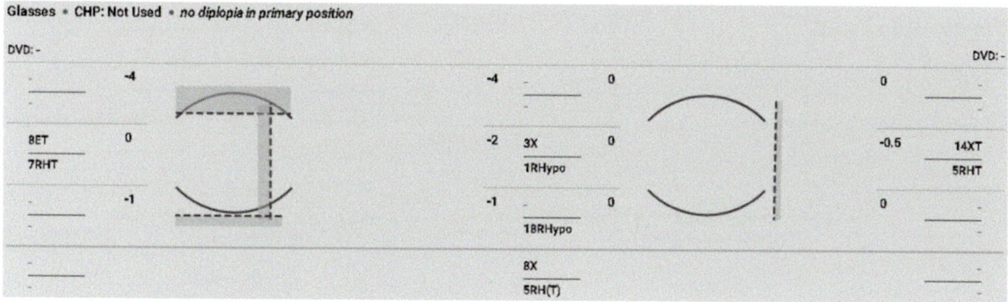

Fig. 8 Post-operative orthoptic report for case 2

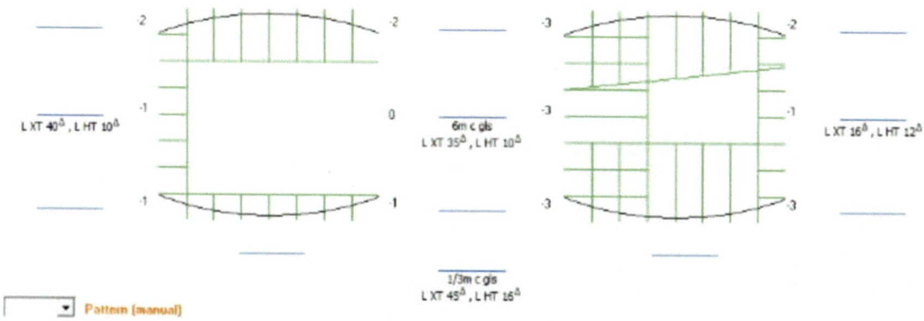

Fig. 9 Preoperative orthoptic report for case 3

Post operatively the patient had no diplopia in primary position and went on to have successful ptosis surgery.

8.3 *Case 3*

A 40-year-old woman presents with partial left third nerve palsy resulting from a cerebrovascular accident following pituitary tumour resection. She had a 35 PD exotropia and 10 PD left hypertropia, with a – 3 deficit in elevation, adduction, and depression in her left eye. Additionally, her right eye shows a – 2 elevation deficit (Fig. 9).

Surgery was performed on the affected side, involving an 8 mm recession of the lateral rectus and a 7 mm resection of the medial rectus. Following the operation, she now has a residual 6 PD esotropia and 9 PD hypertropia on the left side, which is being managed with a vertical prism (Fig. 10).

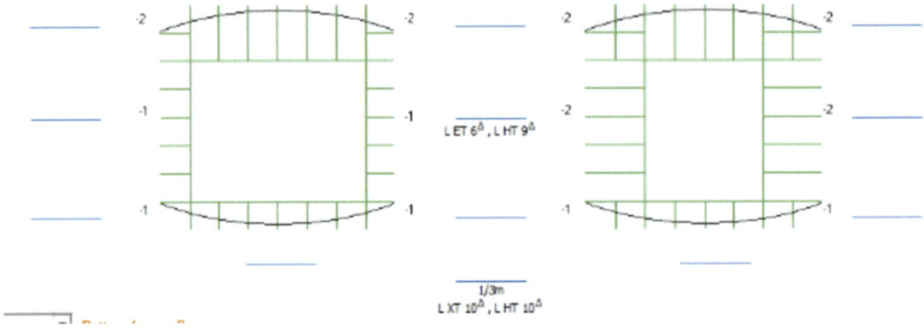

Fig. 10 Post-operative orthoptic report for case 3

References

1. Ansons AM, Davis H. Diagnosis and management of ocular motility disorders. 2013:451–61.
2. Burger DS, London R. Soft opaque contact lenses in binocular vision problems. J Am Optom Assoc. 1993;64(3):176–80.
3. Sukhija J, Kaur S. Treatment options for third nerve paralysis. Adv Ophthalmol Optom. 2020;5:61–70.
4. Bagheri A, Borhani M, Tavakoli M, Salehirad S. Clinical features and outcomes of strabismus treatment in third cranial nerve palsy during a 10-year period. J Ophthalmic Vis Res. 2014;9(3):343–9. https://doi.org/10.4103/2008-322X.143375.
5. Dawson EL, Hancox JC, Lee JP. Use of botulinum toxin in patients with third nerve palsy. J AAPOS. 2011;15(1).
6. Katz BJ, Digre KB. Diagnosis, pathophysiology, and treatment of photophobia. Surv Ophthalmol. 2016;61(4):466–77. https://doi.org/10.1016/j.survophthal.2016.02.001.
7. Kattleman B, Flanders M, Wise J. Supramaximal horizontal rectus surgery in the management of third and sixth nerve palsy. Can J Ophthalmol. 1986;21:227–30.
8. Yahalom C, Hunter DG, Dagi LR. Strategies for managing strabismus from oculomotor nerve palsy. J AAPOS. 2023;27(1):3–9. https://doi.org/10.1016/j.jaapos.2022.11.017.
9. Khaier A, Dawson E, Lee J. Traction sutures in the management of long-standing third nerve palsy. Strabismus. 2008;16(2):77–83. https://doi.org/10.1080/09273970802077474.
10. Eraslan M, Cerman E, Onal S, Ogut MS. Superior oblique anterior transposition with horizontal recti recession-resection for total third-nerve palsy. J Ophthalmol. 2015;2015:780139.
11. Young TL, Conahan BM, Summers CG, Egbert JE. Anterior transposition of the superior oblique tendon in the treatment of oculomotor nerve palsy and its influence on postoperative hypertropia. J Pediatr Ophthalmol Strabismus. 2000;37(3):149–55. https://doi.org/10.3928/0191-3913-20000501-06.
12. Singh A, Pandey PK, Mittal SK, Agrawal A, Bahuguna C, Kumar P. Impact of superior oblique transposition on primary position deviation, a pattern and intorsion in third nerve palsy. Strabismus. 2016;24(4):173–7. https://doi.org/10.1080/09273972.2016.1243136.
13. Oke I, Lorenz B, Basiakos S, et al. Nasal transposition of the split lateral rectus muscle for strabismus associated with bilateral 3rd-nerve palsy. Am J Ophthalmol. 2022;242:165–172. https://doi.org/10.1016/j.ajo.2022.06.010
14. Shah AS, Dodd MU, Gokyigit B, et al. Worldwide outcomes of nasal transposition of the split lateral rectus muscle for strabismus associated with 3rd-nerve palsy. Br J Ophthalmol. 2023;107(5):725–31. https://doi.org/10.1136/bjophthalmol-2021-319667.
15. Sharma P, Gogoi M, Kedar S, Bhola R. Periosteal fixation in third-nerve palsy. J AAPOS. 2006;10(4):324–7. https://doi.org/10.1016/j.jaapos.2006.02.005.

16. Saxena R, Phuljhele S, Sharma P, Pinto CN. Periosteal fixation procedures in the management of incomitant strabismus. Middle East Afr J Ophthalmol. 2015;22(3):320–6. https://doi.org/10.4103/0974-9233.159736.
17. Saxena R, Sinha A, Sharma P, Phuljhele S, Menon V. Precaruncular approach for medial orbital wall periosteal anchoring of the globe in oculomotor nerve palsy. J AAPOS. 2009;13(6):578–82. https://doi.org/10.1016/j.jaapos.2009.11.003.
18. Salazar-León JA, Ramírez-Ortíz MA, Salas-Vargas M. The surgical correction of paralytic strabismus using fascia lata [published correction appears in J Pediatr Ophthalmol Strabismus. 1998;35(5):269. https://doi.org/10.3928/0191-3913-19980101-10
19. Tsai CB, Fang CL. Fascia lata augmented nasal transposition of split lateral rectus in complete oculomotor nerve palsy with a previous failed surgery. Eur J Ophthalmol. 2020;30(3):608–11. https://doi.org/10.1177/1120672119871456.
20. Shah AS, Prabhu SP, Sadiq MA, Mantagos IS, Hunter DG, Dagi LR. Adjustable nasal transposition of split lateral rectus muscle for third nerve palsy. JAMA Ophthalmol. 2014;132(8):963–9. https://doi.org/10.1001/jamaophthalmol.2014.756.
21. Lincoff H, Stopa M, Kreissig I, et al. Cutting the encircling band. Retina. 2006;26(6):650–4. https://doi.org/10.1097/01.iae.0000236475.01938.c4.
22. Tasman W. Jaeger EA Duane's ophthalmology. Lippincott, Williams and Wilkins (on CD ROM); 2013.
23. Scott AB. The faden operation: mechanical effects. Am Orthopt J. 1977;27:44–7.
24. Cuppers C. The so-called "Fadenoperation.". In: Fells P, editor. Transactions of the 2nd congress. International Strabismological Association; 1974. p. 395–400.
25. Nishida Y, Inatomi A, AokiY, et al. A muscle transposition procedure for abducens palsy, in which the halves of the vertical rectus muscle bellies are sutured onto the sclera. Jpn J Ophthalmol 2003;47: 281–6.
26. Knapp P. Incomitant exodeviations and their treatment. In: Manley D, editor. Symposium on horizontal ocular deviations. St. Louis: Mosby; 1978. p. 350–57.
27. Kushner BJ. Surgical treatment of paralysis of the inferior division of the oculomotor nerve. Arch Ophthalmol. 1999;117(4):485–9. https://doi.org/10.1001/archopht.117.4.485.
28. Fouad HM, Kamal AM, Awadein A, Del Monte MA. Contralateral surgery for the treatment of third nerve palsy with aberrant regeneration. Am J Ophthalmol. 2021;222:166–73.

The Management of Superior Oblique Paresis

Anthony J. Vivian

Abstract Superior oblique paresis may present acutely or as a congenital or insidious onset condition. Investigation of acutely presenting causes is important. Careful assessment of the ocular motility and deviation in all positions of gaze enables various patterns of presentation to be identified. This allows the appropriate surgical treatment to be targeted. This chapter outlines the important features of the assessment and choices of surgical intervention and detailed surgical techniques involved in the various surgical options.

Keywords Strabismus · Superior oblique paresis · Inferior oblique surgery · Superior oblique surgery

1 Introduction

- The superior oblique is responsible for intorsion, depression and abduction.
- Superior oblique paresis can therefore cause torsional, vertical and horizontal diplopia.
- It may present either acutely due to damage to the nerve or nuclei in the midbrain, or insidiously as a congenital abnormality or later onset idiopathic paresis.
- The two groups have different characteristics of incomitance and so need different investigation and management strategies.
- This highlights the importance of careful measurement of deviations in nine positions of gaze, version measurements, deviation on head tilting, analysis of torsion and abnormal head posture.
- This thorough orthoptic assessment will inform which surgical approach is most appropriate.

A. J. Vivian (✉)
Cambridge University Hospitals, Cambridge, UK
e-mail: vivianeye@aol.com

S. Jain (ed.), *Surgical Management of Strabismus*,
https://doi.org/10.1007/978-3-031-80633-9_9

2 Aetiology

2.1 Congenital/Idiopathic Superior Oblique Paresis

- Little is known about the underlying causes of congenital or idiopathic superior oblique paresis.
- It presents in infancy or childhood or later as an insidious progression of abnormal head posture and eventually intermittent vertical diplopia.
- Sometimes, looking back at old photos, an abnormal head tilt can be seen to be present many years before any symptoms develop.
- It is likely that these represent a heterogenous collection of vertical deviations with different mechanisms:
  - Structural abnormality or absence of the trochlear (fourth) nerve and hypoplasia of the superior oblique muscle: This can sometimes be seen on high resolution MRI scan and probably represents a dysinnervation syndrome
  - Familial superior oblique paresis is unusual but is occasionally reported
  - As yet no genetic defects have been associated with isolated superior oblique paresis but mutations in the *ARIX* (PHOX2A) gene have been associated with congenital fibrosis of the extraocular muscles (CFEOM) Type 2 which is characterised by trochlear and oculomotor nerve dysinnervation. Some polymorphisms in the ARIX gene have been reported in familial superior oblique paresis [1]
  - In some cases the insertion of the superior oblique tendon is found to be abnormal suggesting a congenital abnormality of muscle development rather than nerve development.

2.2 Acquired/Neurological Superior Oblique Paresis

- The trochlear nerve has a convoluted course from the dorsal midbrain to the orbit, including decussating from one side of the brain to the other, and has the longest intracranial course of any cranial nerve
- It is also very delicate as it only supplies one small muscle
- For these reasons, it is very susceptible to damage and although it is less common as an acquired acute isolated cranial nerve paresis than third or sixth nerve paresis in most series, it is difficult to manage
- Trauma:
  - The nerve can be damaged by rotational traumatic injuries because it wraps around the midbrain
  - This occurs particularly in closed head trauma as a result of road traffic accidents, and falling off motorbikes and horses

  - The damage is often bilateral in closed head trauma, although usually asymmetric
  - In bilateral cases, the torsional component is often the most difficult aspect to manage
  - Some recovery is to be expected in the first six months at least.

- Vascular:

  - Causes include microvascular damage, probably to the nerve itself, associated with conditions such as diabetes, hypertension, and atherosclerosis and, less commonly, vasculitis (including Giant Cell Arteritis)
  - Midbrain cerebrovascular accidents (CVA) can cause isolated trochlear paresis or trochlear paresis can be part of a collection of signs.
  - Isolated trochlear nerve paresis is not commonly caused by aneurysm but has been reported in association with intracavernous carotid aneurysm or fistula and posterior communicating artery aneurysm [2].

- Other compressive causes include intracranial or intra-orbital tumours and intracranial hypertension
- Inflammatory causes include multiple sclerosis, sarcoidosis and bacterial meningitis
- Mimics/differential diagnoses:

  - Clinical features such as fatigability or variability raises the suspicion of myasthenia gravis and should be investigated
  - Thyroid eye disease (TED) should always be ruled out if there is any evidence of restriction or other features of TED
  - Vestibular or neurological symptoms or other inconsistencies in the orthoptic assessment such as incyclotorsion of the hypotropic eye or variability in the vertical deviation should raise suspicions of a skew deviation. The "upright-supine" test can help distinguish the two diagnoses [3].

2.3 Assessment of Fourth Nerve Paresis

Many surgical and non-surgical options exist in the management of fourth nerve paresis. Therefore, once the cause of the paresis has been established and, if necessary, investigated, careful measurement is essential to target treatment appropriately. This includes assessing abnormal head posture, measurements of deviations in nine positions of gaze, versions, vertical deviation on head tilting, and torsion.

Only when all this information is available can a strategic management plan be formulated. This is because superior oblique paresis presents with different patterns depending upon the cause, the duration, and the reaction of the other extra-ocular muscles in response to the superior oblique being weaker. For instance, in congenital fourth nerve paresis the inferior oblique overaction is often the most predominant feature and the deviation is worse in upgaze whereas, in traumatic fourth nerve paresis it is the weakness of the superior oblique with accompanying torsional deviation which is prominent with the deviation being worse in downgaze. Without nine positions of gaze measurements and measuring vertical deviation on head tilting to each side it is difficult to detect bilateral involvement in traumatic fourth nerve paresis which is often subtle. For the most effective management, the choice of operation is different in all of these cases.

Below is a structured approach to such patients:

1. Ask the relevant history

    - A head tilt from childhood without initial diplopia is suggestive of a congenital cause
    - A history of trauma should always raise suspicions of a bilateral case, which may be masked
    - The timing of onset of diplopia in vascular cases will guide how long the surgeon waits to allow for resolution
    - Careful characterisation of the diplopia will suggest where the barrier to fusion may be and help direct the orthoptic assessment
    - Similarly, asking where or when the patient's diplopia is most troubling will help establish the aims of management
    - The clinical features of myasthenia gravis, skew deviation and thyroid eye disease should be ruled out.

2. Assess for an abnormal head posture (AHP)

    - AHPs are used to help maintain single vision and give clues to the diagnosis
    - A significant AHP alone may merit intervention
    - This is particularly true of long-standing congenital fourth nerve paresis when the many years of AHPs can cause musculo-skeletal neck problems
    - Typically the head is tilted away from the affected superior oblique (a left superior oblique paresis presents with a right head tilt).
    - A chin down AHP may be associated with a traumatic bilateral fourth nerve paresis as torsional diplopia is worse in downgaze and is a barrier to binocular vision
    - AHP can be measured with a simple orthopaedic goniometer, a device such as the CROM tool or computer image analysis devices [4].

3. Tilt test

It is not enough to establish that the deviation is worse on tilting the head to one side compared to the other. The difference should be measured with as full a tilt of the head as possible. In bilateral fourth nerve paresis it is important to notice that the deviation is reversed which is very obvious if prisms are being used to measure the vertical deviation.

4. Characterise the deviation and assess the motility: nine positions of gaze measurements and versions

   - Nine positions of gaze: the horizontal and vertical deviation should be measure in the nine positions of gaze to help target management. This can be accomplished by using prisms in free space with distance fixation. By asking the patient to fix on a distance target, and moving their head into the most appropriate position, it is possible to produce accurate and reproducible measurements in the extremes of gaze. This can also be achieved by using the synoptophore
   - Versions: it is important to assess ocular motility to identify the over- and under-acting muscles. This helps confirm the diagnosis, evaluate the muscle sequelae, and formulate the appropriate management plan. A nine point scale can be used for assessing versions paying attention to the action of all six muscles in each eye [5].
   - Muscle sequelae: A fourth nerve paresis will initially manifest as an incomitant deviation due to the primary under-action of the superior oblique. With time, especially in congenital fourth nerve paresis, deviations become more comitant (known as 'spreading comitance'). This is important because it may influence the choice of surgical technique. Sequelae occurs in the following order:
     a. **Overaction** of the *inferior oblique in the same eye*
     b. **Overaction** of the inferior rectus *in the opposite eye*
     c. **Underaction** of superior rectus in the opposite eye
     d. **Overreaction of the superior rectus in the same eye**: There may be overaction of the ipsilateral Superior rectus in long-standing superior oblique paresis. This is because the superior rectus compensates for the loss of intorsion caused by superior oblique weakness and as it's intortion function is inseparable from its role as an elevator, the eye becomes hypertropic.

5. Assess the vertical fusion range in primary position.

Measuring the vertical fusion range in primary position is a good measure of how long- standing the deviation is. Normal vertical fusion range is usually only 2–3 prism-dioptres so if it is increased to 5–6 prism dioptres or more, it is likely that the deviation has been present for a number of years.

6. Assess the degree of torsion

   - The superior oblique muscle is an incyclorotator
   - In a fourth nerve paresis, patients may experience significant torsional diplopia due to excylorotation. It can be the most troubling form of diplopia experienced by the patient and the hardest to overcome.
   - There are many ways to measure torsion, none of them particularly accurate or reproducible
   - It is important to measure torsion in downgaze in fourth nerve paresis as this is where it is often worse and where it causes the most problems

- To estimate the torsional deviation in real life situation, the most effective way of measuring is using Bagolini lenses in a trial frame. This is because it does not dissociate the two eyes and allows cyclofusion
- The head can be tilted upwards to measure torsion in downgaze
- Maddox rods in a trial frame can also be used but this is dissociative and will exaggerate the deviation.
- Otherwise, torsion can also be measured using a synoptophore, a torsionometer or using fundus images

7. Consider using HESS chart

A HESS chart can be useful to confirm the diagnosis, particularly in subtle cases, where there has been spread of comitance or to rule out other causes such as restrictive pathology. It may help guide the surgical decision making. A Hess chart does not measure torsional deviation.

2.4 Surgical Decision Making in Fourth Nerve Paresis

- Non-surgical management

Non-surgical management of fourth nerve paresis is largely restricted to prisms to reduce the vertical deviation or occlusion to eliminate diplopia. Occasionally a comitant deviation can be treated with botulinum toxin treatment to the contralateral inferior rectus but this is a rare scenario.

- Surgical principles

There are a number of fundamental principles when deciding on the appropriate surgical intervention in fourth nerve paresis:

- Incomitant deviations are best treated with oblique surgery, comitant deviations with rectus muscle surgery
- Torsion is a significant barrier to fusion, and addressing torsional deviation is a priority
- More than one operation may be necessary. The deviations may well evolve over time requiring multiple interventions
- Traumatic fourth nerve paresis is nearly always bilateral although the damage to each nerve is often asymmetrical. The least affected nerve damage may be masked
- Patterns of presentation

The pattern of deviation in 9 positions of gaze will be different for each patient and depends on the underlying cause and the duration of paresis. Recognising these different patterns is important because it will influence the choice of operation for each patient.

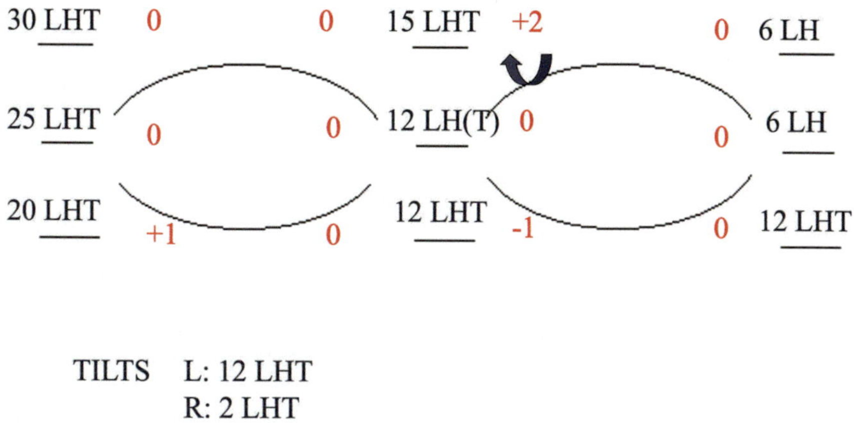

Fig. 1 Positions of gaze and version measurements where inferior oblique overaction is predominant

The pattern and the amount of deviation will determine whether it is appropriate to operate on the overacting antagonists (either the ipsilateral inferior oblique, contralateral inferior rectus or, rarely, ipsilateral superior rectus) or whether strengthening of the paretic superior oblique itself would be the most effective intervention.

It is not helpful to formally categorise presentation patterns as each patient is different; it is about assessing which muscle/s are most responsible for the deviation and deciding on surgery options.

1. *Inferior oblique overaction is predominant*: This is the most common presentation of congenital superior oblique paresis.
    a. The inferior oblique overaction causes the maximum deviation to be in contralateral upgaze (Fig. 1)
    b. Superior oblique weakness on versions is often not very apparent, it is only on tilt testing that the diagnosis of superior oblique paresis can be made
    c. The vertical deviation is incomitant, being much greater in contra-lateral gaze than in primary position or ipsilateral gaze
    d. The deviation is greater in contra-lateral upgaze than in contralateral downgaze

2. *Superior oblique weakness is predominant*: This is a more common presentation in traumatic or other neurological causes of superior oblique paresis.
    a. The vertical deviation is incomitant but it is significantly worse in downgaze than upgaze (Fig. 2)
    b. In general, a superior oblique strengthening operation is preferred
    c. The exception to this rule is if the primary position deviation is large, because superior oblique tuck is not a very powerful operation in terms of correcting primary position deviation (inferior oblique surgery will correct a much larger deviation). In this situation, it may be prudent to perform an inferior oblique

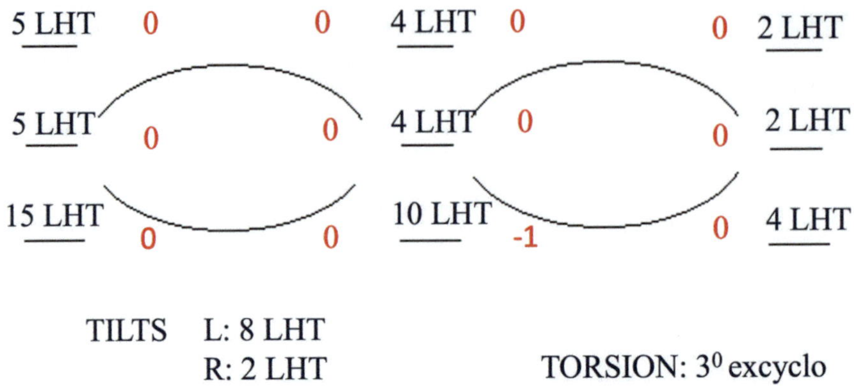

Fig. 2 Positions of gaza version measurements where left superior oblique weakness is predominate

operation first, and only if there is a significant residual downgaze incomitant deviation, perform a superior oblique strengthening operation.

3. *Contralateral inferior rectus overaction is predominant*: This is the most typical presentation of long-standing superior oblique paresis when the deviation becomes more comitant. Often, the patient will have had previous ipsilateral inferior or superior oblique surgery in the past.
   a. The deviation is greater in downgaze, and the difference between right and left downgaze deviation is minimal (Fig. 3).
   b. In this case, weakening of the contralateral inferior rectus is the preferred approach.

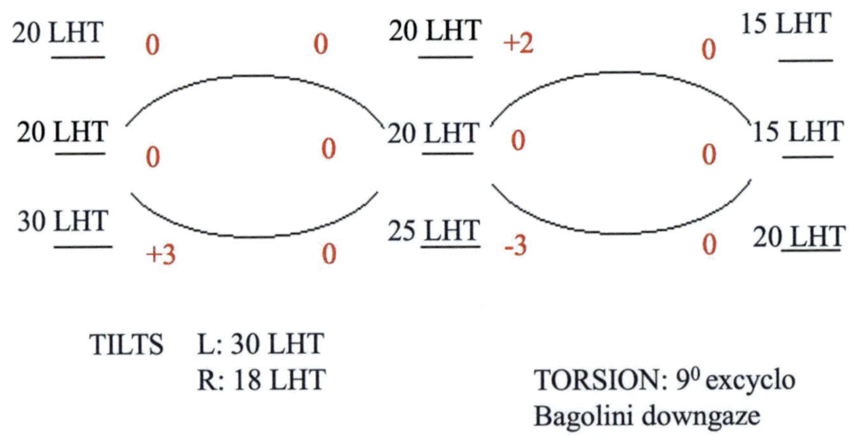

Fig. 3 Measurements of a patient who has become much more comitant over time with contralateral inferior rectus overaction

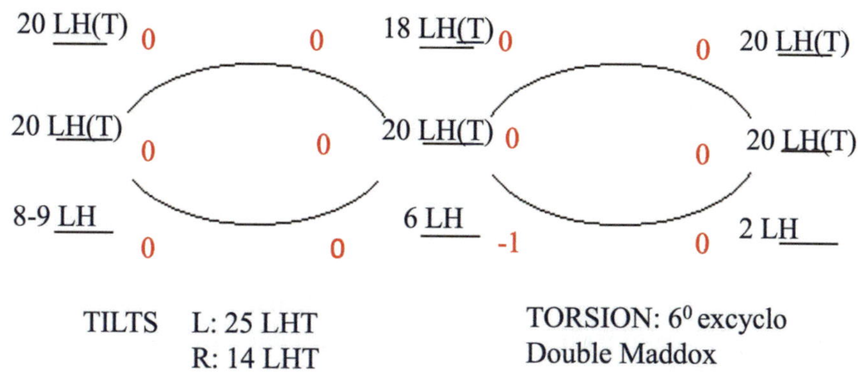

Fig. 4 This patient's measurements have become more comitant, mainly in upgaze. She is well controlled in downgaze so the operation of choice would be recession of the left superior rectus

   c. Occasionally, operating to weaken the contralateral inferior rectus is the only option if the superior oblique has already been strengthened in the past and the deviation is greatest in downgaze, even if there is some incomitance.

4. *Ipsilateral superior rectus overaction is predominant*: This is an unusual presentation of very long-standing deviations where the deviation has become comitant but the deviation is greater in upgaze than downgaze (Fig. 4). Often these patients have been managed with prisms and have large vertical fusion ranges.
5. *Torsion is predominant feature*: This is commonly the presentation of traumatic superior oblique paresis.

   a. It is worse if it is bilateral paresis
   b. It may be accompanied by minimal deviation in primary position, but alternating height in right and left gaze and alternating tilt tests (Fig. 5)
   c. Bilateral paresis is characterised by a small amount of esotropia in downgaze (V pattern) which will be revealed on the 9 positions of gaze measurements
   d. Torsion is less commonly a feature of congenital superior oblique paresis, but maybe a feature in neurological causes (such as MS or compressive lesions)
   e. The presence of a significant torsional component in a unilateral fourth nerve paresis of unknown cause should raise suspicions and trigger further investigations.

2.5 *Surgical Portfolio*

1. *Inferior oblique recession or myectomy*

The most common two ways of weakening the inferior oblique are by recession or myectomy. There is little evidence that one is more effective than the other, but the advantage of recession is that the final position of the muscle is controlled and

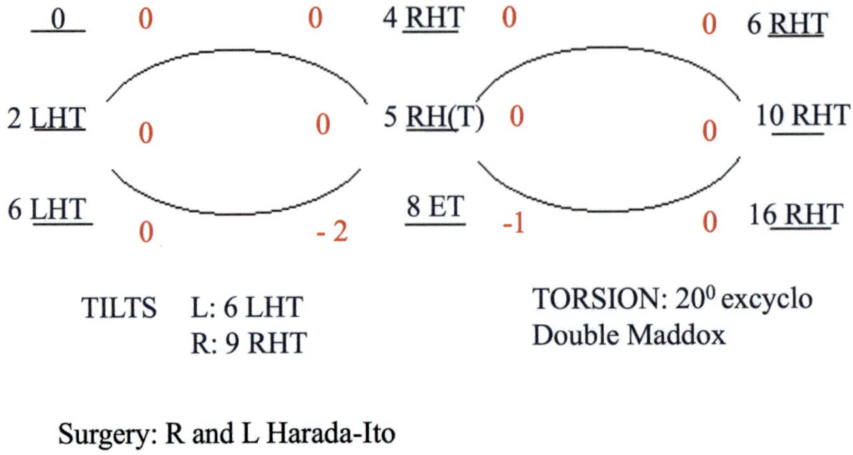

Fig. 5 This patient had head trauma resulting from a horse riding accident and has developed a large torsional deviation due to bilateral lvth nerve paresis with minimal vertical deviation. Notice that the head tilt tests show LHT on left tilt and RHT on right tilt and that there is a small ET in downgaza

modification (such as reversal) is possible. The rare complication of myectomy is fibrosis of the cut end either onto the globe, or more commonly onto the inferior rectus and its connective tissues which can cause hypotropia and torsion problems especially on adduction of the eye. This is probably associated with haemorrhage post-operatively and is extremely difficult to treat effectively. So, although both operations effectively weaken the inferior oblique overaction, recession may be the safer option.

Video 3.5: Inferior oblique myectomy

2. *Inferior oblique anterior transposition*

This is an operation that has two roles: It weakens the inferior oblique but also exerts a passive down-force on the eye. This helps the weakened superior oblique in downgaze so is additive to a simple inferior oblique weakening procedure. The operation became unpopular because of the complication of "anti-elevation syndrome" which was characterised by a limitation of elevation in abduction as well as adduction. However, with modification of the technique, anti-elevation can be avoided and it is a very effective operation for managing superior oblique paresis and may well reduce the need for subsequent contralateral inferior rectus recession [6]. The way the operation works, there is always some limitation of elevation in adduction (as there is with inferior oblique recession to a lesser degree) and patients should be warned about this. Although patients may be aware of this initially post-op, particularly when performing functions requiring chin depression (such as riding a drop-handlebar bike or playing snooker) it rarely causes long term symptomatic problems.

3. *Inferior rectus recession*

Contralateral inferior rectus recession is an operation to correct more comitant deviations worse in downgaze. It is helpful to be able to adjust the recession but conventional hang-back recessions are not appropriate for the inferior rectus. This is because there are a number of forces intent on pulling the muscle away from the globe: gravity, the lower lid retractors (which are attached to the inferior rectus), and the inferior oblique (which shares a sheath with the inferior rectus). This means that the muscle on a hang-back suture hangs below the globe, and although fibrous attachments form between the muscle and globe, when the vicryl resorbs, the muscle slips back a little and late over-correction becomes a problem. Although this is more an issue in patients with thyroid eye disease, it can affect any inferior rectus recession and so alternative techniques are required. A "semi-adjustable" inferior rectus technique will be discussed in Chap. 3 on surgical techniques.

4. *Superior oblique tuck*

The superior oblique has a complicated insertion which is curved and extends far back on the globe. The anterior part of the tendon is more involved with incyclotorsion, the posterior part affecting vertical movement. For this reason, a resection is not really feasible. To maintain the complex insertion in situ, the tendon can be tucked without having to disinsert it. This does not strengthen the muscle but shortens it, so it becomes more effective in it's weakened state. It is essentially an "all or none" operation and is self-titrating, the same amount of tuck correcting more deviation in patients with larger deviations than those with smaller deviations [7]. It corrects more deviation in contra-lateral downgaze than in the primary position. It also corrects some amount of torsional deviation if torsion is present (between 6 and 10°), but does not cause torsion if there is none pre-operatively. Like inferior oblique surgery, superior oblique tuck limits elevation in adduction to some degree and patients should be made aware. In patients who require both a superior oblique tuck and an inferior oblique anterior transposition, this limitation in adducted upgaze is not additive [7].

Video 3.10: Superior Oblique Tuck

5. *Fells modified Harada Ito procedure*

Harada and Ito described splitting the superior oblique tendon and moving the anterior half of the tendon anteriorly without disinserting it [8]. Peter Fells modified this technique to take the anterior half of the tendon, disinsert it and transpose it laterally and anteriorly towards the upper insertion of the lateral rectus [9]. Some vary this to take only a quarter or a third of the tendon. This is an effective operation for correcting excyclotorsion without significantly affecting vertical deviation. It is most commonly used in patients who have suffered closed head trauma and have significant torsion. A single Fells modified Harada Ito procedure will correct approximately 10 degrees of excyclotorsion [10]. Greater amounts will require bilateral surgery. Some favour adjustable surgery, but it often takes several weeks for the full effects of the surgery to be realised and the brain to come to terms with the new eye position, so adjustable surgery may not be advantageous.

Video 3.13: Harada Ito Procedure

6. *Superior rectus recession*

Some patients with long-standing superior oblique paresis develop comitant deviation in upgaze and require ipsilateral superior rectus recession. This may benefit from adjustable hang-back recession.

3 Surgical Technique

1. *Inferior oblique anterior transposition*

This operation involves disinserting the inferior oblique and transposing it to the lateral border of the inferior rectus insertion. 'Anterior' refers to the fact that the inferior oblique would normally cross the inferior rectus a long way posterior to the insertion and is being brought forward. It does not refer to transposing the inferior oblique anterior to the inferior rectus insertion which will increase the risk of anti-elevation syndrome.

There are some steps in the operation that are important to get right to reduce the risk of complications:

(a) Avoid splitting the inferior oblique muscle (it is best to hook it under direct visualisation) (Fig. 6)
(b) Avoid damage to the vortex vein and the neurovascular bundle supplying the inferior oblique. The inferior rectus/inferior oblique complex is uniquely sensitive to haemorrhage and responds by becoming fibrosed (Fig. 7)
(c) Disinsert the inferior oblique as close to the sclera as possible. It is important not to shorten the oblique by resecting a portion of it (Fig. 8)
(d) Attach the suture right at the end of the inferior oblique tendon so as not to shorten the muscle (Fig. 9)
(e) Attach the inferior oblique in a point (do not spread it out) at the lateral margin of the inferior rectus insertion
(f) Do not bring it anterior to the inferior rectus insertion (Fig. 10).

2. *Superior oblique tuck*

This operation involves a tuck in the superior oblique tendon lateral to the superior rectus insertion. It is effectively an "all or none" operation but the tuck size can be varied if the tendon is particularly lax or particularly tight at force duction testing.

(a) The tendon can be approached through a limbal incision but a fornix incision gives good exposure and is quicker and more comfortable for the patient

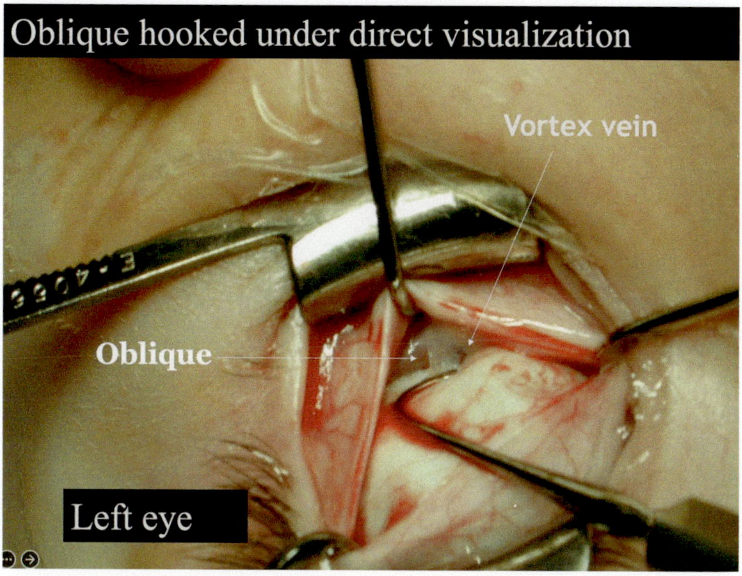

Fig. 6 The inferior oblique (IO) is hooked under direct visualisation

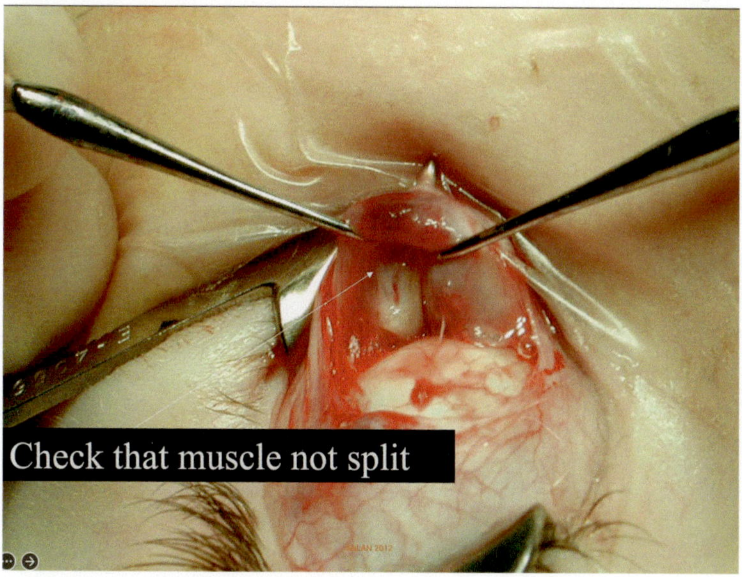

Fig. 7 It is essential to ensure the IO is not split by retracting the muscle under the posterior border and the 'white triangle' is visible

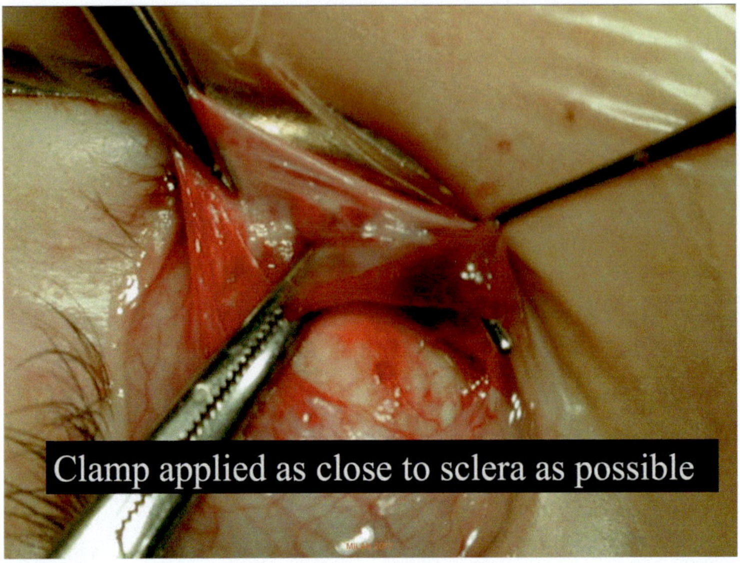

Fig. 8 The IO is clamped using an artery forceps as close to the insertion as possible and then detached

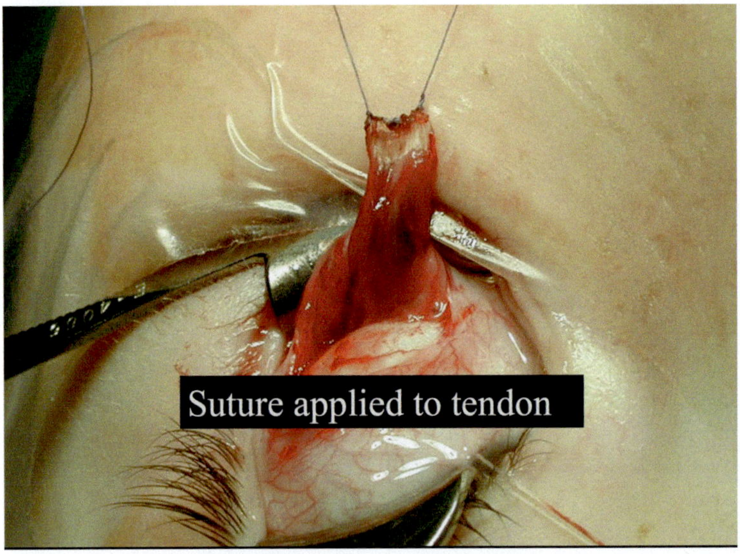

Fig. 9 The detached IO is isolated onto a double ended 6/0 vicryl suture ensuring both ends are included

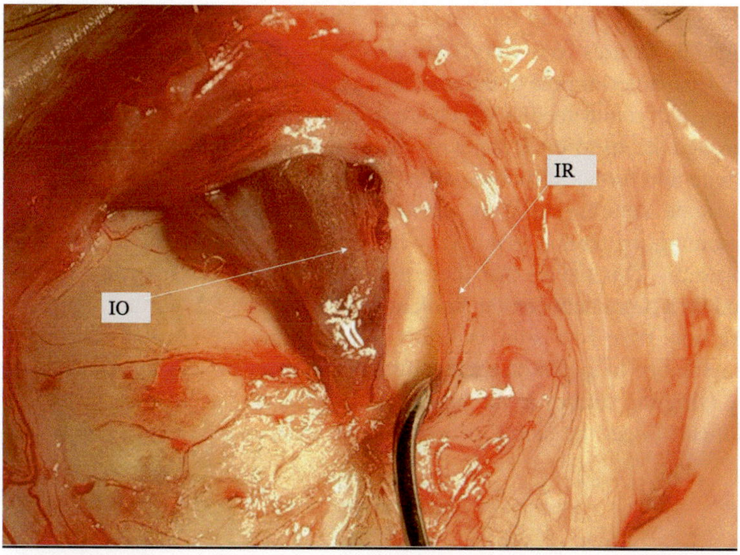

Fig. 10 The detached IO is attached next to the IR ensuring the fibres are bunched up to avoid antielevation syndrome

(b) The superior oblique tendon is almost invisible on the sclera and the insertion is under the superior rectus. The superior rectus has to be moved medially to expose the tendon which can be hooked with a small tenotomy hook. It is important to ensure that the whole tendon is hooked
(c) Better exposure can be gained by removing the speculum altogether and using the retractor to give good visualisation (Fig. 11)

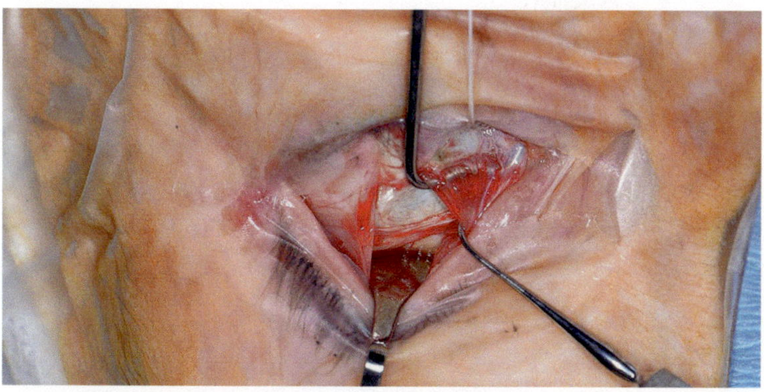

Fig. 11 Left eye: View of superior oblique can be improved by removing speculum and using retractor (Fison's retractor in this case)

(d) It is easiest to spread the tendon on a hook such as a Green hook (Fig. 12). Separate sutures (6/0 vicryl) are attached with a double pass to the posterior pole and anterior pole of the insertion as close to the sclera as possible. It is best to use half round needles which are easier to retrieve once they have been passed through the insertion. It is not necessary to pass the sutures through sclera which would add further difficulty, especially for the posterior pole
(e) Separate sutures are then attached at the tuck position. Most commonly, assuming the tendon is not very lax, I put these sutures in at 10mm from the insertion. This means that there are 5mm between the insertion and the hook and then 5mm between the hook and the position of the sutures (Fig. 13)
(f) We now have four sutures firmly attached and the needles can be removed leaving one long end on each suture and one end short. We now make our tuck by tying the sutures at the insertion to the sutures at the tuck position. If it is difficult to get the tuck together, an artery clip can be used to oppose the two

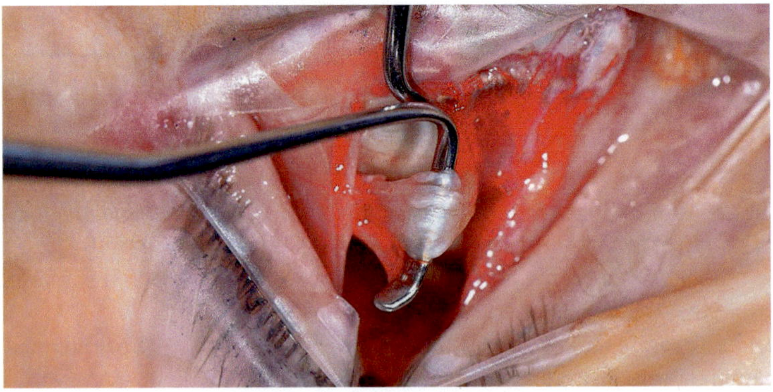

Fig. 12 Spreading the tendon on a Green's hook

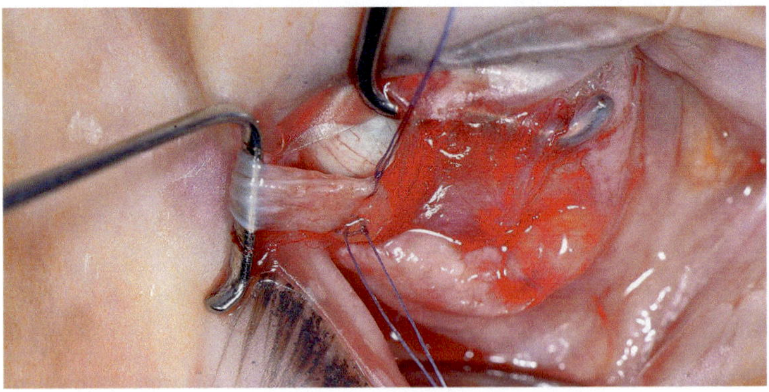

Fig. 13 Separate sutures attached at the tuck position 10mm from the insertion

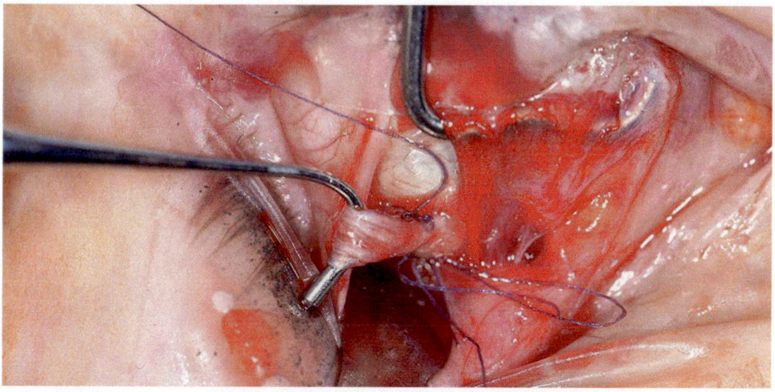

Fig. 14 If the FDT shows that the tuck is appropriate, the bow sutures can be converted to knots

sides. The sutures are tied in a bow at this stage because we need to perform a force duction test (FDT) to make sure that the tuck is not too tight or too loose

(g) The FDT is an important part of the operation because the tuck needs to be not too tight and not too loose. This is quite a difficult judgement and takes some experience. The tuck is too tight if the eye cannot be moved much above the midline on FDT. The tuck is too loose if there really isn't much resistance to FDT and the eye can be moved right up into elevation in adduction. There should be a springiness so that when you let go of the eye it springs back to primary position briskly

(h) If the FDT seems right, the bows can be made permanent by cutting the loop of the bows, removing the free bit of suture and putting one more turn on them to compete the knots (Fig. 14)

(i) If the FDT is too loose or too tight, the bows can be undone. The ends of the proximal suture can be cut off, but leave the knot as an indicator. New sutures can then be applied (with bows) one side of the knot or the other depending on whether the tuck needs to be tighter or looser. The FDT is then repeated.

3. *Fells modified Harada Ito procedure*

This operation is performed to the superior oblique tendon lateral to the superior rectus insertion (the same as the tuck procedure) either through a limbal or fornix based conjunctival incision.

(a) Hook the superior oblique tendon in the same way as for a tuck procedure and spread the tendon on an appropriate hook

(b) Split the tendon longitudinally somewhere between 1/3 and 1/2 into a smaller anterior portion and a larger posterior portion. The tendon should be split from the insertion right up to the superior rectus margin (which can be done with one blade of a small pair of scissors or with a tendon hook) (Fig. 15)

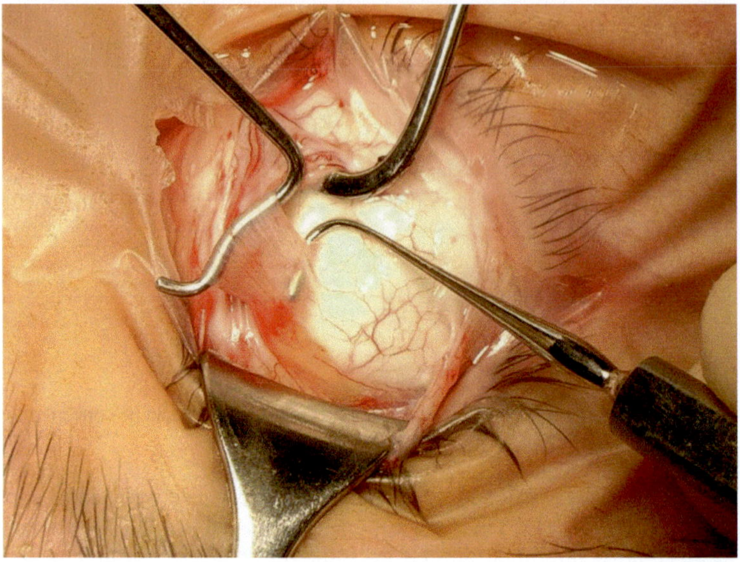

Fig. 15 Right eye: Fell's modification of Harada Ito procedure. The tendon is split into anterior and posterior halves

(c) Separate sutures are now inserted into the anterior 1/3 of the tendon at the insertion. There does not seem to be much room for two sutures but there is just enough
(d) The anterior part of the tendon is now disinserted and the posterior portion is left attached at the insertion (Fig. 16)
(e) The anterior part of the tendon is now advanced to upper pole of the lateral rectus insertion and the two needles inserted into the sclera, being sure not to twist the tendon (Fig. 17)
(f) Some surgeons like to mark the sclera to determine how much incyclotorsion is being achieved and titrate the surgery accordingly

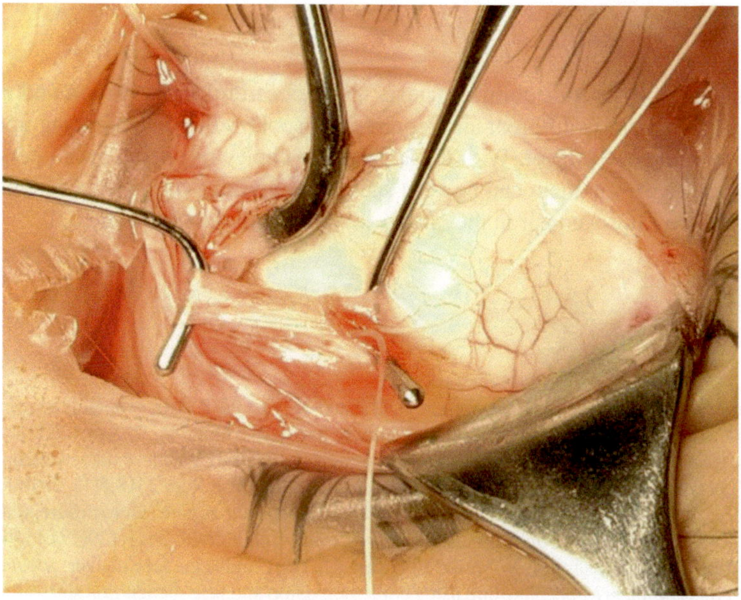

Fig. 16 Once the sutures have been inserted into the anterior tendon it can be dis-inserted

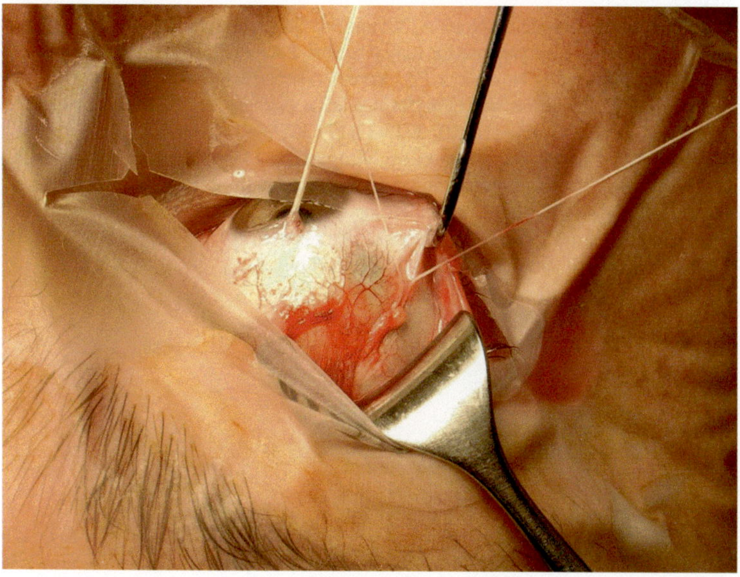

Fig. 17 The anterior part of the tendon is advanced to the superior margin of the lateral rectus

4 Conclusion

Management of superior oblique paresis requires careful investigation and assessment. Each patient is different and requires a bespoke solution depending upon the outcome of the assessment. With the appropriate choice of operation or operations, the outcomes of treatment can be very successful giving a useful area of binocular vision and an improvement in the quality of vision and quality of life.

References

1. Jiang Y, Matsuo T, Fujiwara H, Hasebe S, Ohtsuki H, Yasuda T. Arix gene polymorphisms in patients with congenital superior oblique muscle palsy. Br J Ophthal. 2004;88:263–7.
2. Durgam A, Hussain H, Nakatsuka AS, Raghuram K. Isolated trochlear nerve (cranial nerve IV) palsy in a patient with carotid-cavernous fistula. BJR Case Rep. 2018;5(1): 20180028.
3. Wong AM, Colpa L, Chandrakumar M. Ability of an upright-supine test to differentiate skew deviation from other vertical strabismus causes. Arch Ophthalmol. 2011;129(12):1570–5.
4. Thomas PB, Baltrušaitis T, Robinson P, Vivian AJ. The Cambridge face tracker: accurate, low cost measurement of head posture using computer vision and face recognition software. Transl Vis Sci Technol. 2016;5(5):8.
5. Vivian AJ, Morris RJ. Diagrammatic representation of strabismus. Eye (Lond). 1993;7(Pt 4):565–71.
6. Clifford L, Roos J, Dahlmann-Noor A, Vivian AJ. Surgical management of superior oblique paresis using inferior oblique anterior transposition. J AAPOS. 2015;19(5):406–9.
7. Malem AH, Somner JE, Novitskya ES, Vivian AJ. Superior oblique tuck-effectiveness in reducing vertical deviations when performed as a primary versus secondary procedure in superior oblique paresis. Eye (Lond). 2023;37(17):3656–60.
8. Harada M, Ito Y. Surgical correction of cyclotropia. Jpn J Ophthalmol. 1964;8:88–96.
9. Fells P. Management of paralytic strabismus. Br J Ophthalmol. 1974;58:255–65.
10. Flodin S, Karlsson P, Rydberg A, Andersson Grönlund M, Pansell T. Surgical outcome of graded Harada-Ito procedure in the treatment of torsional diplopia—a retrospective case study with long-term results. Strabismus. 2022;30(1):8–17.

Surgical Management of 6th Nerve Palsy

G. G. W. Adams

Abstract This chapter discusses the surgical management of 6th nerve palsy. It emphasises the importance of determining whether the palsy is partial or complete as this defines both the surgical plan and the likely outcome. The use of diagnostic botulinum toxin can be helpful in determining lateral rectus function. If the palsy is partial then horizontal surgery on the rectus muscles should be undertaken, usually a recession of the medial rectus muscle and resection or plication of the lateral rectus muscle. If the palsy is complete a transposition procedure will be required. The various transposition operations available are described. Second stage management for residual palsy or over correction is also discussed.

Keywords Partial lateral rectus palsy · Complete lateral rectus palsy · Assessment of lateral rectus function · Botulinum toxin · Transposition procedures · Nishida procedure · Faden procedure · Scott procedure · Overcorrection

1 Introduction

- Congenital 6th nerve palsy is extremely rare and, in most cases, will resolve spontaneously. Surgical treatment is therefore unlikely to be required.
- There are other causes of congenital abduction failure which are not covered in this chapter.
- Intervention is therefore usually only required for acquired 6th nerve palsies, many of which will resolve with time and may not require surgery.
- Undertaking surgery before natural resolution has occurred can lead to an overcorrection.
- Appropriate investigation of an acquired 6th nerve palsy will depend on the age of the patient and any other associated findings e.g., papilloedema. Investigate children and young adults. In all older adults check BP, blood sugar and ESR.

G. G. W. Adams (✉)
Moorfields Eye Hospital, London, UK
e-mail: gill.adams5@nhs.net

S. Jain (ed.), *Surgical Management of Strabismus*,
https://doi.org/10.1007/978-3-031-80633-9_10

Investigate older adults with vascular risk factors, but no other concerns, if no improvement after 3 months.

- Recovery varies. Knowledge of the underlying aetiology will help define the possible need for, and timing, of any surgical intervention e.g., transection of 6th nerve during neurosurgery is unlikely to recover and is likely to be complete. 6th nerve palsy following a stroke is less likely to recover than one caused by a microvascular ischaemic event.

2 Early Management

- **Await resolution**: Many acquired 6th nerve palsies will resolve in about 3 months e.g. in children with post viral palsies or in adults with microvascular palsies. In such cases the management is supportive whilst awaiting recovery.
- **Supportive measures**, whilst awaiting resolution, include Bangerter foil, patch or Fresnel prism. A prism will need to be changed as the squint reduces, probably once a month and is not very helpful if large angle or significant abduction deficit where a foil or patch is of more use.
- **Botulinum toxin** has little role to play in the early management of microvascular palsy as its use does not speed up recovery and adds a changing dynamic to the underlying, hopefully resolving, microvascular problem. It does however reduce the compensatory head posture which can develop following an acute 6th nerve palsy which patients may find beneficial [1]. Botulinum toxin therapy may help in prevention of medial rectus contracture in traumatic cases where recovery is unlikely. Consider toxin therapy from 3 months if no resolution.
- **Consider surgery** if there is no improvement in the situation after 6–12 months. If surgery is undertaken too early in the recovery process an overcorrection can occur.
- **Prisms**: If the angle is small consider prismatic incorporation in glasses.

3 Surgery

- **Aims of surgery:** The aim of surgery is to provide the widest area of single vision in primary position and improve abduction.
- **Pre operative counselling:** The patient should be warned that they may still have some diplopia in side gaze following their procedure; this is more likely with a complete nerve palsy than with partial palsies. They should be advised that if they have a unilateral palsy there is an approximately 1 in 3 probability of needing second stage treatment and that if the palsy is bilateral this rises to 2 in 3. As well as the usual surgical risks the patient should be warned of the risk of anterior segment ischaemia if intervention is required on 3 rectus muscles and of induced vertical diplopia and potentially torsion if undertaking some transposition

procedures. It should be explained and emphasized that restoration to complete normality is unlikely.

- **Assess lateral rectus function:** Selection of the appropriate operation depends on the function of the lateral rectus muscle. Choosing the incorrect intervention leads to a poor outcome. If the palsy is partial the eye can abduct beyond the midline. If the eye cannot abduct beyond the midline, then this is a complete or total lateral rectus palsy.
- **Surgical procedure selection**: is based on LR function.
  - If the eye can abduct beyond the midline, then a MR recess and LR resect or plicate procedure can be undertaken.
  - If there is no abduction beyond the midline a transposition procedure will be required.
  - If the patient is over 21y do not operate on 3 rectus muscles at the same operation because of the risk of anterior segment ischaemia. This is a rare complication of surgery but does occur even in the middle aged.
  - If the patient has bilateral 6th nerve palsies treat each eye individually i.e. identify if there is a complete palsy on both sides or is one complete and the other incomplete, and offer the appropriate intervention. Surgery can be staged by doing one eye first or bilateral surgery can be undertaken.
- **Anaesthesia**: in children a general anaesthetic is required. In adults if undertaking an adjustable suture as part of the process then a general anaesthetic is usual. In adults who do not wish or are unfit for a general anaesthetic consider surgery under a local block. This will likely influence the surgical choices.
- **Post operative management**: standard strabismus management.

4 Assessment of Lateral Rectus Function

Assessment of lateral rectus function is vital as this defines the surgical plan. There is little benefit to operating to try and strengthen a non-functioning lateral rectus muscle. A paralytic muscle will still have no power after surgery and the patient will continue to be left with no abduction even if the deviation in primary position has been improved.

The options for assessing lateral muscle function include:

- **Diagnostic botulinum toxin injection**: can be helpful in clarifying the lateral rectus function. This can be identified by injection of botulinum toxin into the ipsilateral medial rectus which will weaken the adducting effect of the medial and allow the lateral, even if weak, to exert an abduction effect. If the eye can then abduct beyond the midline proceed as for a partial palsy.
- **EMG of the lateral rectus**: this is most appropriately undertaken at the same time as performing a toxin injection to see if there is any abduction power (use the injecting EMG needle but with a syringe filled with saline, do this test first

then swap over the syringe to one filled with toxin for the medial injection. Do not perform the EMG with the toxin loaded syringe in case any seeps into the lateral rectus). After inserting EMG needle into the lateral rectus ask the patient to abduct the eye as fully as possible. If there is lateral rectus function you will see an EMG recording as the lateral rectus muscle contracts and if the lateral rectus muscle is completely palsied there will be no or virtually no muscle signal generated as the eye attempts to move laterally.

- **Forced generation test**: can be used to assess the function of the lateral rectus. The test requires an awake and cooperative patient and therefore it is of limited use in children or anxious adults. Topical anaesthetic is instilled and the eye is held by forceps in full adduction and the patient is asked to abduct the eye. The amount of tug or pull generated, on a scale normal to no force, is then used to assess lateral rectus function and whether the lateral rectus palsy is partial or total. Assessment of the outcome requires significant experience and in practical terms this test is not as useful as diagnostic toxin or EMG.
- **Assessment of saccades**. Analysis of saccades requires significant experience to differentiate partial from complete lateral rectus weakness. In 6th nerve palsy there is slow saccadic velocity on side gaze; a floating saccade on abduction is reported in complete palsies.

Partial palsy: If the eye can abduct beyond the midline, then plan surgical management as for a convergent squint.

See Chap. 3 for details on horizontal strabismus surgery techniques and conjunctival incisions.

- **Horizontal muscle surgery** is the standard intervention; most commonly an ipsilateral recession of the medial rectus and an ipsilateral resection or plication of the lateral rectus muscle. An adjustable suture can be used on the medial rectus muscle but care should be taken not to over recess the muscle or this can result in reduced adduction as well as reduced abduction of the eye. This will result in exotropia with diplopia in contra lateral gaze and will reduce the patient's binocular field. Whilst in theory an adjustable can be used on the LR, the muscle is weak and a large resection/plication is usually needed so titrating with an adjustment is not often required. Check the pre op angle in primary and right and left gaze at distance. Calculate the amount of LR strengthening procedure on the angle of deviation on abduction. Less weakening of MR may be needed if there is only a small angle for near. In a child or adult who does not wish adjustable suture surgery plan for fixed surgery. Most patients prefer to be left minimally exophoric rather than with a small esotropia as fusional control is usually much better in an exophoria.
- Alternatively consider **ipsilateral LR strengthening and contralateral MR weakening**. Theoretically this will allow more MR recession and greater improvement in comitancy on side gaze.
- **If the angle of deviation in primary is small** and the patient does not wish to use prims consider an ipsilateral single medial rectus recession alone on an adjustable suture. Alternatives are to consider a central tenotomy or Z plasty on the medial

rectus but these are difficult to grade; an adjustable recession is more likely to give a good outcome.
- **Minimal deviation in primary and reduced abduction** with diplopia on side gaze consider:
  - A unilateral ipsilateral LR resection (safest using an adjustable suture). Consider a 7mmm resection and hang the muscle 2-3 mm back from the insertion on the adjustable suture. At adjustment if over corrected loosen the suture and if under corrected pull it up. A plication is difficult to adjust and the option is to cut the sutures and let the muscle return to the original position if overcorrected but finessing the result is not possible.
  - Contra lateral medial rectus Faden or Scott procedure.

5 Complete Palsy

If there is no abduction beyond the mid line then a transposition procedure is required. These operations move one or both normally functioning vertical muscles, in whole or in part, temporally to improve abduction when there is no or very little lateral rectus function. There are many types of transposition operation in the literature [2]. This suggests that there is no one perfect surgical procedure. Transposition can be combined with additional procedures for improved efficacy:

- Augmentation sutures on the transposed vertical muscles to increase the abducting effect.
- MR weakening either ipsilaterally or contra laterally. As there may be some ipsilateral MR contracture it is more appropriate to consider ipsilateral MR surgery.
- Lateral rectus plication or resection.

6 General Surgical Points When Undertaking Transposition Surgery

- **Forced duction test**: do this at the start of the operation to assess if the medial rectus is tight. This may affect the surgical plan as a tight medial rectus will need releasing as part of the procedure.
- **Traction sutures**: these are helpful to gain good exposure.
- **Good muscle exposure is vital**: When planning transposition surgery make sure to have good exposure of the muscles to allow muscle cleaning and movement out of its normal trajectory. Open the conjunctiva 180–270 degrees, from the superior nasal quadrant to the inferior nasal quadrant for 3 muscles including the vertical recti and lateral rectus. If also operating on the medial rectus a larger 360 conjunctival incision will give best exposure and closure. Multiple separate conjunctival

openings tend to provide poorer exposure and are often more difficult to close neatly. For one vertical muscle transposition surgery a fornix-based approach in either the superotemporal or inferotemporal quadrant can be used. Marking the conjunctival edges with gentian violet can assist in optimal closure. Carefully clean all attachments between the vertical muscles and superior and inferior obliques and any attachments to the lid retractors. Depending on the procedure being undertaken you may need to clear any attachments around the lateral rectus e.g. using a Foster augmentation suture.

- **Pre operative BTXA to the MR**. This weakens any adducting effect and allows the transposed muscles to attach in the new position without any inward pull. The toxin injection can be given pre operatively or peri operatively. Pre operative toxin injection is best performed 2 weeks pre surgery to allow the toxin to take effect. It also allows the surgeon to assess for any induced height created by the toxin injection. This is helpful post operatively to differentiate toxin induced from a surgical induced vertical deviation. If toxin is injected peri operatively it will likely leak out of the muscle and can induce complications of a vertical deviation and ptosis. If toxin is required at the time of the procedure e.g., in a child, then ***inject the toxin before opening the conjunctiva*** as this will reduce toxin leakage out of the muscle and reduce the risk of side effects. The injection can be performed under EMG but there will be a low signal under anaesthesia or without EMG guidance using Mendonca forceps to grasp the muscle which has been reported as a safe and effective alternative method to identify the MR (Fig. 1).
- **Augmentation sutures**: also called Foster, lateral fixation or myopexy sutures [3]. These can be used in conjunction with vertical muscle transpositions, either on one or both vertical rectus muscles. They 'close the gap' between the vertical recti and the lateral rectus muscles and improve the abducting force. It has been suggested that this reduces the need for an ipsilateral medial rectus recession and so reduces the possibility of anterior segment ischaemia. A modification of the Foster augmentation suture has been described by Struck [4].

  – Foster sutures: After undertaking the vertical muscle tendon transposition to the LR border the fixation sutures are attached from the transposed vertical rectus muscles into the sclera adjacent to the superior or inferior border of the lateral rectus muscle at 8 mm posterior to the LR insertion /16 mm from the limbus. Use a non absorbable suture (eg 5/0 or 6/0 mersilene, Ethibond or prolene) and take a bite of 1/3 muscle width of the vertical rectus muscle. If placing these sutures on both SR and IR take care to mirror their placement

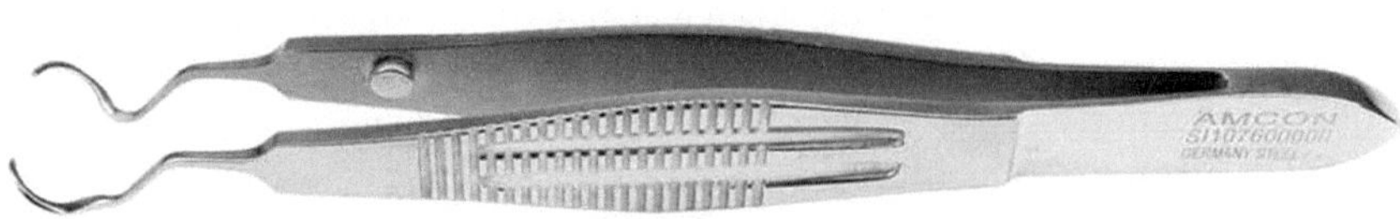

Fig. 1 Mendonca Strabismus Forceps

and put both sutures at the same place to avoid any twisting effect which can result in torsion. Some surgeons have reported that despite balancing the 2 augmentation sutures they still have patients with post-operative torsion and vertical deviation. A way of checking for intra operative torsion is to mark the limbus at 12 and 6 o'clock with gentian violet (put the dye on the end of a caliper or use a skin marker pen) [5]. Monitor the dots as the sutures are placed. SR augmentation alone may result in intorsion of the eye which should be balanced by the extorting effect of the IR augmentation suture. Place a bow knot on the IR and adjust to achieve dot balance before finally tying the suture. The Struck modification involves using a single fixation suture, not two as used in the standard Foster technique. The 5/0 polyester suture is placed in the sclera under the lateral rectus 15 mm posterior to the limbus after a full tendon width transposition of the vertical recti. The suture is then passed into the superior and inferior rectus muscles and tied. The lateral rectus muscle needs to be well mobilised, (detaching the lateral rectus to place the suture was described in Duane patients). In practice it can be difficult to obtain an adequately clear view under the lateral rectus muscle and it only reduces the scleral passes by one bite.

- **Conjunctival closure**: must be meticulous; you may have to do second stage surgery on the eye!

7 Transposition Procedures

Operations involving both vertical recti

(1) **Partial double vertical tendon transposition**

Hummelsheim procedure

The Hummelsheim is the original transposition procedure [6]. It is a half tendon transposition of both vertical recti. The superior and inferior rectus muscles are split in half for 12–15 mm and the temporal portions of the superior rectus and inferior rectus are detached from the globe and moved temporally adjacent to the lateral rectus muscle. Hummelsheim advised not incising the muscles more than 12 mm to avoid damage to their nerve supply but other authors have suggested up to 15 mm splits. The lateral rectus muscle is not split in this procedure.

Variations on the procedure include augmentation with resection of the transposed vertical rectus muscle sections, posterior fixation sutures on the transposed muscles, addition of a plication of the lateral rectus, a medial rectus recession or medial rectus toxin injection. In a surgical 3D simulation, the Hummelsheim achieved 28 prism dioptres (pd) of correction [7]. If combined with medical rectus recession and augmentation sutures an average correction of 37pd has been reported. A Hummelsheim procedure combined with resection of the transposed muscle slips has been reported to produce a mean 54pd correction in esotropia.

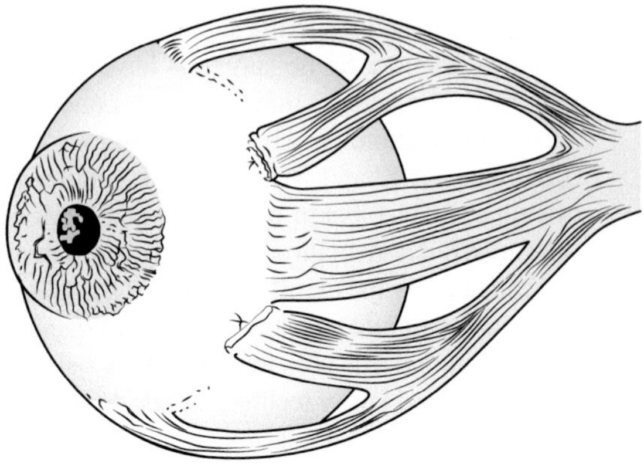

Fig. 2 Hummelsheim: temporal half of the tendons of the SR and IR muscles detached from the globe and moved to the LR muscle border

Good exposure of all 3 muscles is essential. After exposing and cleaning the muscles divide the muscles equally, best done by making a button hole in the muscle near the insertion and extending the incision backwards with small scissors. The muscle portions are usually sutured into place, on the spiral of Tillaux, using 6/0 vicryl. Consider operating on the IR first. If the SR is the initial muscle undergoing surgery, then bleeding may seep into the surgical field and make IR surgery more difficult. Take care to split the muscles equally as induced vertical deviation has been reported with unequal tendon splitting.

Surgery on the LR and MR is usually undertaken with 6/0 vicryl, although a thicker suture may be used for plication. See Chap. 3 for details on horizontal strabismus surgery techniques.

The procedure preserves some blood supply to the superior and inferior rectus muscles but causes scarring which makes can make revision surgery challenging (Fig. 2).

(2) **Muscle Union Procedure**

Jensen procedure

The original Jensen operation described a medial rectus recession (3–5 mm) followed by a transposition procedure which involved looping together split muscle slips of both vertical and lateral rectus muscles [8]. The muscles are not detached from the globe but all 3 muscles (both vertical and lateral rectus muscles) are split in half. Variations on the procedure include splitting the LR into 3 leaving an unoperated central LR section attached to sclera which is thought to reduce the risk of ASI. A correction of about 30-34pd appears to be an average outcome for a Jensen and medial rectus recession. This is similar to a 34pd correction reported on 3D modelling.

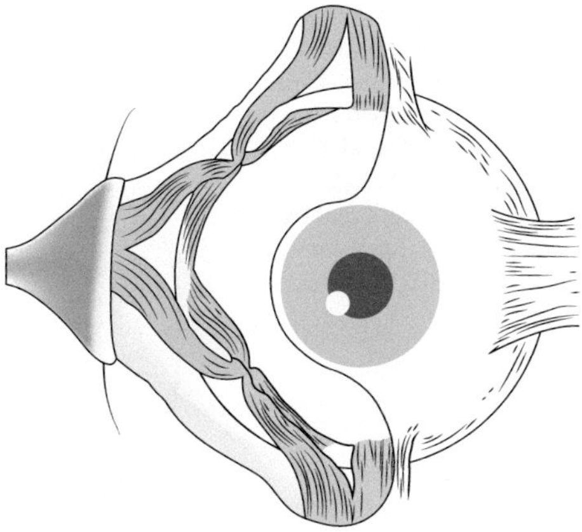

Fig. 3 Jensen procedure: SR and IR muscles are divided into two equal parts, transposed and united with the split LR muscle slips. The muscles are not detached from the globe- from David K. Coats, Scott E. Olitsky. Strabismus Surgery and its Complications. Springer Berlin 2007. Rights obtained

Jensen reported recessing the medial rectus first then operating on the vertical muscles. The conjunctiva was opened separately over the medial rectus then a 180° incision was made temporally to expose the vertical and lateral rectus muscles which were then cleaned and mobilised. The superior, inferior and lateral rectus muscles are then split in half for 15 mm from the insertion. The temporal half of the split SR is then looped to the upper half of the split LR with a non-absorbable suture and the temporal half of the inferior rectus is looped to the lower half of the split lateral rectus muscle. Care should be taken to place the sutures at the same point to avoid any vertical deviation. This can be achieved by using gentian violet to mark the muscles at the mirror points. The operation can be done without medical rectus recession and with the transposition alone. The procedure does create scarring and it is very difficult to re-operate if further surgery is required (Fig. 3).

(3) **Double full vertical rectus tendon transposition procedures (VRT procedures)**

This procedure involves detaching the SR and IR from the globe and moving them to the LR border. This procedure is best combined with pre operative BTXA to the MR, or medial rectus recession. Augmentation sutures are commonly used [9, 10].

Induced vertical deviation post-surgery have been reported, both hyper (higher) and hypo (lower) with hyper-deviations being more common. This can be reduced by precise alignment of the transposed muscles and augmentation sutures if used.

The range of correction has been given as 20–36 pd (average 35pd) without the use of augmentation sutures and 25.8–43 (average 38) with augmentation sutures. Full tendon transfer with toxin augmentation has been reported to correct 30–66 pd of esotropia, with an average of 42 pd. Double vertical tendon transposition with augmentation and MR recession has been reported to correct 40pd (Figs. 4 and 5).

After opening the conjunctiva and cleaning the vertical muscles place two 6/0 Vicryl sutures one into each side of each vertical rectus muscle and detach the muscle from the globe and move it temporally. For the inferior/superior rectus muscle the

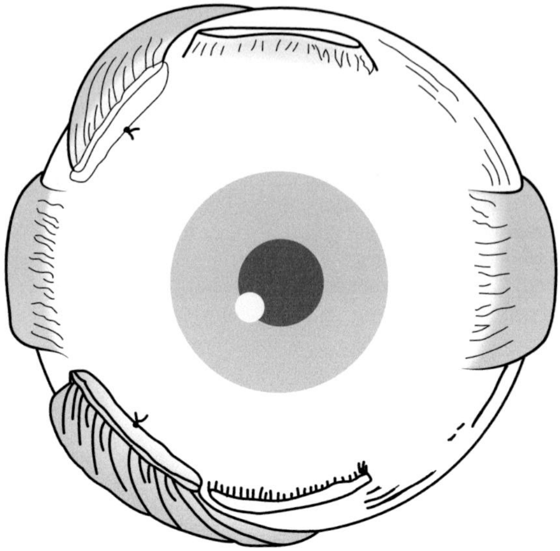

Fig. 4 Full transposition of both SR and IR muscles to the LR muscle border, both muscles are detached from the globe-from David K. Coats, Scott E. Olitsky. Strabismus Surgery and its Complications. Springer Berlin 2007. Rights obtained

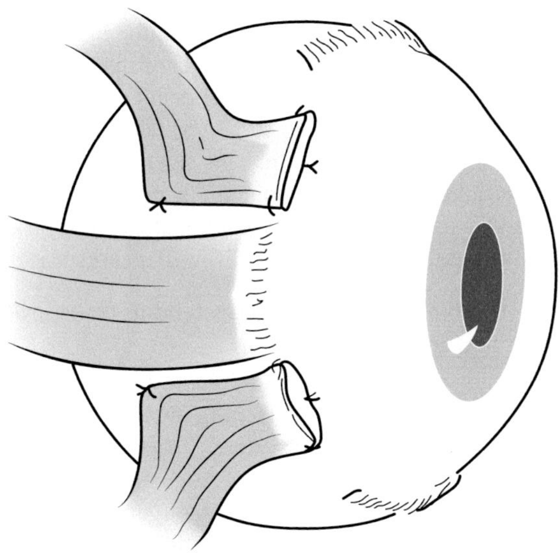

Fig. 5 Full transposition of both SR and IR muscles to the LR muscle border augmented with posterior fixation sutures from David K. Coats, Scott E. Olitsky. Strabismus Surgery and its Complications. Springer Berlin 2007. Rights obtained

temporal muscle edge will insert into the sclera at the inferior/superior border of the lateral rectus and the nasal pole will insert into the temporal corner of the inferior/superior rectus muscle insertion. The muscles are sutured into place on the spiral of Tillaux between the lateral rectus edge and the temporal border of the vertical muscle insertion.

Post op there may be over correction if pre op toxin has been used. This will wear off over about 3 months. Pre op counselling is essential to warn the patient of this possibility and the fact that this is a good sign and not an indication of a bad outcome.

(4) **Double vertical muscle transposition without tenotomy or splitting**

These procedures move the vertical muscles temporally without splitting them or removing them from the globe and as such are thought to produce less risk of vascular compromise.

Nishida procedure

The Nishida procedure is sometimes erroneously referred to as a modified Nishida procedure. The procedure has not been modified but evolved from another operation the Inatomi procedure in which the vertical rectus muscle bellies were split and transposed. In the Nishida procedure the SR and IR muscles are transposed laterally without splitting them hence the description of a no tenotomy and no splitting procedure [11]. It can be combined with medial rectus recession and/or toxin to the medial rectus.

The conjunctival approach can either be at the limbus with relieving incisions over the superior and inferior recti or placed nearer the fornix with the conjunctiva folded forwards for exposure. Mark the incisions with gentian violet to allow good closure at the end of the procedure. Expose both muscles before starting to insert the sutures to ensure that the operation is mirrored in each muscle. The vertical recti are exposed and cleaned and then a suture is placed to move the muscle temporally sideways. A non-absorbable suture (e.g. 6/0 prolene or mersilene; some authors have described 5/0 Ethibond as an alternative suture) is used and placed 8–10 mm from the insertion of the superior or inferior rectus muscle and knotted in the muscle. The bite should be a minimum of 1/3 of the muscle width and the same on each muscle. Each suture is then placed through the sclera 10–12 mm from the limbus, at the halfway point between the superior and inferior and lateral rectus muscles in the superotemporal and inferotemporal quadrants and tied. If it is difficult to move the muscles slide a 240 retinal band under the vertical muscle being operated upon and the lateral rectus and then pull the muscles together using the band before suturing the vertical muscle into position.

It is important to obtain a good and equal bite of each vertical rectus muscle to ensure that an abduction effect is achieved. Use gentian violet or equivalent to mark the muscles to ensure the muscle bites are identical in positioning and width. Mark the point of temporal scleral positioning with gentian violet or a cautery mark to ensure a good temporal movement is achieved.

This procedure can be combined with a medial rectus recession or toxin to MR combined with MR recession. The amount of correction obtained varies. A comparison study has reported a Nishida alone correcting almost 30pd, the addition of a medial rectus recession correcting an average of 62pd and the addition of both MR recession and botulinum toxin correcting 95pd [12] (Fig. 6).

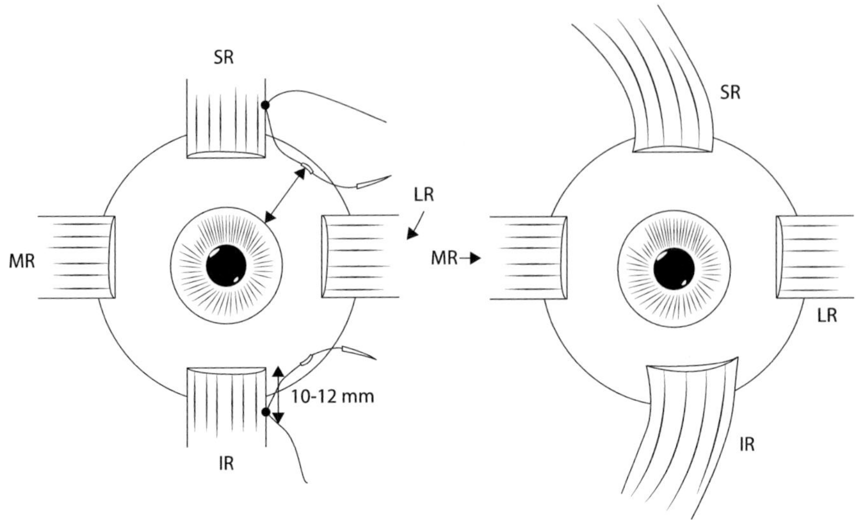

Fig. 6 The modified muscle transposition procedure of Nishida and associates, where a 6–0 or 5–0 nonabsorbable suture is inserted through each temporal margin of vertical recti at approximately one third of the width from the edge at a distance of 8–10 mm behind the insertion. The same suture also is inserted through each scleral wall at a distance of 10–12 mm behind the limbus at the superotemporal or inferotemporal quadrant

Marcon procedure

A variant of the no tenotomy no splitting muscle transposition technique involves placing a non-absorbable suture through the temporal side of each vertical rectus muscle and tying the sutures over the lateral rectus muscle. This has been combined with MR recession and also LR plication.

Operations involving one vertical rectus muscle

Single tendon transposition of either SR or IR to LR border.

This has been reported to be very successful. Can be combined with MR recession so only involves two rectus muscles. The chosen vertical rectus muscle is moved temporally to the lateral rectus border and in most cases transposition will be combined with augmentation sutures. The operation can induce post operative torsion as well as height. This can be reduced by precise alignment of the transposed muscle and augmentation sutures.

SR transposition: post operative intorsion and an induced vertical deviation (both hyper and hypo) have been described, but most commonly hypertropia [13].

IR transposition: extorsion has been reported and vertical deviation especially hypotropia. It can therefore be beneficial to consider in patients with hypertropia and incyclotorsion as well as abduction deficit [14].

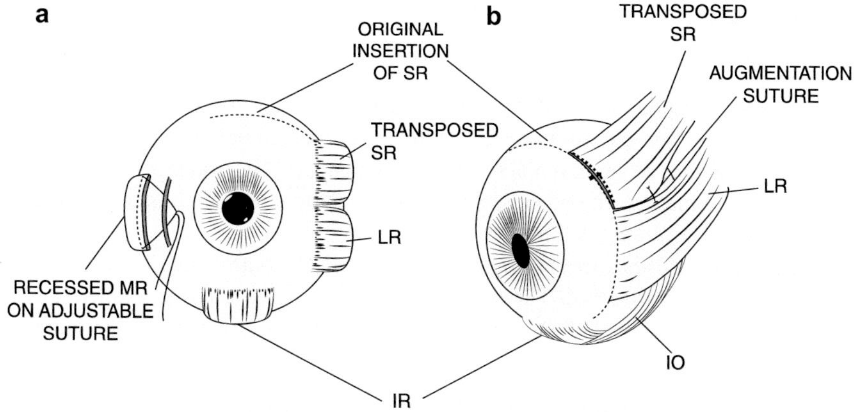

Fig. 7 Superior rectus transposition (SRT) plus medial rectus recession procedure demonstrating a) Medial rectus recession with adjustable sutures; b) SRT technique with augmentation suture

Single vertical rectus transposition with medial rectus recession is reported to provide an average of 44 pd of correction. A single transposition and Foster suture is reported to correct an average correction of 27 pd. A combined single vertical transposition, medial rectus recession and Faden is to is reported to correct 43 pd on average (Fig. 7).

8 Summary

The older muscle splitting transposition procedures such as Hummelsheim or Jensen are likely to result in significant scarring which can limit further intervention.

Full tendon transfer (with augmentation sutures, pre or peri op toxin or medial rectus recession) of both vertical rectus muscles works well but can induce height and torsion if care is not taken. Three muscle surgery carries the risk of anterior segment ischaemia in the older patient.

Single vertical muscle transposition can be very successful and can be combined with medial rectus recession but there is a small risk of inducing a vertical deviation and torsion which is troublesome in the binocular patient.

The Nishida procedure works well but does need attention to detail to ensure that equal bites of SR and IR are taken and that the muscles are moved adequately temporally. This appears to be a very effective procedure with the least risk of vascular compromise, induced vertical deviation or torsion. It can be combined with medial rectus weakening or medial rectus recession and toxin injection to augment the surgical outcome. The published outcomes show correction of the largest angles with a Nishida in combination with other procedures.

9 Second stage management

Second stage procedures may be needed as part of planned management, to manage a progressive 6th nerve palsy or to deal with a sub optimal outcome.

If the patient has bilateral 6th nerve palsies which are being managed sequentially then proceed to manage the other eye with an appropriate intervention depending on the amount of lateral rectus function.

If the patient still has troublesome diplopia after 6 months, then a second stage procedure can be considered. The time lapse is to allow the anterior segment circulation to become optimal if intervention on the previously operated eye is being planned.

Second stage surgery after initial horizonal muscle surgery

(1) **Residual esotropia**

This can be needed if the angle of deviation was initially large and unilateral intervention was insufficient.

- In this case the next operation will most helpfully be horizontal surgery on the contra lateral eye. Undertake an MR recession/LR resect or plicate as required.
- If the residual deviation is small and the patient does not wish contra lateral surgery the options are to further recess the MR (be careful not to make divergent in contra lateral side gaze) or to consider an MR central tenotomy or Z plasty. A tenotomy or Z plasty is difficult to grade and cannot be undertaken on an adjustable suture. Even a small recession of the MR beyond the equator can have a significant effect on adduction inducing divergence on nasal gaze. If possible, it is best undertaken with an adjustable suture.

(2) **Diplopia on side gaze but none in primary position with small residual limitation in abduction**

If the deviation in primary is small with no double vision but the issue is diplopia on side gaze consider:

- Faden or Scott procedure on the contra lateral MR. If undertaking a Scott procedure this can be done using an adjustable suture technique.
- If diplopia persists in side gaze and the contra lateral MR has been previously operated upon a further recession risks producing incomitance with divergence in primary position so a Faden would be the optimal approach rather than a Scott.

(3) **The patient has undergone a previous ipsilateral recess of the MR and resect of the LR but remains with no abduction beyond the midline**

This may occur if there is progression of a 6th nerve palsy or if the palsy was complete not incomplete. The following options can be considered:

- Nishida procedure. This is probably the best approach with the least risk to the vascular circulation or of producing an induced vertical deviation.
- A single muscle vertical transposition could be used.
- A full tenon transfer of both SR and IR should be avoided otherwise all 4 rectus muscles will have had surgery with a risk of vascular compromise.
- If the patient has reduced abduction with diplopia on side gaze but is divergent in contra lateral gaze consider a Nishida to improve the abduction, and advancing the medial rectus muscle to manage the consecutive divergence. It may be best to undertake this in two procedures.

Second stage procedures after initial transposition procedure

(1) **Residual esotropia with diplopia in primary position as well as residual abduction deficit**

If still a significant deviation in primary position consider:

- MR recession. This can be on the ipsilateral eye if the MR was not operated on at the initial surgery or the contralateral MR if the ipsilateral MR has had surgery. If the deviation is small and patient has had a previous ipsilateral MR recession and does not wish contra lateral surgery the options are to further recess the MR (be careful not to make divergent in contra lateral side gaze) or to consider an MR central tenotomy or Z plasty.
- If the angle is large a combined contra lateral MR- and LR+ could be considered to reduce the primary position angle which will reduce the diplopia in primary position but would be expected to leave residual diplopia on abduction. This can be undertaken using fixed or adjustable sutures. Then tackle any residual diplopia in side gaze with a contra lateral MR Faden at a later procedure.
- If previous surgery was one vertical rectus transposition consider transposing the second vertical muscle and a MR recession.

(2) **Residual abduction defect with diplopia on side gaze but none in primary position**

Consider:

- Contra lateral MR Scott or Faden. Plan carefully the amounts of recession and resection if undertaking a Scott procedure. If the angle in primary is minimal a larger recession than resection may leave the patient divergent in primary and convergent on side gaze which is a poor outcome. An adjustable suture would be useful in this setting. If the MR has previously been operated upon a further recession risks producing incomitance with divergence in primary position so a Faden would be the optimal approach.
- Transposition of second vertical muscle: If the previous procedure was a single muscle vertical transposition consider transposing the other vertical. Use the same technique as for the first muscle (i.e. augmentation suture or not) to avoid inducing

a vertical deviation with diplopia. If this were to result in a vertical deviation it would present considerable difficulties to resolve.

(3) **Divergence after transposition procedure**

If there is over correction with full abduction this suggests it was initially an incomplete palsy.

- If the operation was a toxin and transposition procedure it may be over 3 months before the over correction wears off. Do not intervene before this time and the deviation will slowly settle as the weakened MR regains function.
- If divergent in primary but still reduced abduction and if surgery was a transposition procedure and MR recession then consider readvancing the MR muscle alone. This can be undertaken using a fixed or adjustable suture but a fixed suture avoids the risk of muscle slippage.
- If divergent in primary but patient still has reduced abduction but no MR surgery was undertaken, undoing the transposition may reduce the primary angle but will worsen the abduction defect therefore consider an ipsilateral MR plicate or resection. Alternatively consider a contra lateral divergent squint operation.
- If a Nishida without MR recession was performed open up the conjunctiva and identify the scleral/muscle sutures. This can be done by sliding a flat muscle hook or a 240 retinal band under the muscles until the site of the scleral attachment is identified. Then cut the sutures off the globe and gently massage the muscles back to their original position (if necessary, a single 6/0 vicryl to bind the muscles back into place can be useful but do not attach the suture to sclera).
- If a full tendon transfer was the previous procedure the options are to remove any augmentation sutures if used or reverse the transposition. Simple removal of augmentation sutures may not be very helpful. Replacing the SR and/or IR to their original position may make the patient convergent again. Part replacement back to the original position is not likely to be successful and could result in a vertical deviation. If revision is required it is best to replace the vertical muscles back to their original position and reevaluate the position. If still convergent after vertical muscle replacement consider a recession of MR and either a resection or plication of LR. A LR plication is likely to be preferable to a resection as this will then be 4 muscle rectus surgery which may well cause ASI.
- If the original procedure was a Jensen muscle union procedure remove the sutures binding the muscles sections together and move the superior and inferior muscle slips back to their original muscle path; pull together and if necessary suture the LR if it is still split apart.
- If a Hummelsheim was the previous procedure, carefully identify the transposed vertical muscle strips, the lateral rectus and the vertical rectus muscles. Clean the transposed vertical muscle strips of any attachments and place two 6/0 vicryl sutures in each segment. Detach from the globe and move back to the original insertion site. It may, in addition, be necessary to suture the replaced vertical muscle strips to the body of the SR and IR to ensure muscle repositioning.

10 Anterior segment ischaemia

The patient will complain of deep orbital pain, which is different from the muscle and surface pain from squint surgery. The patient will have reduced vision, a mid dilated and irregular pupil, folds in Descemet's membrane, and slit lamp examination will show cells and flare in the anterior chamber. The patient is likely already to be on post-operative medication, most commonly a combination of antibiotic and steroid. The patient should be changed to preservative-free hourly topical steroid with a cycloplegic (e.g. cyclopentolate 1% three times a day) and if the situation does not resolve promptly consider starting oral steroid (40 mg per day prednisolone would be a reasonable starting dose). If the situation does not settle involve colleagues who are expert in inflammatory ocular disease management as other modulators may have to be considered (eg intravenous methylprednisolone, methotrexate or cyclophosphamide). The vision should return, but the patient may be left with a persistently dilated pupil with some iris atrophy which gives glare and glaucomflecken may be present in the lens.

11 Case Study

A patient involved in a road traffic accident sustained a traumatic right 6th nerve palsy which did not improve with time. Neuroimaging with MRI was undertaken as part of the patient management. The patient was initially managed with a Bangerter foil on one spectacle lens. At 9 months after the accident the patient had a convergent 40pd esotropia with no abduction beyond the midline and troublesome diplopia. The patient requested surgical treatment. Diagnostic toxin was performed and confirmed no movement beyond the mid line, indicating a complete palsy of the lateral rectus muscle. The patient underwent a Nishida on the ipsilateral eye with good result. However, the patient still had diplopia on right gaze and wished this to be improved and therefore underwent a left Faden procedure. This had a good effect leaving the patient with diplopia only on extreme right gaze which did not interfere with day-to-day life.

12 Key Points

- Investigate an acquired 6th nerve palsy as appropriate
- Wait for resolution/stability before planning potential intervention
- Assess lateral rectus function before planning any surgical procedure
- If the eye can abduct beyond the midline undertake horizontal squint surgery
- If the eye cannot abduct beyond the midline a transposition procedure is required

- Older operations involving muscle splitting are more destructive and considerably more difficult to reverse should the deviation be over corrected

13 Clinical Pearls

The key to surgical management of 6th nerve palsies is knowledge of LR function.

References

1. Lee J, Harris S, Cohen J, Cooper K, MacEwen C, Jones S. Results of a prospective randomized trial of botulinum toxin therapy in acute unilateral sixth nerve palsy. J Pediatr Ophthalmol Strabismus. 1994;31(5):283–6.
2. Sen S, Dhiman R, Saxena R, Phuljhele S, Sharma P. Vertical rectus transposition procedures for lateral rectus palsy: a systematic review. Indian J Ophthalmol. 2019;67(11):1793–9.
3. Foster R. Vertical muscle transposition augmemnted with lateral fixation. J Aapos. 1997;1:20–30.
4. Struck MC. Augmented vertical rectus transposition surgery with single posterior fixation suture: modification of foster technique. J AAPOS. 2009;13(4):343–9.
5. Holmes J, Hatt S, Leske D. Intraoperative monitoring of torsion to prevent vertical deviations during augmented vertical rectus transposition surgery. J Aapos. 2012;16(2):136–40.
6. Hummelsheim E. Weitere Ertahunger mit partiellar Sehnenuberpflanzung an der Augenmuskln. (abstract). Arch Augenheilkd 62:71
7. Lee JY, Lim HW, Yoon J, Oh JE, Park KA, Oh SY (2018) Comparison of the efficiency of various muscle transposition procedures using a novel three-dimensional model. Published online, pp 1–11. https://doi.org/10.1371/journal.pone.0204078
8. Jensen C. Rectus muscle union: a new operation for paralysis of the rectus muscles. Trans Pac Coast Otoophthalmol Soc Annu Meet. 1964;45:359–87.
9. Schillinger R. A new type of tendon transplant operation for abducens paralysis. J Int Coll Surg. 1959;31(5):593–600.
10. Rosenbaum AL, Kushner BJ, Kirschen D. Vertical rectus muscle transposition and botulinum toxin (oculinum) to medial rectus for abducens palsy. Arch Ophthalmol. 1989;107(6):820–3.
11. Nishida Y, Hayashi O, Oda S, et al. A simple muscle transposition procedure for abducens palsy without tenotomy or splitting muscles. Jpn J Ophthalmol. 2005;49(2):179–80.
12. Hernandez-García E, Burgos-Blasco B, Özkan SB, et al. A comparative multicentric long-term study of un-augmented modified Nishida procedure vs augmentation in unilateral sixth nerve palsy. Eye. 2023;37(1):170–5.
13. Mehendale R, Dagi LR, Wu C, Ledoux D, Johnston S, Hunter DG. Superior rectus transposition and medial rectus recession for Duane syndrome and sixth nerve palsy. Arch Ophthalmol. 2012;130(2):195–201.
14. Velez F, Chang M, Pineles S. Inferior rectus transposition: a novel procedure for abducens palsy. Am J Ophthalmol. 2017;177:126–30.

Management of Strabismus in Thyroid Eye Disease

Richard Harrad

Abstract Thyroid eye disease (TED) is an auto-immune condition characterised by an acute inflammatory phase followed by a fibrotic phase which sometimes leads to restricted eye movements and diplopia. Medical treatment with systemic steroids with or without orbital radiotherapy and immunosuppression can control the inflammatory response. Strabismus surgery should be carried out only after the inflammation is no longer active and after any decompression surgery. Surgery comprises recession of tight muscles using adjustable sutures so as to maximise the area of binocular single vision. There is debate as to whether adjustable sutures should be used for the inferior rectus muscle. Patients should be encouraged to have realistic expectations since binocular single vision (BSV) may not be achievable in all directions of gaze and lid retraction may be made worse by surgery.

Keywords Strabismus · Surgery · Thyroid eye disease

1 Pathogenesis

TED is an auto-immune condition characterised by auto-antibodies to the TSH receptor and the insulin-like growth factor (IGF1) receptor. In the initial acute phase, there is lymphocytic infiltration and oedema of the extra-ocular muscles with deposition of glycosaminoglycans and hyaluronic acid as well as adipogenesis [1]. These processes can lead to an increase in the volume of the contents of the orbit with resultant proptosis, optic nerve compression and raised intra-orbital pressure. Later the inflammation subsides but there may be fibrotic change in the orbit leading to tightness and restriction of movement of the extra-ocular muscles. The inferior rectus is most commonly affected followed by the medial and superior rectus [2]. Involvement of extra-ocular muscles may be bilateral or unilateral. Sometimes only one

R. Harrad (✉)
Bristol Eye Hospital, Bristol, UK
e-mail: r.a.harrad@bristol.ac.uk

S. Jain (ed.), *Surgical Management of Strabismus*,
https://doi.org/10.1007/978-3-031-80633-9_11

muscle is affected. It is not known why some muscles are more commonly involved than others. The inferior rectus is the bulkiest and most tonically active extra-ocular muscle, it may be that the degree of muscle activity and hence blood supply is a factor.

2 Clinical Assessment and Non-surgical Management

The presence of lid-lag or lid retraction in an adult presenting with recent onset of strabismus is highly suggestive of TED. Thyroid function tests are usually diagnostic, but a small proportion of patients with TED have normal thyroid function tests. Patients with TED are assessed for disease severity and activity and treatment in the form of immunosuppression is given depending on the degree of disease activity according to a clinical scoring system [3]. MRI scan of the orbits, particularly STIR [4] sequence is useful in gauging disease activity and demonstrating muscle involvement and optic nerve compression (Fig. 1).

It is useful to know which muscles are affected as this may affect the outcome of surgery. If a hypotropic eye has an enlarged superior rectus, and inferior rectus recession surgery is planned there may be a larger than normal effect of recession. Patients should be advised to stop smoking; smokers with TED are twice as likely to need strabismus surgery [5]. Systemic steroids are prescribed with or without additional immunosuppression in the form of Azathioprine or Cyclosporin or low-dose radiotherapy. Biological agents such as Rituximab are now sometimes employed and there is some evidence that cyclo-oxygenase (COX) inhibitors such as Indomethacin may be effective [6]. Studies of medical treatment of TED have mostly been retrospective with small numbers and a tendency to include both active and inactive disease. RCTs of radiotherapy have produced conflicting results. The CIRTED study, a multi-centre double armed RCT of radiotherapy v placebo and Azathioprine immunosuppression v placebo for patients on treatment with steroids for active TED found no significant additional benefit from radiotherapy or Azathioprine. Although post hoc analysis showed benefit from Azathioprine at 48 weeks [7]. It is widely observed that strabismus surgery is now carried out less frequently over recent years in TED patients as a result of better medical management.

3 Timing of Surgery

Surgery for strabismus in TED should not be carried out until the condition has become inactive and any orbital decompression has been performed. Patients who have already had a prolonged course of treatment and who are disabled by diplopia are understandably keen to have their strabismus corrected as soon as possible. However, measurements of the strabismus should be stable for at least 6 months prior to surgery: one study has reported a significant change in the strabismus in 30% of patients after

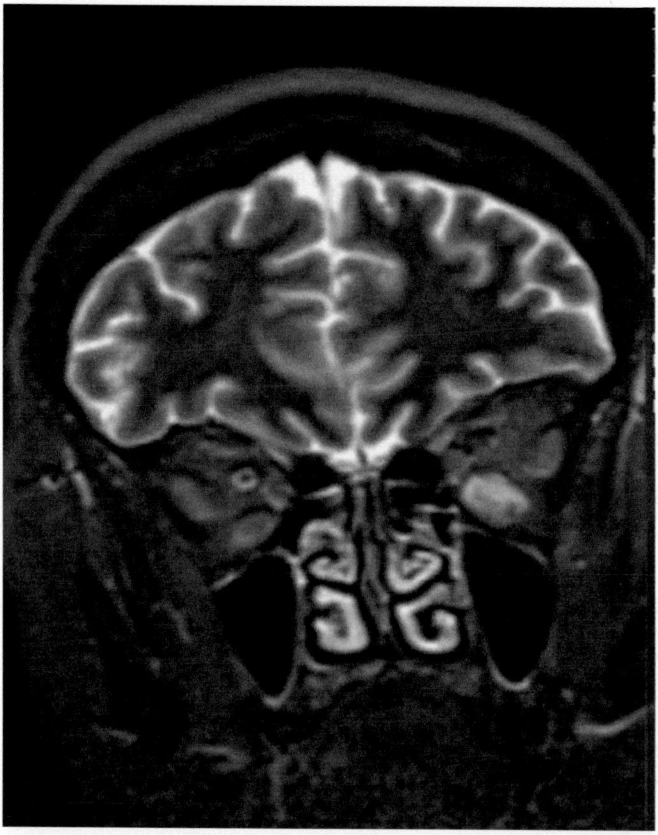

Fig. 1 STIR MRI scan of the orbits showing enlarged and oedematous left inferior rectus muscle

6 months of stable measurements [8]. Eyelid surgery should be delayed until after strabismus surgery. Some authors advocate the use of Botox in the acute phase and prisms can be helpful if there is a small deviation.

4 The Surgical Plan

At surgery the affected extra-ocular muscles are usually tight and fibrotic. Gaining access to the muscles can be challenging. Following decompression muscles may be incarcerated in bone. Where a deviation has increased significantly following decompression it advisable to repeat the MRI scan of the orbits.

Case 1. A 43 year old man presented with a left esotropia following left 3 wall orbital decompression for proptosis and corneal exposure. There was 55 prism dioptres of esotropia and the left eye was fixed in adduction. MRI scan showed adhesion

between the medial orbital wall and the medial rectus muscle along almost its entire length (Fig. 2). At surgery it was impossible to free the medial rectus muscle, which was recessed 7 mm on an adjustable suture using the relaxed muscle technique and recessed a further 2 mm on adjustment. 3 months later there was a good result with 5 prism dioptres of esotropia, with BSV in the primary position.

Surgery is carried out with the patient paralysed under general anaesthetic and an experienced assistant is recommended. A forced duction test should be carried out in order to assess the tightness of all the muscles of both eyes. A Fison's retractor is helpful to expose the muscle. Sometimes when the muscle is very tight it may be necessary to divide it using a scalpel while protecting the globe with the squint hook. The position of the muscle insertion should be measured prior to dividing it and again after division. The insertion of a very tight muscle may move up to 2 mm anteriorly after division of the muscle and unless this is recognised the muscle may be under-recessed.

Surgery usually comprises recession of the tight muscles. Resection is rarely carried out unless the tight muscles have already been maximally recessed, in which case success has been reported with lateral rectus resections [9]. In a series of 8

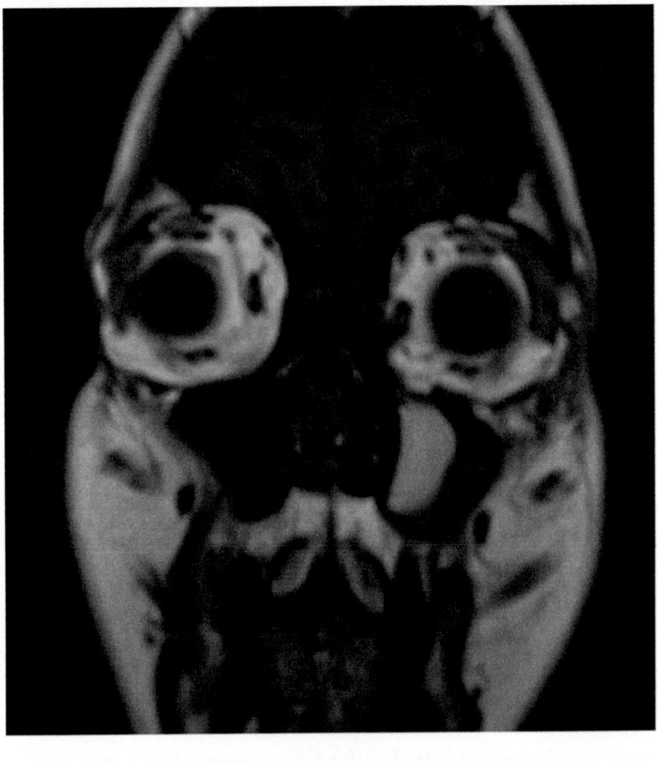

Fig. 2 MRI scan of the orbits showing incarceration of the left medial rectus muscle in the medial orbital walling following orbital decompression in Case 1

patients with vertical muscle resections the majority had a successful outcome [10]. Some authors advocate fixing the recessed muscle in the "relaxed muscle position" [11]; this is where the muscle lies at surgery with the eye centrally placed. There is some controversy over the use of adjustable sutures when recessing the inferior rectus muscle. Several authors have described late over-correction using this technique [12, 13]. The effects of gravity and the downward pull of the inferior oblique and the lower lid retractors combined with a short arc of contact can prevent the formation of a strong adhesion between the inferior rectus and the globe. However, a recent study found no significant difference between fixed recession and adjustable sutures [14, 15]. Some surgeons use non-absorbable sutures to reduce the risk of late over-correction, but these sutures have a higher risk of infection and a tendency to erode through the conjunctiva. Kushner reported 100% success in abolishing muscle slippage by employing a semi-adjustable suture technique [16]. This procedure involves suturing the corners of the muscle to the sclera and putting the centre of the muscle on an adjustable suture. An alternative approach is to recess the inferior rectus using a fixed suture while recessing the contralateral superior rectus muscle on an adjustable. This technique also has the advantage of reducing the amount of surgery on each of the vertical rectus muscles making surgically-induced upper and lower lid retraction less likely.

Case 2. A 60 year old woman with thyroid eye disease developed diplopia with a 30 prism dioptre right hypotropia. An MRI scan showed enlarged extraocular muscles and she was treated with radiotherapy and steroids (Figs.* 3 *and* 4*). After 1 year there was no change in her ocular alignment and surgery comprising a 6mm fixed right inferior rectus recession and a left superior rectus recession of 3mm using adjustable sutures was performed. Immediately post-surgery there was 10 prism dioptres of right hypotropia but no adjustment was made in anticipation of late upward drift of the right eye. 3 months later the eyes were straight for near and distance with no diplopia and the patient was pleased with the outcome (Fig.* 5*).

There are no published randomised controlled trials comparing adjustable and non-adjustable sutures in TED. Recession of an inferior rectus muscle results in between 3 and 4 prism dioptres of effect per mm of surgery [12, 15].

When recessing a vertical muscle, it should be sagittalised [17], that is moved in a nasal direction by half an insertion width in order to reduce the "A" or "V" pattern induced by weakening its adducting power. There is a risk that this will induce incyclotorsion.

Recession of a vertical muscle carries the risk of exacerbating lid retraction since there are fibrous connections between the superior rectus and the levator complex in the upper lid and the inferior rectus and the lower lid retractors. At the time of strabismus surgery it is advisable to divide these fibres as far posteriorly as possible. The lower lid retractors and Lockwood's ligament can be advanced to reduce lower lid retraction and sometimes the introduction of a spacer may be necessary. Conversely, recessing a tight inferior rectus may reduce the extent of ipsilateral upper lid retraction where this is due to Hering's law and secondary to increased tone in the superior rectus, so-called pseudo lid retraction.

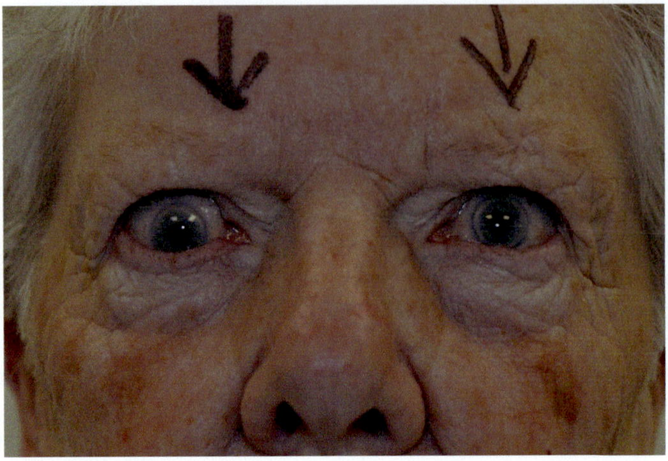

Fig. 3 Case 2. Right hypotropia and bilateral upper lid retraction

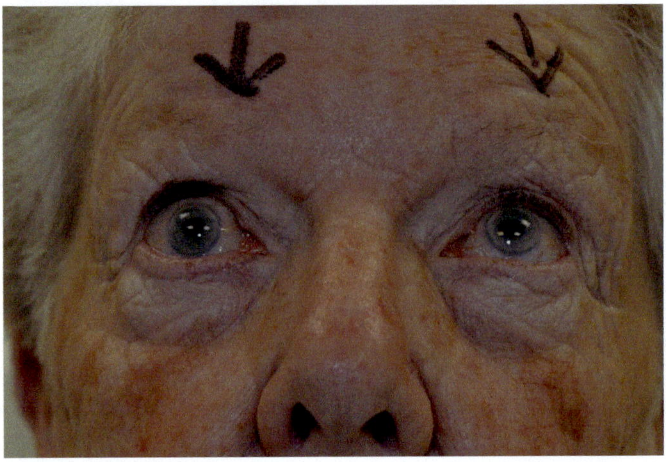

Fig. 4 Case 2. Limited right upgaze

Several authors advise aiming to under-correct a vertical deviation to allow for a late over-correction [14]. The aim should be to achieve single vision with both eyes in about 10 degrees of downgaze. This facilitates reading and walking down steps while requiring only a minimal chin-up head position for distance vision. Where there is no excyclotorsion in the presence of a tight inferior rectus muscle a tight superior oblique should be suspected and if present it will be tight on traction testing following division of the inferior rectus and per-operative measurement will show incyclotorsion. Torsion can be measured at surgery by inking the 6 and 12 o'clock positions at the limbus and measuring change using the Mendez ring. If tight, the

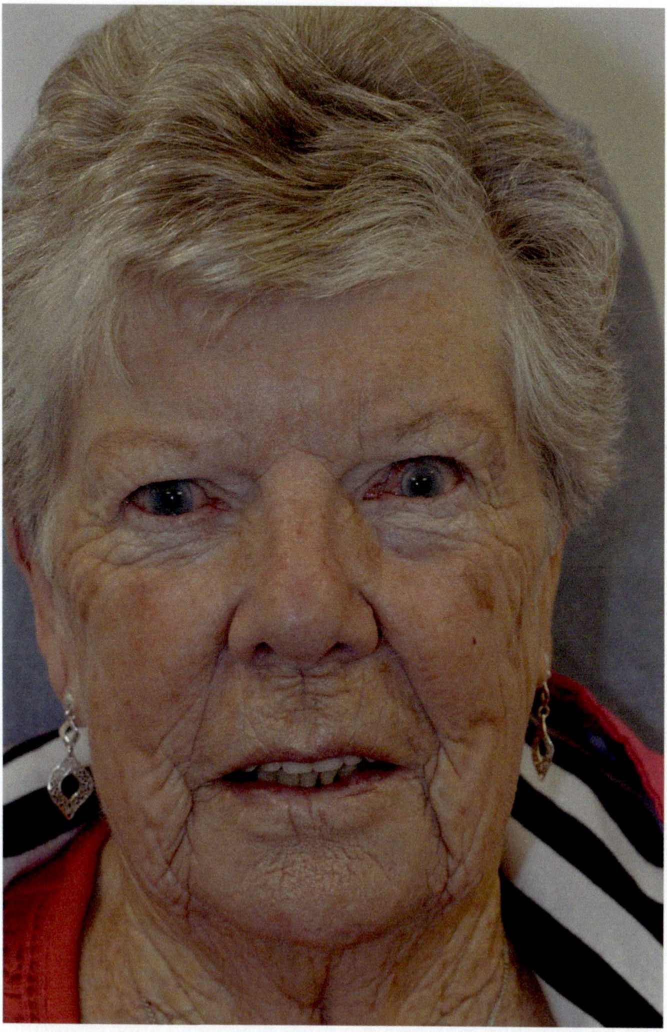

Fig. 5 Case 2. Good eye alignment with residual bilateral upper lid retraction

superior oblique should be recessed [18, 19]. If both inferior rectus muscles are tight this usually results in a chin-up abnormal head posture and may necessitate bilateral inferior rectus recessions. Patients' expectations must be carefully managed: it is usually possible to achieve single vision in the primary position with or without the aid of prisms in one operation, however the patient may have to get used to moving their head in order have single vision in other directions. Sometimes more than one operation may be necessary to achieve a satisfactory outcome, a 24.8% re-operation rate has been reported [20]. Fortunately many patients develop an impressively large fusion range which helps to reduce their diplopia. Patients need to be warned that their

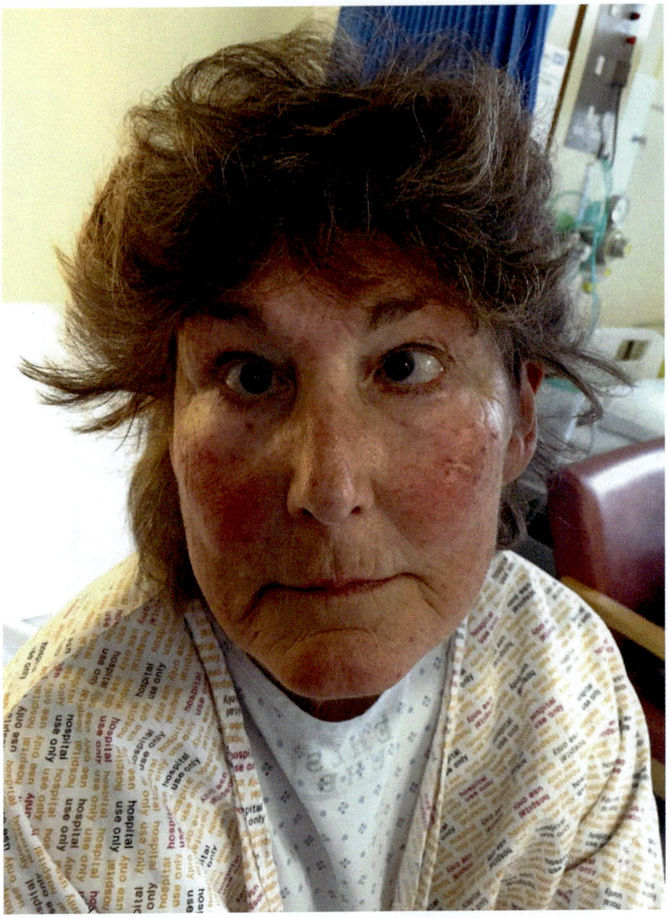

Fig. 6 Case 3. Large left esotropia

proptosis and lid retraction may become more noticeable after strabismus surgery: recession of 2 tight rectus muscles may lead an increase in proptosis of 2–3 mm.

Case 3. A 70 year old woman was treated with steroids and Cellcept for thyroid eye disease. She developed optic nerve compression and had bilateral medial and inferior wall decompression. She developed post-operative diplopia with a left esotropia of 40 prism dioptres (Fig. 6)***. Measurements were stable for 6 months and both medial recti were recessed by 5 mm using an adjustable suture. Post operatively there was an esotropia of 4 prism dioptres and no adjustment was made. At 3 months the eyes were straight without diplopia (Fig.*** 7)*.*

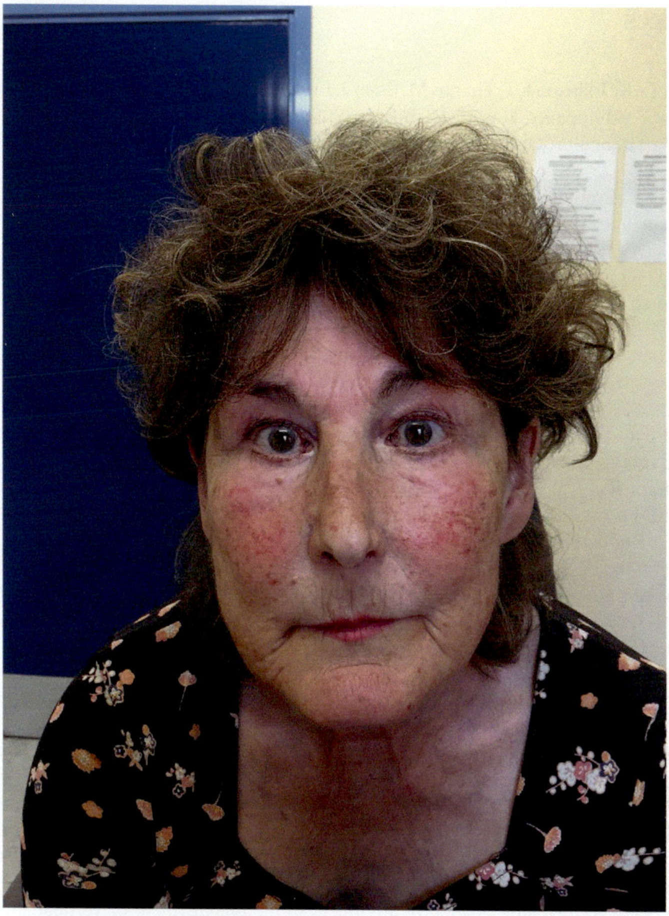

Fig. 7 Case 3. Orthotropia 3 months after surgery

5 Conclusion

Strabismus surgery in TED should be carried out once the disease is inactive and after any orbital decompression. Measurements should be stable for at least 6 months. Recession of those muscles that are tight on forced duction test using adjustable sutures brings about the best results. Although some authors report good results using this technique, the use of adjustable sutures on the inferior rectus is probably best avoided.

References

1. Eckstein AK, Johnson KT, Thanos M, Esser J, Ludgate M. Current insights into the pathogenesis of Graves' orbitopathy. Horm Metab Res. 2009;41(6):456–64.
2. Dyer JA. The oculorotary muscles in Graves' disease. Trans Am Ophthalmol Soc. 1977;74:425–56.
3. Mourits MP, Prummel MF, Wiersinga WM, Koornneef L. Clinical activity score as a guide in the management of patients with Graves' ophthalmopathy. Clin Endocrinol (Oxf). 1997;47(1):9–14.
4. Laitt RD, Hoh B, Wakeley C, Kabala J, Harrad R, Potts M, et al. The value of the short tau inversion recovery sequence in magnetic resonance imaging of thyroid eye disease. Br J Radiol. 1994;67(795):244–7.
5. Rajendram R, Bunce C, Adams GG, Dayan CM, Rose GE. Smoking and strabismus surgery in patients with thyroid eye disease. Ophthalmology. 2011;118(12):2493–7.
6. Kuriyan AE, Woeller CF, O'Loughlin CW, Phipps RP, Feldon SE. Orbital fibroblasts from thyroid eye disease patients differ in proliferative and adipogenic responses depending on disease subtype. Invest Ophthalmol Vis Sci. 2013;54(12):7370–7.
7. Rajendram R, et al. Combined immunosuppression & radiotherapy in thyroid eye disease (CIRTED) a multi-centre, 2 × 2 factorial double-blind randomised controlled trial. Lancet Diabetes Endocrinol. 2018;6:299–309.
8. Lee YH, Oh SY, Hwang JM. Is 6 months of stable angle of strabismus enough to perform surgery in patients with strabismus related to thyroid ophthalmopathy? Br J Ophthalmol. 2010;94(7):955–6.
9. Akbari MR, et al. Management of thyroid eye disease related strabismus. J Curr Ophthalol. 2020;32:1–13.
10. Tacea, et al. Rectus muscle resection for vertical strabismus in thyroid eye disease. Strabismus. 2018;26:71–6.
11. Dal Canto AJ, Crowe S, Perry JD, Traboulsi EI. Intraoperative relaxed muscle positioning technique for strabismus repair in thyroid eye disease. Ophthalmology. 2006;113(12):2324–30.
12. Scott WE, Thalaker JA. Diagnosis and treatment of thyroid myopathy. Ophthalmology. 1981;88:493–8.
13. Sprunger DT, Helveston EM. Progressive overcorrection after inferior rectus recession. J Pediatr Ophthalmol Strabismus. 1993;30:145–8.
14. Jefferis, et al. Prioritising downgaze alignment in the management of vertical strabismus for thyroid eye disease: principles and outcomes. Eye. 2020;34:906–14.
15. Peragallo JH, Velez FG, Demer JL, Pineles SL. Postoperative drift in patients with thyroid ophthalmopathy undergoing unilateral inferior rectus muscle recession. Strabismus. 2013;21(1):23–8.
16. Kushner BJ. An evaluation of the semi-adjustable suture strabismus surgical procedure. J AAPOS. 2004;8:481–7.
17. Harrad RA. Management of strabismus in thyroid eye disease. Eye. 2015;29:234–7.
18. Thacker NM, Velez FG, Demer JL, Rosenbaum AL. Superior oblique muscle involvement in thyroid ophthalmopathy. J AAPOS. 2005;9(2):174–8.
19. Holmes JM, Hatt SR, Bradley EA. Identifying masked superior oblique involvement in thyroid eye disease to avoid postoperative A-pattern exotropia and intorsion. J AAPOS. 2012;16(3):280–5.
20. Hwang B, Heo H, Lambert SR. Risk factors for reoperation after strabismus surgery among patients with thyroid eye disease. Am J Ophthalmol. 2022;238:10–5.

Restrictive Strabismus and Reoperations

Kevin Falzon and Ian Simmons

Abstract This chapter discusses the surgical management of restrictive strabismus and principles and strategies for reoperations. The causes of restrictive strabismus are multi-factorial and the treatment options are often complex and unpredictable. In general, surgical management includes relieving any restriction in the affected eye and/or creating a matching limitation in the fellow eye. A reoperation may be needed due to an under-correction, over correction or a newly created motility problem. Reoperation surgery offers its own challenges and problems.

Keywords Restrictive strabismus · Reoperations · Congenital cranial dysinnervation disorders · Brown syndrome · Orbital fractures

1 Restrictive Strabismus

1.1 Introduction

Restrictive strabismus is caused by factors that either interfere with muscle contraction or relaxation, or otherwise prevent free movement of the globe [1]. Management of restrictive strabismus is challenging because both muscle and surrounding tissue is involved. The causes are multifactorial, and the treatment options are often complex and unpredictable [1–4].

K. Falzon
Eye Clinic, York Hospital, York, UK
e-mail: kevinfalzon@nhs.net

I. Simmons (✉)
Leeds Teaching Hospitals NHS Foundation Trust, Leeds, UK
e-mail: i.simmons@nhs.net

S. Jain (ed.), *Surgical Management of Strabismus*,
https://doi.org/10.1007/978-3-031-80633-9_12

1.2 History

A history of head or facial trauma can be associated with blow-out fractures [3]. Pain on eye movements may suggest active thyroid orbitopathy and orbital myositis. It is important to remain vigilant for non-painful restrictive causes such as neoplastic orbital infiltration. It is also important to take a careful medication and general history from patients including the use of anticoagulants or anti-platelet medications.

1.3 Examination

Inspection may identify a manifest tropia, hypoglobus, enopthalmos and eyelid changes including eyelid retraction and ptosis. A positive forced duction test is one of the hallmarks of restrictive strabismus. Ductions and versions are equally limited with normal saccadic velocity up to the point of limitation. Movement in the opposite direction of gaze and muscle sequalae are often limited. Pain on eye movement and globe retraction may be present.

1.3.1 Investigations

It is important to assess for subjective and objective torsion preoperatively to avoid any potential suboptimal outcomes postoperatively. A post-operative diplopia test done pre-operatively can be valuable in guiding the amount of surgical correction that is safe to perform. A Hess test can also help identify a restrictive strabismus. Hess tests and BSV charts can both be helpful to document any spontaneous improvement following trauma. A BSV chart is also useful post-operatively to demonstrate to patients that surgery was beneficial, or on the contrary, to identify that surgery has not been successful and to then offer better prognostic advice regarding any further intervention.

1.3.2 Forced Duction and Forced Generation Tests

A forced duction test is important to quantify the amount of restriction. This is easily performed intraoperatively at the start of surgery in theatre or can also be performed preoperatively in clinic; the authors' preference is to perform an intra-operative forced duction test in theatre. It is important to determine the amount of limitation in both directions for each muscle e.g. elevation and depression in an orbital floor fracture with inferior rectus involvement. It is also important to avoid retropulsion when performing a forced duction test on a rectus muscle; however, it is essential to perform retropulsion when performing forced duction tests on oblique muscles. Another useful test is the forced generation test; this can help determine whether there is a paretic component in restrictive strabismus.

1.3.3 Ocular Examination

Careful slit lamp examination may reveal conjunctival scars and/or scleral changes (e.g. darker sclera from thinning associated with medial rectus recession) consistent with previous strabismus surgery. Care should be taken to identify the presence or absence of existing suture material i.e. patients may have had surgery utilizing non-absorbable sutures many years previously. It is important to remember that previous ocular, orbital or sinus surgery can have a significant effect on the tissue surrounding the extraocular muscles and globe.

1.4 Expectation Management and Consent Process

Patients with restrictive strabismus need particularly careful consenting and detailed discussions to manage expectations. In general, surgical management includes relieving any restriction in the affected eye and/or creating a matching limitation in the fellow eye. Operating on the unaffected eye to create a matching limitation can understandably be a difficult decision to make by the patient.

Elimination of a restriction is usually achieved with muscle weakening procedures e.g. recessions. This can create an undesirable effect in the field of action of the recessed muscle e.g. inferior rectus recession in thyroid orbitopathy can help eliminate diplopia in primary gaze but can cause limited downgaze resulting in diplopia when looking down. Where patients have restrictive strabismus in the context of a blow-out fracture or iatrogenic cause e.g. inferior oblique adherence, it may be advisable to consider surgery to the fellow eye due to concerns about extensive fibrotic scarring or muscle damage in the affected eye.

The use of posterior fixation sutures with or without a recession of the muscle is a useful and effective surgical option, however, should be considered with care. A combined resection and recession of a rectus muscle, a technique described by Alan B. Scott, with or without adjustable sutures may be an alternative option [5].

2 Reoperations

The need for reoperation strabismus surgery may be apparent soon after surgery or not until many years later. A reoperation may be needed due to an under-correction, over correction or a newly created motility problem. Reoperation surgery offers its own challenges and problems. There may be no pre-operative history either from medical records or patient and/or carers. Surgical dose table are not as useful e.g. the effect per millimeter of a medial rectus readvancement in a consecutive exotropia is more unpredictable. Although surgical planning is as important, the patient and surgeon need to understand that the surgery performed may need to be modified based on the intraoperative findings; this is relevant to the consent process.

One of the most common indications for reoperations in adults is a consecutive exotropia following esotropia surgery in childhood. Adults with a history of infantile esotropia may have had bilateral medial rectus recessions in early childhood whilst adults with significant amblyopia may have undergone unilateral medial rectus recession and lateral rectus resection in childhood. Assessment of any medial rectus duction deficits and careful slit-lap exam for any conjunctival scars can again help identify what surgery may have been carried out previously. Recently, anterior segment optical coherence tomography has been shown to accurately identify post-surgical horizontal muscle insertion if the insertion is less than 8 mm from the limbus. However, the extraocular muscle insertion was undetectable if the distance to the limbus was greater than 10 mm, which is typical for a medial rectus recession for esotropia in childhood [6].

2.1 Intraoperative Forced Duction Tests

An intraoperative forced duction test is essential to identify any limitation of adduction in a consecutive exotropia. Limitation of adduction may be due to either a large medial rectus recession, slipped medial rectus or contracture following lateral rectus resection. Readvancement of a previously recessed medial rectus alone may be sufficient; however, recession of the lateral rectus may also be needed. In adults, it is important to consider the natural changes of both conjunctiva and tenon capsule with age when performing forced duction tests, placement of incisions and choice of traction sutures or fixation forceps (Fig. 1). Anticoagulants or antiplatelet medications can also increase the risk of bleeding. If the conjunctiva is likely to tear and bleed when performing the forced duction test, this will make placing the traction suture more challenging. A useful tip is to place the traction suture first and then perform the forced duction test.

2.2 Slipped Muscle

When performing a readvancement of the medial rectus it is necessary to assess the muscle for any pseudo-tendon and slipped muscle. A slipped muscle occurs when, during initial surgery, the muscle inside the tenon sheath is insufficiently transfixed allowing it to recess within the capsule over time. A slipped muscle has a thin, translucent capsule (pseudo-tendon) through which the muscle hook is visible. Repair of a slipped muscle necessitates securing the skeletal muscle portion with sutures and excision of the pseudo-tendon prior to readvancement (Fig. 2).

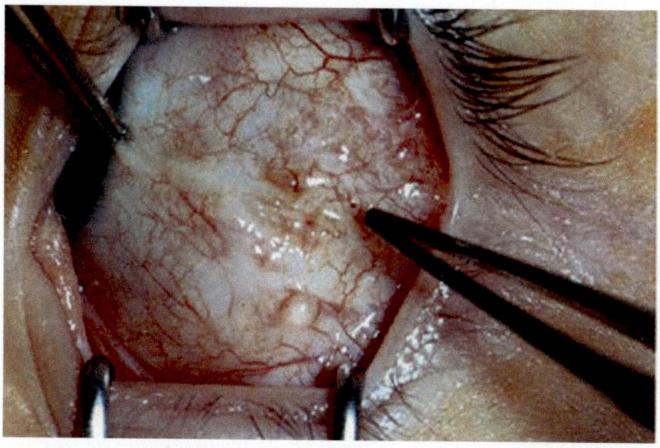

Fig. 1 Conjunctiva causing restriction due to scarring from prior surgery. Note stringlike indentation of conjunctiva with forced duction into field of restriction. The forceps on the left is grasping the eye at the limbus. The forceps on the right is pointing to the stringlike indentation of the globe (photo courtesy of Art Jampolsky, MD) Burton Kushner. Strabismus. Springer Inc 2017. Rights obtained

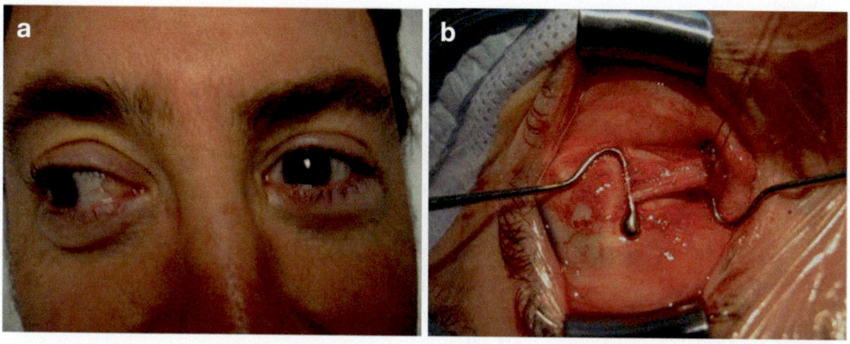

Fig. 2 (**a**) Patient with a slipped left medial rectus muscle after medial rectus recession. This patient is looking to the right, demonstrating a large exotropia with the left eye showing limited adduction and lid fissure widening. (**b**) Surgical exploration shows a translucent, avascular capsule connecting the globe to the medial rectus muscle. Note that the capsular attachment is so thin that the large Jameson hook can be seen through the overlying capsule [7]. Rights obtained

2.3 *Adjustable Sutures*

Adjustable surgery is an additional consideration. Adjustable sutures can be used with either a muscle recession or resection. However, it is important to remember that an adjustable recession can be further recessed or readvanced postoperatively whilst a resected muscle can only be recessed with no option of readvancement. Some patients may choose not to have adjustable surgery and care must be taken when discussing the option of an awake adjustment with patients.

2.4 Botulinum Toxin

Botulinum toxin may have a role in restrictive strabismus. A trial of botulinum toxin may be helpful in a consecutive exotropia following a unilateral medial rectus recession and lateral rectus resection. A botulinum toxin injection of the lateral rectus can help differentiate between a tight lateral rectus or weakened/slipped medial rectus. It is sometimes difficult to distinguish muscle contracture from fibrosis in thyroid orbitopathy and botulinum toxin can be considered to eliminate diplopia and restore alignment and may obviate the need for strabismus surgery [8]. It can be used intraoperatively with a muscle recession (e.g. inferior rectus recession following an orbital floor fracture) as an alternative to or in combination with traction sutures. Botulinum toxin can also be useful in post-traumatic strabismus, iatrogenic adherence problems and following orbital or retinal detachment surgery.

3 Congenital Cranial Dysinnervation Disorders

The discovery of the genetic basis of syndromes and the availability of clinical molecular testing has allowed the resolution of conflicting opinions about clinical diagnoses [9]. Congenital cranial dysinnervation disorders are one group of related conditions that has received a lot of attention in recent years because of the discovery of several of the genes that cause individual clinical entities [10]. These disorders result from aberrant innervation of the ocular and facial musculature. They are congenital, the primary findings are non-progressive, and they generally arise from abnormal development of individual or multiple cranial nerve nuclei or their axonal connections [11]. Congenital cranial dysinnervation disorders describe related conditions including Duane syndrome, Congenital Fibrosis of the Extraocular Muscles (CFEOM), Möbius syndrome, and others.

4 Duane Syndrome

Duane syndrome is a congenital condition with a wide clinical spectrum. There is congenital aberrant innervation of the lateral rectus by the third cranial nerve. Duane syndrome is usually sporadic and isolated but there are reports of a familial tendency. It is usually unilateral, predominantly affecting the left eye, but it has been reported to be bilateral in up to 20% of cases [1, 4]. There is a female predisposition and Duane syndrome probably represents between 1 and 5% of strabismic patients in clinical practice [1]. There is a high incidence of Duane syndrome in adults with thalidomide embryopathy [12].

It is well understood that Duane syndrome is primarily an innervational disorder with secondary restrictive problems. Electromyographic studies have demonstrated

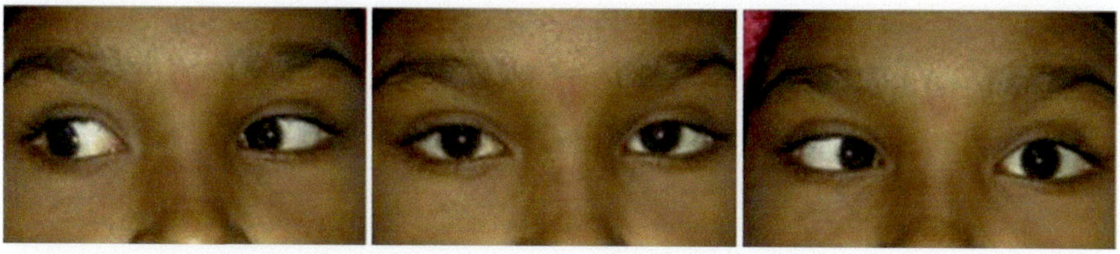

Fig. 3 Duane syndrome Type I left eye. Note the anomalous head posture, small-angle deviation in primary position, narrowing of palpebral fissure on adduction and gross limitation of abduction in the left eye. S. Agrawal Strabismus [14]. Rights obtained

anomalous recruitment of the lateral rectus most commonly on attempted adduction. It can be associated with hypoplasia of the sixth cranial nerve nucleus. An observational study reviewing thin section magnetic resonance images has showed that the abducens nerve was absent in patients with Type I Duane syndrome but present in patients with Type 2 Duane syndrome [13].

4.1 Clinical Features

The clinical features of Duane syndrome are globe retraction and narrowing of the palpebral fissure on adduction. Up-shoots and down-shoots on adduction are caused by co-contraction of the lateral rectus slipping up (causing an up-shoot) or down (resulting in a down-shoot) [4] (Figs. 3 and 4). Patients may adopt an abnormal head posture, typically a face turn to allow fusion. In esotropic Duane syndrome there is a face turn *towards* the affected eye whilst in exotropic Duane syndrome there is a face turn *away* from the affected eye [4].

There are systemic associations with Duane syndrome. Patients can have a hearing impairment and for this reason it's important to consider referring any infant with Duane syndrome to audiology [4]. Other recognized associations include Goldenhar Syndrome, Klippel-Fell Anomaly and Wildervanck Syndrome.

4.2 Classifications

There have been several attempts to classify Duane Syndrome. The balance of medial rectus innervation and lateral rectus anomalous innervation results in either an esotropia, an exotropia or orthophoria in the primary position. Huber's classification (1974) describes Duane syndrome as Type I, 2 or 3, depending on whether there is an esotropia or an exotropia in primary position and the main gaze limitation is abduction, adduction or both abduction and adduction respectively [1]. All types of

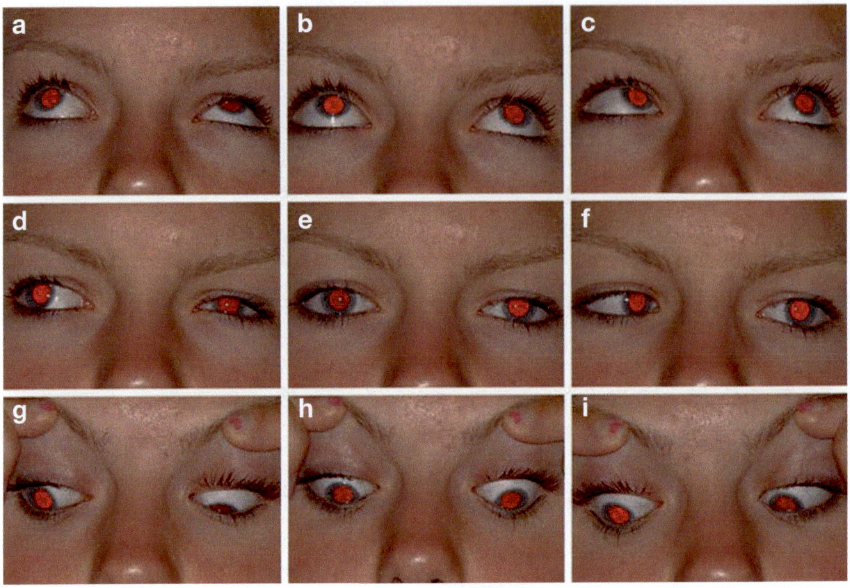

Fig. 4 Motility of a patient with Duane syndrome OS with a lot of lateral rectus muscle co-contraction. (**a**) up right; (**b**) straight up; (**c**) up left; (**d**) middle right; (**e**) middle straight; (**f**) middle left; (**g**) down right; (**h**) straight down; (**i**) down left. On attempted adduction above the midline there is an upshoot, below the midline there is a downshoot, and on direct horizontal side gaze there is substantial globe retraction. Burton Kushner. Strabismus. Springer Inc 2017. Rights obtained

Duane syndrome may present with orthophoria in the primary position. This classification system however doesn't incorporate the variables that may influence the surgical strategies [4].

Atypical Duane syndrome, also described as types 4, 5 and 6 include synergistic divergence, vertical retraction syndrome and a Y-pattern deviation respectively [15]. In synergistic divergence there is simultaneous abduction on attempted adduction. Vertical retraction syndrome is characterized by horizontal Duane syndrome, globe retraction on vertical gaze with or without limitation of vertical movements. Y-pattern Duane syndrome is associated with co-contraction of the lateral recti with the superior recti resulting in a "pseudo-inferior oblique over action" and Y-pattern in upgaze [4].

It is important to consider the differential diagnosis of Duane syndrome including sixth cranial nerve palsy, medial wall blow-out fracture, orbital inflammation, Moebius Syndrome and iatrogenic causes e.g. recession of the lateral rectus [1].

4.3 Surgical Management

The treatment of children with Duane syndrome should, as with all patients, start with correcting any refractive error and any amblyopia [1]. Amblyopia is less common in Duane Syndrome, particularly those who are orthophoric in primary position.

Most patients do not require further treatment. It is common for patients to adopt a slight abnormal head posture. Indications for surgery are to improve ocular alignment and to reduce a significant abnormal head posture. The surgical approach to Duane Syndrome involves consideration of the variables seen [4]. These include the degree of co-contraction of the lateral rectus, the presence of up-shoots or down-shoots, the presence of any lateral rectus function from an existing 6th cranial nerve and the size and direction of the deviation in adduction [4].

4.3.1 Esotropic Duane Syndrome

- An *ipsilateral medial rectus recession* is the most performed operation for unilateral esotropic Duane syndrome. It can reduce the esotropia in primary position and the abnormal head posture. It can, however, lead to limited adduction and narrowing of the area of binocular single vision [4].
- An alternative approach is *bilateral asymmetric medial rectus recessions* with a *larger* recession in the non-Duane eye.
- *Transpositions* can also be considered. This can expand the area of binocular single vision but may be more prone to adverse effects [4]. One approach is a full tendon transposition of the superior rectus and inferior rectus (vertical rectus transposition) to the upper and lower border of the lateral rectus respectively with or without Foster augmentation sutures. To allow for medial rectus recession at the same time, an alternative approach is to transpose the superior rectus alone with an augmentation suture [16].
- *Lateral rectus resection* in the Duane eye is commonly avoided. This can be considered in an esotropic Duane syndrome with limited abduction, minimal globe retraction and a negative forced duction test but any resection is limited to a maximum of 3.5 mm [17].

4.3.2 Exotropic Duane Syndrome

- *Unilateral or bilateral recession of the lateral rectus* can be performed with or without resection of the medial recti. A large ipsilateral lateral rectus recession can be performed to relieve mechanical restriction. An even larger contralateral lateral rectus recession with or without posterior fixation suture may widen the field of binocular single vision as it will create a compensatory duction limitation of the normal eye [2].
- An *ipsilateral lateral rectus recession with Y-splitting* may help to eliminate up and downshoots; a 7–9 mm recession is performed with the insertion separated

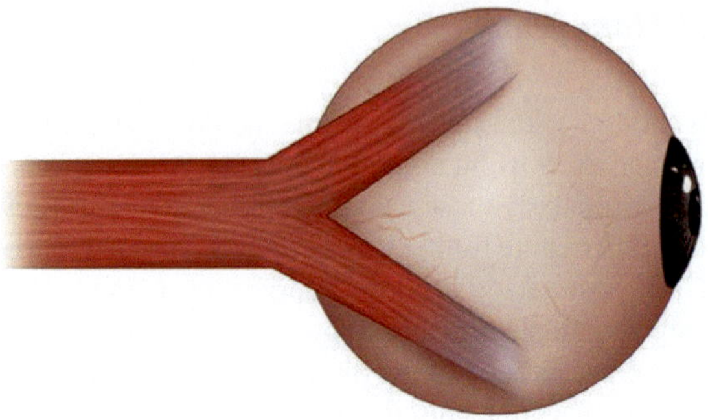

Fig. 5 Depiction of Y-splitting of the lateral rectus muscle (LR) with 20 mm separation between the split halves and a recession of 8 mm. Prior to Y-splitting and recession the co-contracting LR causes an upshoot or a downshoot of the globe as depicted in Fig. 1. After Y-splitting and recession the two split halves will anchor the LR from slipping up or down. Burton Kushner. Strabismus. Springer Inc 2017. Rights obtained

by 20 mm [18] (Fig. 5). Vertical rectus transposition surgery can be considered with full tendon superior rectus and inferior rectus transposition with posterior fixation suture to the medial rectus [19].

4.3.3 Botulinum Toxin

Botulinum toxin can be used diagnostically in Duane syndrome to determine whether reduction of the angle of deviation will improve binocular function, reduce abnormal head posture or reduce diplopia [20]. It can also be considered an option for maintenance therapy as an alternative to surgery [15].

5 Congenital Fibrosis of the Extra Ocular Muscles

Congenital fibrosis of the extra ocular muscles (CFEOM) classically presents with bilateral ptosis, marked limitation of up-gaze, convergence on attempted up gaze and limited horizontal eye movements [2]. There is often a positive family history and is commonly bilateral (Fig. 6). The hallmark is thin fibrotic muscles at the time of surgery [21]. Ptosis is due to levator muscle fibrosis. Patients may adopt a compensatory chin up head posture. Refractive errors and amblyopia are common and early intervention is required. Getting glasses to fit effectively is technically difficult because of the abnormal head posture. Refractive errors can, however, be effectively managed with contact lenses [21]. The phenotypes and associated genes are detailed in Tables 1 and 2 respectively [22].

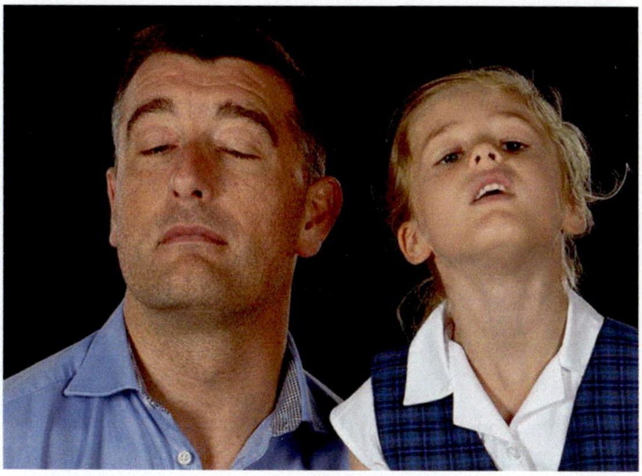

Fig. 6 A father and daughter with CFEOM type 1, both with ptosis and restriction of elevation of the eyes and a chin-up abnormal head posture Vivian [21]. Rights obtained

Table 1 Classification of CFEOM types [22]

Type	CFEOM1	CFEOM2	CFEOM3	CFEOM5
Inheritance	AD	AR	AD	AR
Laterality	Bilateral	Bilateral	Bilateral or unilateral	Bilateral or unilateral
Findings	Hypotropia and exotropia	Exotropia Bilateral 3rd and 4th nerve paresis	Hypotropia	Exotropia
Ptosis	Present	Present	Present	Present
Other findings	Usually no systemic findings	Small, sluggish pupils Occasionally retinal dystrophy	Often associated CNS abnormalities	

Table 2 Genetic causes of CFEOM [22]

Inheritance	Gene	% of all CFEOM	CFEOM1	CFEOM2	CFEOM3	CFEOM5
AD	KIF21A	55	+++		+	
	TUBA1A	< 1	+		+	
	TUBB2B	< 1			+	
	TUBB3	35	+		+++	
AR	COL25A1	< 1				+
	PHOX2A	10		+		

The differential diagnosis includes monocular elevation deficiency (also known as double elevator palsy), myasthenia gravis, third cranial nerve palsy and Brown syndrome.

5.1 Surgical Management

The treatment of CFEOM is challenging. It is usually not possible to restore useful ocular rotations because all the muscles are involved. The aim of surgery is limited to alignment in primary gaze and down gaze and to reduce any symptomatic abnormal head posture that in the long term can lead to significant neck problems. This requires addressing the ptosis and the extraocular muscle restriction. Levator function is usually minimal and correction of the ptosis requires brow suspension [21]. There may be horizontal and vertical misalignment, usually exotropia and hypotropia.

- The fundamental problem is that there may be virtually no superior rectus or medial rectus function and so relieving the restrictive element (by inferior rectus and/or lateral rectus recession) only allows the eyes to achieve a fixed position close to the midline at best [21].
- With very significant limitation of up gaze, the inferior recti are usually tight. *Large recessions of the inferior recti* of more than 6mm improve the hypotropia but under-correction is common [2]. These are, however, fibrotic and extremely thin muscles and are prone to snapping during recession surgery (pulled in two syndrome—PITS).
- A *small superior rectus resection* may enhance the effect of an inferior rectus recession but this can limit down gaze.
- *Large recessions of the lateral recti* are often needed if an exotropia is present and sometimes the lateral recti require disinsertion. Medial rectus resection might be considered but this can worsen convergence in up gaze [2].

6 Möbius Syndrome

Möbius syndrome is a rare, congenital and usually sporadic condition. It is characterised by a bilateral (but may be asymmetrical) facial nerve palsy and absent abduction caused by hypoplasia of one or more cranial nerves. Bilateral facial weakness is present with lack of facial expression. Reduced lid closure can lead to corneal exposure and the mouth is often kept open [3]. An esotropia is present due to reduced lateral rectus muscle function and medial rectus muscle contracture. Recognised associations include difficulty with speech, feeding and reduced corneal sensation. Skeletal and limb abnormalities may also be present.

6.1 Surgical Management

Correction of refractive errors, amblyopia treatment and management of exposure keratopathy is important.

- *Bilateral medial rectus recession* may be successful in correcting mild to moderate esotropia. In patients with larger esodeviations, bilateral medial rectus recession alone may be disappointing.
- *Combined bilateral medial rectus recession and superior rectus muscle transposition*, either simultaneous or as staged procedures, may result in better postoperative results in patients with larger preoperative angles [23].

7 Orbital Wall Fractures

Orbital wall fractures can occur following facial trauma. Diplopia and limitation of ocular movement is common, and the resultant strabismus can be quite complex. These patients are usually managed in coordination with the maxillofacial team.

7.1 *Types of Orbital Wall Fractures*

- *Orbital floor fractures* are the most common. The location of the fracture (anterior or posterior) and the presence or absence of muscle entrapment determine the severity. They may result in a hypotropia (or orthotropia) and limitation of elevation due to a restriction. A limitation of depression simulating an inferior rectus weakness may also occur; this may be due to a posterior entrapment or a flap tear of the inferior rectus [3] (Fig. 7).

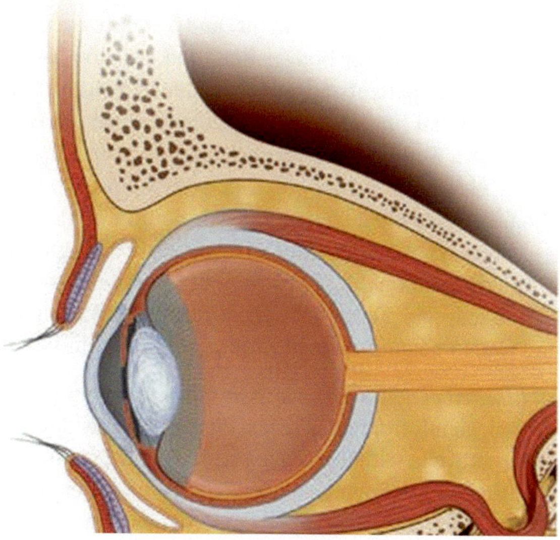

Fig. 7 Posterior orbital floor fracture can not only restrict upgaze, but also alter the torque vector of the inferior rectus muscle, weakening its depressing action. Burton Kushner. Strabismus. Springer Inc 2017. Rights obtained

- *Medial wall fractures* in isolation are uncommon and typically occur in combination with an orbital floor fracture. They may result in an esotropia or othotropia in primary gaze with an increasing esotropia on attempted ipsilateral lateral gaze due to restricted abduction. Limitation of adduction may also occur due to paresis or flap tear of the medial rectus [2, 3].
- *Superior and lateral wall fractures* are less common [2].

7.2 Examination

Examination includes assessment of the range of movement for any leash effect, involvement of surrounding tissue and current area of binocular single vision. The leash effect describes relatively normal initial movement with a sudden stop and represents scarring in and around the muscle. Hess charts and plots of binocular single vision are commonly performed. Computed tomography can accurately identify the site and extent of an orbital fracture and the degree of entrapment. Magnetic resonance imaging may provide better definition of the extent of any soft tissue injury [3].

7.3 Surgical Management

Initial observation is reasonable in most patients. The restrictive strabismus following an orbital fracture can be due to oedema, and to a lesser extent haemorrhage, and may resolve spontaneously. Recovery of inferior rectus function following a paresis also may occur after several months. Two specific indications for prompt intervention, often seen in children, include the oculocardiac reflex (nausea, vomiting, bradycardia and syncope due to entrapment) and a 'white eyed' trap door fracture [3].

It is important for both patient and surgeon to remember, that for vertical deviations, many patients adapt to a reduced field of binocular single vision in upgaze and a residual limitation in upgaze is less troublesome than creating a limitation in downgaze. Surgery on both eyes may be necessary to improve the field of binocular single vision and it may also be reasonable to avoid surgery on the involved eye altogether and create a matching limitation in the unaffected eye.

Three types of motility disorders are recognized after orbital floor fractures. Limited elevation due to restriction, limited depression due to inferior rectus paresis or flap tear and a combination of limited elevation and depression. Forced ductions and forced generation tests are important in guiding the decision-making process.

- ***Limited elevation***: If a hypotropia in primary gaze is present with marked restriction, an inferior rectus recession can be considered; this may create a postoperative hypertropia with limited depression and a contralateral inferior rectus recession or posterior fixation may be needed. If the patient is orthotropic in primary gaze and/or a mild restriction is present with contralateral superior rectus overaction, then a

contralateral superior rectus recession in combination with posterior fixation may be an alternative to an inferior rectus recession of the involved eye [2].
- ***Limited depression***: if there is no spontaneous recovery, forced generation testing reveals a paresis, and no restriction is present on forced duction, a resection of the ipsilateral inferior rectus may be considered; this may cause restriction of elevation [2]. Alternatively, an inverse Knapp procedure (transposition of the medial and lateral recti to the inferior rectus) or a recession of the contralateral inferior rectus with or without posterior fixation [2, 3].
- ***Limited elevation and depression***: if the patient is hypotropic in primary gaze and forced duction shows restriction in elevation but not depression, a recession of the inferior rectus to relieve the restriction to restore binocular single vision in primary gaze may result in a hypertropia on downgaze. An inverse Knapp procedure of the ipsilateral eye or posterior fixation of the contralateral inferior rectus may be necessary [2, 3].

With medial orbital wall fractures, the aim is to restore single vision in the primary position, improve the amount of horizontal eye movement and widen the area of binocular single vision.

- ***Limited abduction***: if the patient is esotropic (or orthophoric) in primary gaze an ipsilateral medial rectus recession can be performed to improve abduction. This may result in an exotropia on contralateral gaze and a lateral rectus recession of the contralateral unaffected eye may be necessary to help widen the area of binocular single vision.
- ***Limited adduction***: suggests either a medial rectus muscle flap tear, involvement of the muscle pulley in the fracture site or paresis. This may need exploration of the medial orbital wall and the management and repair of a flap tear considered [15]. Medial rectus paresis is managed similarly to a partial or complete palsy.

8 Brown Syndrome

Brown syndrome presents with limited elevation in adduction due to restriction of the superior oblique tendon or the tendon-trochlear complex [2]. Brown syndrome is usually congenital and sporadic but may be acquired. Heritable Brown syndrome has been reported. Congenital Brown syndrome is usually unilateral (90% of cases) but can be bilateral and may be asymptomatic (Fig. 8).

8.1 Causes of Acquired Brown Syndrome

Causes include trauma, surgery, and inflammation.

- *Trauma* to the trochlea–superior oblique tendon complex by penetrating injury or orbital fracture are recognised causes.

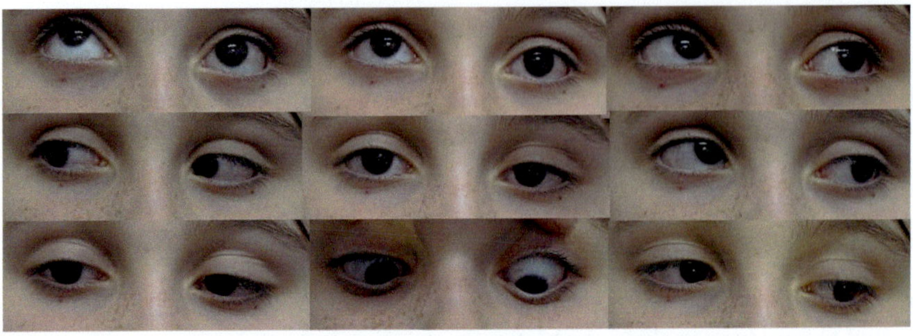

Fig. 8 A 10 year old girl with a small left hypotropia in primary position associated with a pseudoptosis. There is limitation of elevation of the left eye, more marked in adduction that abduction (from Simplifying Strabismus 2nd Edition. S. Jain, Springer)

- *Iatrogenic* causes for an acquired Brown Syndrome include previous superior oblique tuck, the use of a scleral buckle, glaucoma drainage surgery and surgery on the orbit or sinuses.
- *Auto-immune inflammatory conditions* associated with Brown syndrome include granulomatosis with polyangiitis (formerly known as Wegener granulomatosis) and rheumatoid arthritis. Inflammatory conditions affecting the sinuses and orbit can also lead to Brown syndrome.

8.2 Clinical Features

Patients may be orthophoric in primary gaze with limited elevation in adduction. Elevation may be normal in abduction. There is a hypotropia on attempted elevation in adduction and there can be a hypotropia in primary gaze. Patients may present with a down shoot in adduction. There can be an upshoot of the contralateral unaffected eye in up gaze. Pain or tenderness may be present in attempted elevation in adduction. Patients may feel or hear a click. In order to preserve binocular function, patients may adopt an abnormal head posture including a chin-up posture or a face turn *towards* the unaffected eye [4].

8.3 Differential Diagnosis

The differential diagnosis of Brown syndrome includes inferior oblique palsy, monocular elevation deficiency (double elevator palsy), congenital cranial nerve dysinnervation syndromes, blow-out fractures, thyroid orbitopathy or traumatic and surgical causes [1, 3]. Patients with Brown syndrome will often have a V-pattern compared to an A-pattern in inferior oblique palsy. Inferior oblique palsy is associated with incyclotorsion and a positive Park's three step test. Forced duction tests performed either at the slit lamp or at surgery will be positive for elevation in adduction in Brown syndrome compared to patients who have an inferior oblique palsy [1, 4].

8.4 *Surgical Management*

Most patients with mild Brown syndrome do not require surgery. As children grow taller, the implications of their up-gaze deficit become less of an issue. Brown syndrome can also spontaneously resolve [1]. As with all patients, the first steps in management are to ensure any refractive error is corrected and any amblyopia is treated.

Surgery for congenital Brown syndrome can be considered if there is a significant hypotropia in primary position, particularly if this is associated with a significant abnormal head posture. Surgery, however, carries a potentially significant complication risk. Surgical options described include:

- superior oblique tenotomy
- superior oblique tenectomy with or without an ipsilateral inferior oblique recession
- superior oblique recession
- superior oblique tendon lengthening procedures (chicken wire sutures and silicon spacers) described in Chap. 3.

In inflammatory or acquired Brown syndrome, it is important to fully investigate for an underlying auto-immune disease. Neuroimaging of the orbits with attention to the trochlea can be helpful. Treatment should be considered if there is significant hypertropia in the primary position or troublesome double vision. Oral non-steroidal anti-inflammatory drugs (NSAIDs) can be tried on an empirical basis. An alternative approach is the use of peri-trochlear steroid injection e.g. triamcinolone (Fig. 9).

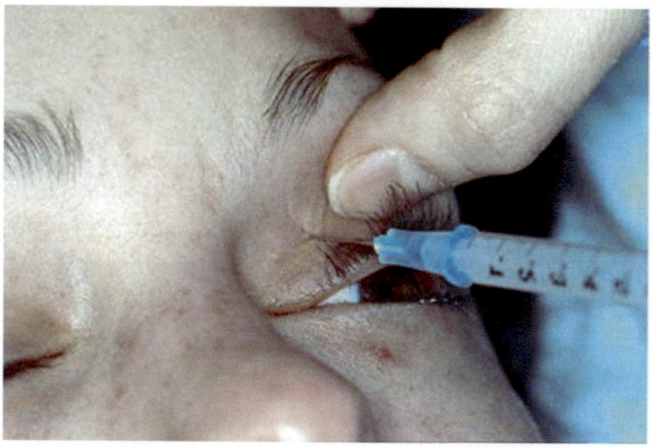

Fig. 9 For treating inflammatory Brown syndrome, 1 cc of corticosteroid is injected through the upper eyelid into the anterior superior-nasal quadrant in the region of the trochlea. Burton Kushner. Strabismus. Springer Inc 2017. Rights obtained

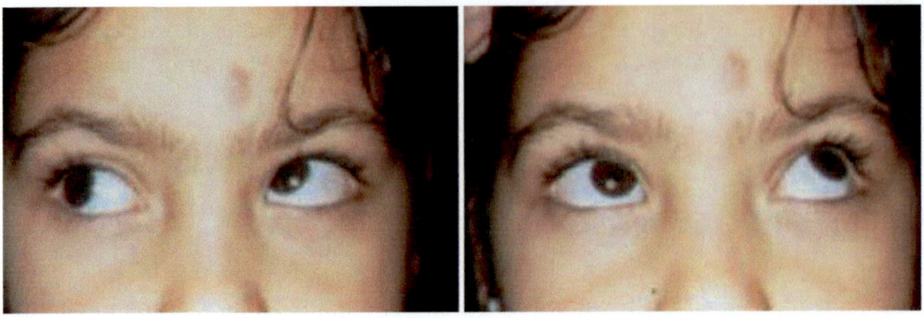

Fig. 10 A right monocular elevation deficiency (double elevator palsy) caused by a paretic superior rectus muscle. Note that the limited elevation is worse in abduction (*left*), compared with elevation in adduction (*right*). Kenneth Wright [7]. Rights Obtained

9 Monocular Elevation Deficiency

Monocular elevation deficiency, previously known as double elevator palsy, implies paresis of both the superior rectus and the inferior oblique muscles. It may be caused by primary inferior rectus restriction, supranuclear causes, superior rectus paresis with or without inferior rectus restriction [4].

9.1 Clinical Features

Clinical features of monocular elevation deficiency include unilateral limitation of elevation in both adduction and abduction (Fig. 10). A hypotropia or orthotropia is usually present in primary gaze and patients may adopt a chin up head posture. True ptosis suggests a superior rectus weakness whilst a pseudo-ptosis suggests inferior rectus restriction [4]. An accentuated lower eyelid crease that increases on attempted up gaze is suggestive of inferior rectus restriction.

9.2 Differential Diagnosis

The differential diagnosis includes Brown syndrome, partial third cranial nerve palsy, myasthenia, congenital fibrosis of the extraocular muscles and restrictive causes including thyroid orbitopathy, orbital fracture, scleral buckle and others [1, 4]. Ocular rotations, vertical saccades, forced duction and generation tests help differentiate these conditions. The elevation deficit is more pronounced in abduction in comparison to Brown syndrome. There is no horizontal muscle involvement in monocular elevation deficiency and Brown syndrome, as opposed to third cranial nerve palsy and myasthenia.

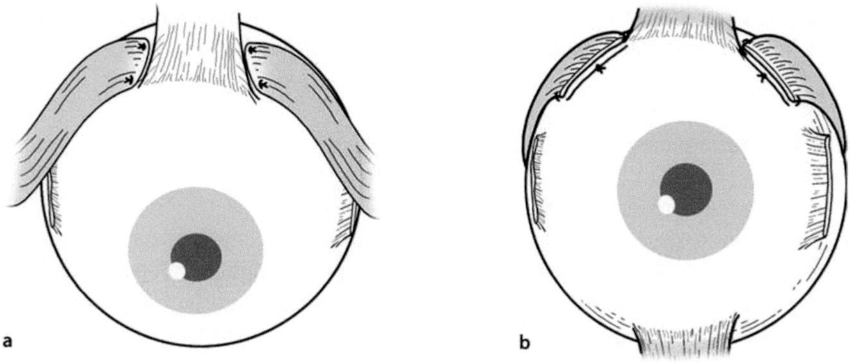

Fig. 11 Knapp procedure for monocular elevator deficiency. **a** As originally described, and **b** modified. David Coats et al. [24] Rights Obtained

9.3 Surgical Management

Indications for treatment include a significant hypotropia in primary gaze or a troublesome chin up head posture.

- *Inferior rectus recession* is indicated if the forced duction test is positive. This may cause a downgaze deficit and contralateral inferior rectus recession with or without posterior fixation may be considered [2].
- A *Knapp transposition* (transposition of the medial and lateral recti to the superior rectus) can be performed if there is no restriction (negative forced duction test) or a residual hypotropia is present following inferior rectus recession [2]. It is important to consider the risk of overcorrection and anterior segment ischaemia. (Fig. 11) A contralateral superior rectus recession is also another option.

10 Iatrogenic Restrictive Strabismus

Restrictive strabismus can occur following various surgical procedures on the eye including retinal detachment surgery, glaucoma drainage device insertion and sinus surgery.

10.1 Retinal Detachment Surgery

Strabismus and/or diplopia following a scleral buckle may be the result of early postoperative inflammation and oedema and tends to resolve. Restrictive strabismus may occur due to adhesions between the extraocular muscles and the explant and/or sclera, mass effect of the scleral buckle restricting movement or redirecting muscle force vectors, or direct muscle injury from excessive stretching.

10.1.1 Management

- Nonsurgical: prisms and occlusion.
- Botulinum toxin can be used both diagnostically and as maintenance treatment.
- Strabismus surgery following scleral buckles is challenging. Preoperatively, it is important to discuss the risks of removing the buckle with both the patient and the vitreoretinal surgeon. Intraoperative findings, including forced ductions, guide the decision making. Removal of the buckle may not be necessary. Removal of a small segment rather than the entire buckle may also suffice to expose the scleral site for muscle reattachment. The muscle over the buckle may be atrophic and it may be preferable to hook the muscle more posteriorly and proceed as though the muscle insertion is at the posterior edge of the buckle [4]. Strabismus surgery on the unaffected eye may also be considered.

10.2 Glaucoma Drainage Device Surgery

Strabismus is usually either restrictive due to mass effect of the device, fibrosis, or muscle weakness from ischaemia or trauma. It is important to discuss further management with the glaucoma surgeon. Removal of the device may correct the strabismus [4]. If this is not possible, it is sensible to avoid surgery in the area of the device, and surgery on the contralateral eye considered.

10.3 Sinus Surgery

Inadvertent medial rectus damage is a recognized complication following endoscopic sinus surgery presenting with a large exotropia and limited or no adduction [4]. Entrapment of the medial rectus in the fracture site, damage to the nerve supply and partial or complete transection of the muscle may occur.

10.3.1 Management

- If orbital imaging suggests the posterior segment of the medial rectus to be intact retrieval and reattachment can be attempted.
- If this is felt unlikely, a nasal transposition of the vertical recti may be considered.
- Optical occlusion, including a black intraocular lens for intractable diplopia.
- Botulinum toxin to the ipsilateral lateral rectus to prevent contracture.

References

1. Rowe FJ. Clinical orthoptics. Wiley-Blackwell; 2012.
2. Plager DA, editor. Strabismus surgery basic and advanced strategies. Oxford; 2004.
3. Ansons AM, Helen D. Diagnosis and management of ocular motility disorders. Wiley-Blackwell; 2014.
4. Kushner BJ. Strabismus: practical pearls you won't find in textbooks. Springer; 2018.
5. Scott AB. Posterior fixation: adjustable and without posterior sutures. In: Lennerstrand G, editor. Proceedings VIIth congress international strabismological association CRC Press, Inc.; 1995. p. 399-402.
6. Saffren BD, Yassin SH, Thau A, Nelson LB, Schnall B, Gunton KB. Anterior segment optical coherence tomography in locating the insertion of horizontal extraocular muscles after strabismus surgery. J Pediatr Ophthalmol Strabismus. 2021;58(1):62–5.
7. Wright KW, Strube YN. Color atlas of strabismus surgery. Springer Inc; 2015. p. 177.
8. Falzon K, Taylor R. Botulinum toxin thyroid eye disease. Helsinki, Finland: Transactions 40th European Strabismological Association; 2019.
9. Traboulsi EI. Congenital cranial dysinnervation disorders and more. J AAPOS. 2007;11(3):215–7.
10. Gutowski NJ, Chilton JK. The congenital cranial dysinnervation disorders. Arch Dis Child. 2015;100:678–81.
11. Gutowski NJ, Bosley TM, Engle EC. 110th ENMC international workshop: the congenital cranial dysinnervation disorders (CCDDs). Naarden, The Netherlands, 25–27 Oct 2002.
12. Miller MT, et al. Curr Opin Ophthalmol. 2011.
13. Kim JH, Hwang JM. Presence of the abducens nerve according to the type of Duane's retraction syndrome. Ophthalmology. 2005;112(1):109–13.
14. Agrawal S. Strabimus. Springer Inc; 2019.
15. Ludwig I. Strabismus surgery: innovative and classic approaches. Thieme Medical Publishers; 2021.
16. Mehendale RA, Dagi LR, Wu C, Ledoux D, Johnston S, Hunter DG. Superior rectus transposition and medial rectus recession for Duane syndrome and sixth nerve palsy. Arch Ophthalmol. 2012;130(2):195–201.
17. Kraft SP. Lateral rectus resection strabismus surgery in unilateral duane syndrome with esotropia and limited abduction. Binocul Vis Strabismus Q. 2010;25(3):149–57.
18. Hoerantner R, Priglinger S, Haslwanter T. Reduction of ocular muscle torque by splitting of the rectus muscle II: technique and results. Br J Ophthalmol. 2004;88(11):1409–13.
19. Snir M, Friling R, Kalish-Stiebel H, Sherf I, Weinberger D, Axer-Siegel R. Full vertical rectus muscle transposition combined with medial posterior fixation sutures for patients with adduction deficiency. Ophthalmology. 2005.
20. Dawson EL, Maino A, Lee JP. Diagnostic use of botulinum toxin in patients with Duane syndrome. Strabismus. 2010;18(1):21–23.
21. Vivian AJ. Congenital fibrosis of the extra-ocular muscles (CFEOM) and the cranial dysinnervation disorders. Eye (Lond). 2020;34(2):251–5.
22. Whitman MC, Jurgens JA, Hunter DG, et al. Congenital fibrosis of the extraocular muscles overview. 2004 Apr 27 [Updated 2021 Aug 12]. In: Adam MP, Mirzaa GM, Pagon RA, et al., editors. GeneReviews® [Internet]. Seattle (WA): University of Washington, Seattle; 1993–2023. Available from: https://www.ncbi.nlm.nih.gov/books/NBK1348/.
23. Farvardin H, Ahmadifar A, Farvardin H, Farvardin M. Long-term results of strabismus surgery for treatment of esotropia in patients with Möbius syndrome. J AAPOS. 2023;27(3):149.e1–5.
24. Coats DK, Olitsky SE. Strabismus surgery and its complications. Springer Inc; 2007.

Strabismus Surgery in Nystagmus

Richard Bowman

Abstract Nystagmus, characterized by involuntary eye movements, may necessitate surgical intervention to mitigate associated abnormal head postures (AHP) and improve visual acuity. Historical pioneers like Anderson and Kestenbaum laid foundational principles for nystagmus surgery. Modern surgical techniques aim to move the eyes AWAY FROM the null point or IN THE DIRECTION of AHP, thereby enhancing visual function and alleviating head posture abnormalities. Surgical planning involves meticulous pre-operative assessment to determine the type and extent of surgery required. Surgical interventions may yield improvements in visual acuity and head posture. Integration of surgical procedures with strabismus corrections, particularly in cases of horizontal AHP and concurrent squint, presents nuanced challenges but offers potential synergistic benefits. Non-surgical interventions such as contact lenses and medications may complement surgical approaches, particularly in optimizing visual function. Despite advancements, counselling and consent processes underscore the importance of managing patient expectations regarding outcomes and potential risks. Understanding the interplay between eye movements, head posture, and surgical techniques remains critical in achieving favourable outcomes for patients with nystagmus.

Keywords Nystagmus surgery · Abnormal head posture · Visual acuity · Surgical technique · Strabismus correction

1 History

The names of Anderson and Kestenbaum are still frequently referred to when considering nystagmus surgery. In 1953 both described operations on the horizontal recti to improve horizontal face turns associated with nystagmus [1, 2]. Anderson described recessing one muscle in each eye whereas Kestenbaum described operating on all 4 horizontal recti (2 recessions and 2 resections). In both cases the muscles surgery was

R. Bowman (✉)
Great Ormond Street Hospital, London, UK
e-mail: Richard.Bowman@gosh.nhs.uk

S. Jain (ed.), *Surgical Management of Strabismus*,
https://doi.org/10.1007/978-3-031-80633-9_13

designed to move both eyes in the direction of the naturally adopted face turn. Less well known are Goti and Pierse. In 1954, Goti described resection of one horizontal rectus muscle in each eye with the same aim of moving the eyes in the direction of the face turn. Pierse, in 1959 described an operation for a chin up head posture. Again the idea was to move both eyes in the direction of the head posture i.e. upwards in this case and he performed weakening of both depressors, inferior rectus and superior oblique.

Most nystagmus surgery performed today is essentially the same as described by these pioneers.

2 Principles of Surgery for Nystagmus

2.1 Move the Eyes Towards the Head Turn

The principle of nystagmus surgery is that many, if not most, patients with nystagmus have a null point where the nystagmus intensity (amplitude x frequency) is minimal and foveal fixation time is maximal and therefore vision is optimal. This null point is often not in primary gaze and the patient will therefore adopt a head turn (particularly when making visual effort) so that their direction of gaze corresponds to the null point. This is called an abnormal head posture (AHP) or torticollis. For instance, if a patient's null point is in left gaze they will adopt a face turn right on visual effort. The surgery would involve moving both eyes to the right. This can be thought of as moving the eyes in the direction of the face turn (rightwards) or moving the null point from the left to the centre (again rightwards). For safety it is probably best to choose one of these ways of thinking about the direction of surgery and stick to it. I prefer to think of moving the eyes in the direction of the AHP—a left face turn—move both eyes to the left, a chin down posture, move both eyes down, a right head tilt—tilt both eyes to the right.

2.2 The Fixing Eye Determines the Head Posture

While all the above descriptions refer to moving both eyes in parallel the same direction and the same amount, this assumes that the patient is straight eyed and binocular. **If patient has a preferred fixing eye with strabismus, it is the fixing eye which determines the head posture** e.g. if a patient has a left esotropia and a right face turn associated with nystagmus (a common scenario in fusion maldevelopment nystagmus where the nystagmus is damped by adducting the fixing eye), the head posture surgery needs to be done on the fixing right eye. It might be possible to correct both the face turn and the esotropia by doing a right esotropia operation in this case (i.e. moving the fixing, right eye to the right).

2.3 *Nystagmus Often Damps on Convergence*

A common feature of infantile nystagmus is that near visual acuity is better than distance visual acuity because convergence damps down the nystagmus. Therefore, in some patients who are binocular with a reasonable fusion range, even without an AHP, surgery to induce a 'artificial divergence' (usually a small bimedial recession) can be considered to stimulate convergence effort, dampen down the nystagmus and improve vision.

2.4 *Does Muscle Surgery Itself Help Damp Nystagmus?*

Finally, Richard Hertle, has shown some benefits in terms of nystagmus pattern from surgically disinserting and reinserting (in exactly the same place) all 4 horizontal recti [3]. The idea is that surgical disruption of the proprioceptive reflexes has a damping effect on the nystagmus. He has advocated the 'tenotomy and reattachment' operation for patients without AHP. This has not gained widespread popularity in the UK and NICE guidelines recommended that it only be performed with special arrangements for clinical governance, consent, and audit or research [4]. Nevertheless the principle that simply disinserting and reattaching the muscles has a damping effect on surgery may explain why sometimes the benefit gained from nystagmus surgery seems to be more than might be expected from just straightening the head. It might also be a relative indication for performing squint surgery earlier in a child with nystagmus and perhaps spreading the surgery over more muscles. Others have suggested large post-equatorial recessions of all 4 horizontal recti in patients with straight eyes and straight heads as a means of damping down nystagmus and improving vision.

3 Visual Benefits of Surgery

Several published retrospective series have reported small improvements in visual acuity in addition to improved head posture. However a recent review conducted on behalf of the American Academy of Ophthalmology examined 22 published papers and concluded that gains in best corrected binocular visual acuity were modest with a range from no improvement to 3 lines of logMAR acuity [5]. The papers in this review included operations for AHP and operations in straight headed patients aimed at improving vision. A Cochrane review of all surgical interventions for infantile nystagmus found no trials comparing surgery with no surgery [6]. Only one randomized controlled trial was identified which included patients with no head posture and compared horizontal tenotomy and reattachment with large recessions of all 4 horizontal recti (9 mm for the medials and 12 mm for the laterals) [7]. They found no improvement in visual acuity in either group.

Hertle responded to the AAO report by pointing out that binocular visual acuity in the primary position is a poor way of assessing the visual benefit from nystagmus surgery. He argues that patients have a broader area of null and better vision in a wider range of gaze positions.

In practice most surgeries for nystagmus in the UK are performed to relieve AHP and therefore the surgeon can counsel the patient that there *might be some modest benefit* to vision as well as to head posture, but it is not guaranteed and may not involve seeing much further down the test chart in clinic. Some young people or adults with nystagmus may feel that they are close to driving level vision and are seeking intervention to get their vision good enough. In these cases, it is advisable to make sure they have tried and passed the hazard perception test which needs to be performed in addition to the vision test. If that is the case it may be reasonable to try surgery on such patients (if they have accompanying torticollis) but with very guarded prognosis and explanation of the uncertain visual benefits as outlined above. Non -surgical interventions can also be considered in this situation instead of or in addition to surgery.

4 Non-surgical Interventions

Although the focus of this chapter is surgery it is important to consider whether any non-surgical interventions might be indicated. Full refraction and correction is of course mandatory. Contact lenses may have a double benefit. First of all, they move with the eyes whereas eye movement under a spectacle lens will induce optical aberrations. Secondly in some patients they seem to have a damping effect on nystagmus, though evidence for this effect is not strong [8].

A variety of medications have been used, mainly in adults. One of the few randomized controlled trials to be performed was for adults with infantile nystagmus and found small improvements in visual acuity, nystagmus intensity and foveation time associated with oral gabapentin and memantine versus placebo [9].

5 Indications for Surgery

Surgery may be considered for a range of nystagmus types (infantile nystagmus with or without concurrent disease), fusion maldevelopment (or manifest latent nystagmus), and acquired neurological nystagmus and the principles are generally the same across the board and are outlined above.

The main indications are.

(1) Abnormal head posture to bring gaze into null point (indication for Kestenbaum/Anderson type procedure). The aim is to improve the head posture and to possibly gain an improvement in nystagmus intensity and functional vision.

(2) Significant improvement in acuity from convergence (indication for artificial divergence surgery). The aim is to improve vision in the distance.

6 Timing

Surgery at almost any age is possible. Hertle feels outcomes may be better if surgery is performed for infantile nystagmus under the age of 2 [10]. The improved head posture and functional vision may have knock on benefits on other areas of development and quality of life.

In some children the extra visual demands of secondary education mean that the head posture is being used more and becoming more tiring for the head and neck muscles and they decide that they want surgery during the teenage years.

7 Assessment

7.1 Preoperative Assessment for Surgery for AHP

A full ophthalmological and orthoptic assessment is required over at least two visits to enable a clear diagnosis of what the type of nystagmus is, where the null point is, whether this corresponds to the head posture. The type and angle of any strabismus is also vital to observe and record in detail. If there is doubt about the cause or type of nystagmus, other texts are available to describe the work up required.

The vision should be tested at near and distance to threshold. Often the full AHP will not become apparent until the visual effort is maximal (at or near threshold acuity). Full AHP can be restricted optically by glasses so if contact lenses are in use the AHP should be measured with both.

The size of the angle of the face turn, head tilt and/or chin up/chin down can be measured either with an adapted orthopaedic protractor or with a special head mounted goniometer. Photos from everyday life are also useful.

The patients should be observed for a few minutes to check that the AHP does not switch to another position. Some children have more than one preferred AHP corresponding to more than one null point. This is not an absolute contra-indication to surgery but may change the surgical plan, so it is important to look carefully for this.

Once you have established the direction of the AHP you can then examine the nystagmus intensity clinically and check that the null point is in the opposite direction to the AHP as would be expected. Sometimes if the nystagmus is subtle, slit lamp viewing can help here.

Once it is established that the null point and the AHP are concordant, a second element to the assessment can be added, which is to put yoked free prisms in front of the eyes mounted on the spectacles with adhesive rings or trial frames. This is conducted again at near and distance with the patient reading an acuity chart at threshold so that the AHP is elicited. The prisms are yoked and the base is in the direction of the AHP e.g. a left face turn both prisms will be base left. The placement of these prisms should bring the head to or near the straight ahead position. This provides further reassurance (to surgeon and parents!) that moving the eyes is going to turn the head in the direction we expect. It also allows some quantification of the head turn. Large face turns require larger prisms whereas smaller face turns may be overcorrected by e.g. 50PD yoked prims. It has been estimated that a 20 degree head turn requires 50PD of yoked prisms to correct it [11]. If the AHP is multiplanar e.g. a face turn with an additional head tilt, the prism test may demonstrate that the horizontal movement of the eyes is enough to correct both dimensions of the AHP in which case horizontal surgery only needs to be done, or it may show that the horizontal prisms correct only the face turn but not the tilt in which case you might plan torsional displacement of the horizontal muscles as well as the recess/resect procedures.

In cases of strabismus, the test prism only needs to be placed in front of the fixing eye to establish the effect on the AHP.

Eye movement recordings in different positions of gaze can provide very helpful evidence to support the surgical plan (Figs. 1 and 2). Not all surgeons have access to this investigation, and it is not essential for all cases. It can be particularly helpful in cases of doubt such as (1) the parents are very aware of an AHP and keen on surgery yet it is not that noticeable in clinic (2) there seems to be more than one clinical AHP (3) the AHP is multiplanar e.g. chin down, right face turn and right head tilt and (4) recurrent AHP after previously successful nystagmus surgery.

7.2 Pre-op Assessment for Artificial Divergence Surgery

Check that near visual acuity is better than distance and that the nystagmus appears to dampen on convergence (can be checked with eye movement recording if necessary). Check that the patient is binocular with reasonable fusion range. It then may be useful to give the patient 7PD BO prisms each eye built into glasses to encourage convergence and a spherical add of − 0.50 to − 1.00DS to their own prescription to counter the accommodation stimulated by the extra convergence. If they are happy and improved in these prism glasses, they may elect to keep them or may choose to undergo artificial divergence surgery, usually bimedial recession of 3 mm.

7.3 Counselling/Consent

I counsel parents that there is about an 80% chance of complete or significant improvement in head posture with one surgery (based on previous audits). I also mention a risk of possible further surgery for under or overcorrection of the head

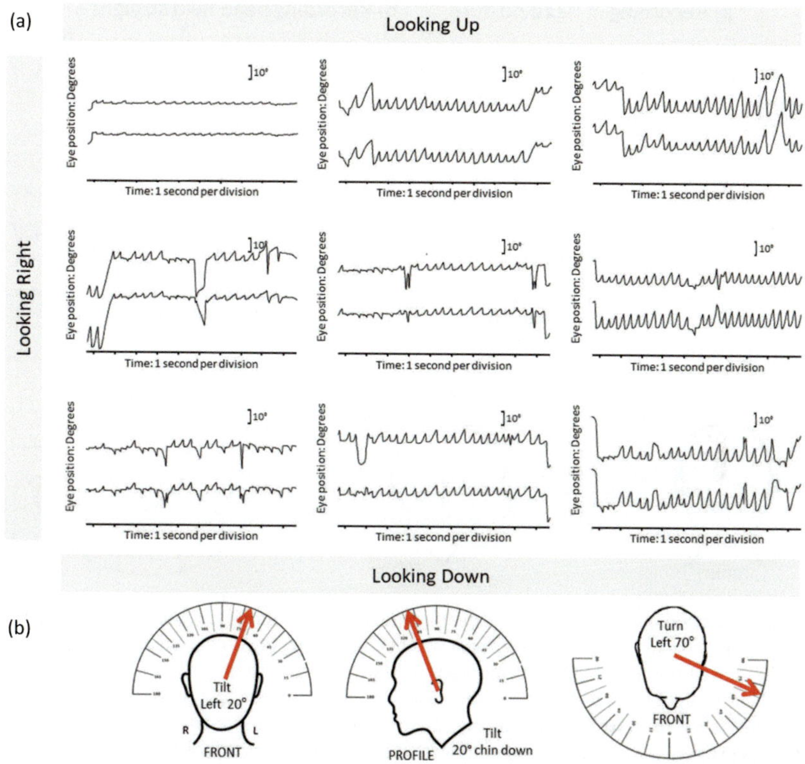

Fig. 1 Examples of preoperative eye movement reports: Eye movement recordings from the right eye (top) and left eye (bottom) carried out in nine positions of gaze (a) showing the nystagmus null point to be in superior-dextroversion. In keeping with the head posture measured (b) of turn and tilt left with chin down. Courtesy of Ms Sian Handley

posture or future recurrence. I also mention a risk of inducing strabismus and, in older patients, double vision. Also, particularly for large head postures, there may be some limitation of gaze in the direction away from the head posture. This does not usually last as a significant issue, and mild restriction contributes to the success of the head repositioning. Otherwise, the counselling is similar to that for strabismus surgery, though the recovery period is longer because the patient is getting a double and large dose of squint surgery.

7.4 Surgical Technique

General points: technique is basically the same as strabismus surgery. It is invariably bilateral and often involving 4 muscles and larger doses than routine strabismus surgery so allow adequate exposure and time. A Desmarres retractor and a surgical

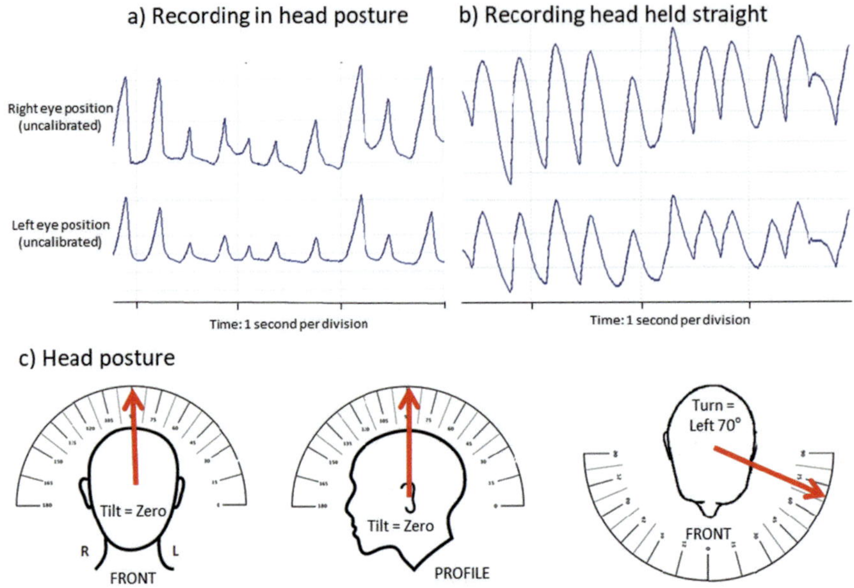

Fig. 2 Examples of preoperative eye movement reports: Eye movement recordings carried out in a 5 year old where the fixation and resulting data was not of sufficient quality to carry out calibration. Recordings carried out to a central static target in chosen head posture of face turn left (a) and with head held straight by parent (b) showing while the frequency of the nystagmus is unchanged there is a difference in nystagmus waveform. There is no foveation periods during the pendular nystagmus in primary position (b), explaining why they are adopting the face turn to the left where there is some evidence of foveation periods (a). The child's co-operation limited data quality but even uncalibrated the data showed changes in the nystagmus when the head posture was adopted and in primary position which supported the clinical picture and development of surgical plan

assistant may be helpful. Plan the surgery in advance and check with a team member that the plan fits the AHP i.e. moving both eyes towards the AHP and write it up in theatre to avoid mistakes of moving eyes in the wrong direction.

8 Types of Operation

Face turn left: Move both eyes to the left.

Anderson: Right LR recess 10 mm and left MR recess 7 mm (usually less than 20 degree face turn).

Kestenbaum: Right LR recess, Right MR resect, Left MR recess, Left LR resect.

Face turn left (deg)	20	20–45	45	50
Recess RLR	8.5	9	9.75	11
Resect RMR	7.25	7.75	8.5	9.5
Recess LMR	6	6.5	7	8
Resect LLR	9.5	10.5	11.25	12.5
Parks augmentation (%)	*20*	*30*	*40*	*60*

*All measurements in mm

Parks originally proposed MR recess 5 mm, LR resect 8 mm in one eye and 6 mm MR resect and 7 mm LR recess in the other eye and these doses in the tables are proportional increases in dose. His original doses are generally thought to be too small. Success has also been reported with doing the same amount of surgery to all 4 muscles rather than variants of the Parks ratio.

Right face turn: Move both eyes to the right.

Anderson: Left LR recess 10 mm, right MR recess 7 mm.

Kestenbaum: Left LR recess, left MR resect, Right MR recess, Right LR resect.

Face turn right (deg)	20	20–45	45	50
Recess RMR	6	6.5	7	8
Resect RLR	9.5	10.5	11.25	12.5
Recess LLR	8.5	9	9.75	11
Resect LMR	7.25	7.75	8.5	9.5
Parks augmentation (%)	*20*	*30*	*40*	*60*

If patients are binocular with a reasonable fusion consider adjusting the above doses to leave a small exophoria because of the added potential benefit of induced convergence but if they are not binocular, err on the side of a small residual esophoria/tropia.

8.1 Chin Down

Traditionally bilateral superior rectus recessions of 8 mm and inferior rectus resections of 4 mm were recommended but it has been realized that this exerts a bilateral extorsional force on the eyes which can produce alphabet patterns and torsional diplopia especially in older patients. So generally weakening of both elevators of the eyes are preferred which balances the torsional response: bilateral inferior oblique recessions and superior rectus recessions. These can be titrated from 5 to 7 mm SR recession and using anteriorization instead of recession of IO for larger AHPs.

8.2 Chin Up

Traditionally bilateral superior rectus resections of 6 mm and inferior rectus recessions of 6 mm were recommended but it has been realized similarly that this exerts a bilateral intorsional force on the eyes which can produce alphabet patterns and torsional diplopia especially in older patients. So generally weakening of both depressors of the eyes are preferred which balances the torsional response: bilateral superior oblique tenotomies and inferior rectus recessions of 5 mm.

8.3 Right Head Tilt

Transpose right superior rectus one tendon width nasally and right inferior rectus one tendon width temporally. Transpose left superior rectus one tendon width temporally and left inferior rectus one tendon width nasally.

This exerts a rightward torsional force on each eye (same principle—move eyes in direction of AHP). An alternative would be to weaken the intorters of the right eye (SR recess 5 mm, SO tenotomy) and the extorters of the left eye (left IR recess 5 mm and IO recess).

When transposing recti muscles torsionally think: (1) disinsert them (2) turn the eyes in the direction of the head tilt and (3) replace muscles in their original position (Fig. 3). This works for horizontal or vertical recti.

8.4 Left Head Tilt

Transpose right superior rectus one tendon width temporally and right inferior rectus one tendon width nasally. Transpose left superior rectus one tendon width nasally and left inferior rectus one tendon width temporally.

This exerts a leftward torsional force on each eye. An alternative would be to weaken the extorters of the right eye (IR recess 5 mm and IO recess to Parks point) and the intorters of the left eye (SR recess 5 mm, SO tenotomy).

8.5 Face Turn Right or Left with Chin Down

If the horizontal bigger: Perform the above horizontal surgery according to above dose and inferotranspose all horizontal muscle one tendon width. If the vertical bigger, chin down surgery as above plus Anderson for face turn.

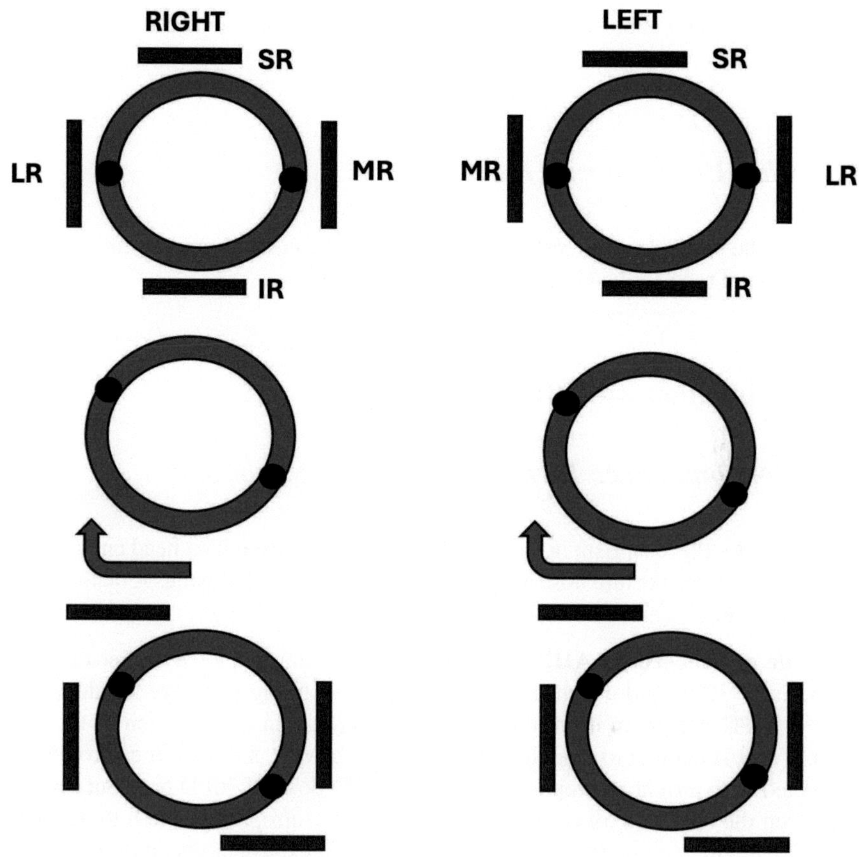

Fig. 3 Torsional transpositions for recti muscles in a case of nystagmus with left head tilt. How to think about direction? Left head tilt. Mentally disinsert (in this case) horizontal recti. Leave muscles where they are and turn eyes in parallel in the direction of the left head tilt

8.6 Face Turn Right or Left with Chin Up

If the horizontal bigger: Perform the above horizontal surgery according to dose and superotranspose all horizontal muscle one tendon width. If the vertical bigger, chin up surgery as above plus Anderson for face turn.

8.7 Face Turn Right/Left with Head Tilt

Perform the above Kestenbaum surgery for the horizontal face turn and for each eye transpose one horizontal rectus upwards and one downwards to exert a torsional force in the direction of the head tilt (same principle as always, move eyes in direction of AHP). If unsure about which way to moves the muscles to exert torsion use the diagram in Fig. 3.

8.8 Chin Up/Down with Head Tilt

Combine the vertical recess resect operations with the nasal /temporal transposition of the vertical recti for head tilt.

9 Combination with Strabismus

9.1 Horizontal Face Turn and Horizontal Strabismus

General rule: Place a prism in front of the fixing eye to straighten head and use this to guide your head posture dose and then correct whatever strabismus remains in the following eye.

Example of concordant AHP and squint: The example quoted earlier of a left esotropia of 30PD and a right face turn to keep the fixing right eye in adduction. Place a 30PD BO prism in front of the right eye (base in the direction of the face turn). If that is enough to straighten head then both AHP and the left esotropia can be treated with a right esotropia operation of 30PD dose. If 30PD base out doesn't straighten the head and 50 is required then a 50PD esotropia operation to the right eye (which will lead to 20PD exotropia) and a 20PD exotropia operation to the left eye will give the best chance of straight head and straight eyes.

Example of discordant AHP and squint: A patient with a left exotropia of 30PD and a right face turn again bringing the fixing right eye into adduction to damp down the nystagmus. Again place a 30PD BO prism in front of right eye and see if the head straightens. If it does, then a right esotropia operation of 30PD is required to correct the AHP. This worsens the strabismus and leaves an exotropia of 60PD so a simultaneous maximal recess resect exotropia operation is required for the left eye. If 30PD does not straighten the head but say 50PD is required, that would leave an 80PD exotropia which is too much to correct with monocular surgery, so normally that means accepting incomplete correction of the AHP (reduce the amount to the right eye) or incomplete or even no correction of the squint depending on the patient's priorities [12].

The danger with the above technique is that it might lead to an undercorrection of the AHP because of the difficulties stacking prisms above 50PD. An alternative way of thinking about combining surgery for horizontal AHP and strabismus (especially for large AHPs and smaller concomitant strabismus is to use the horizontal Kestenbaum formulae above and simply add or subtract your appropriate squint surgery doses to the non fixing eye to address the squint.

For instance say you are doing a 40 degree left face turn and a 30PD right esotropia. You are moving both eyes to the left but you want to reduce the amount that you move the right eye to allow for 30PD esotropia. The Kestenbaum gives RMR resect 5 mm, RLR Recess 9.75, LMR recess 7, LLR resect 11.25. According to my squint tables the right eye surgery is equivalent to 60PD exotropia surgery whereas we want to do 30 so we would convert to RMR resect 5 and RLR recess 7.

9.2 Horizontal AHP and Vertical Squint

Vertical squints which are horizontally incomitant usually require oblique surgery which can be combined with Kestenbaum surgery. Vertical squints which are horizontally concomitant usually require vertical rectus surgery and this may need to be spread across the 2 eyes and combined with an Anderson instead of a Kestenbaum to avoid risk of anterior segment ischaemia.

9.3 Vertical AHP and Horizontal Squint

Smaller head posture: perform horizontal squint surgery with vertical transposition of all 4 horizontal recti in the direction of the AHP.

Larger head posture: Perform the above weakening of both elevators or both depressors as above for the AHP and do horizontal squint surgery with one horizontal rectus muscle in each eye.

9.4 More Than One Head Posture

A number of patients have more than one preferred head posture including the classic periodic alternating nystagmus. Careful history taking and examination is necessary to elicit this. It is not necessarily a contraindication to surgery because the patient may have a dominant AHP which they are keen to improve even if their non dominant one becomes a bit worse.

It might be an indication to wait and delay surgery to see which AHP becomes dominant or to consider non surgical interventions first. I have sometimes used yoked prisms fitted into glasses for a period of time as a diagnostic clue but the size of built in prisms is limited to 7–8PD which may not be enough to help.

Eye movement recordings may help to establish which AHP has maximum effect on the nystagmus waveform.

If intervention is desired it would be possible to use botulinum toxin to the two muscles which would be recessed in a Kestenbaum for the face turn which is thought to be dominant. For instance if there is thought to be a predominant right face turn but an occasional smaller left face turn, toxin could be injected to the right MR and left LR to turn the eyes to the right and see if symptoms are better and to check that the left face turn does not become worse. Doing an Anderson (recession only) as opposed to a Kestenbaum is another option which is fully reversible if problems occur. One child who had face turn in opposite directions for near and distance did well with artificial divergence surgery [13].

Another option if there is more than one significant AHP is large 4 horizontal muscle recession (doses such as MR 9 mm, LR 12 mm).

9.5 Long Term Results

Zheng et al. recently reported long term outcomes with a few of their large series being followed for 10 years. Reoperation rates were 4% for overcorrection (mean 2.7 years) and 5% for undercorrection (mean 3.9 years) [14, 15].

Despite advancements, counselling and consent processes underscore the importance of managing patient expectations regarding outcomes and potential risks. Understanding the interplay between eye movements, head posture, and surgical techniques remains critical in achieving favourable outcomes for patients with nystagmus (Fig. 4) [16, 17].

A.

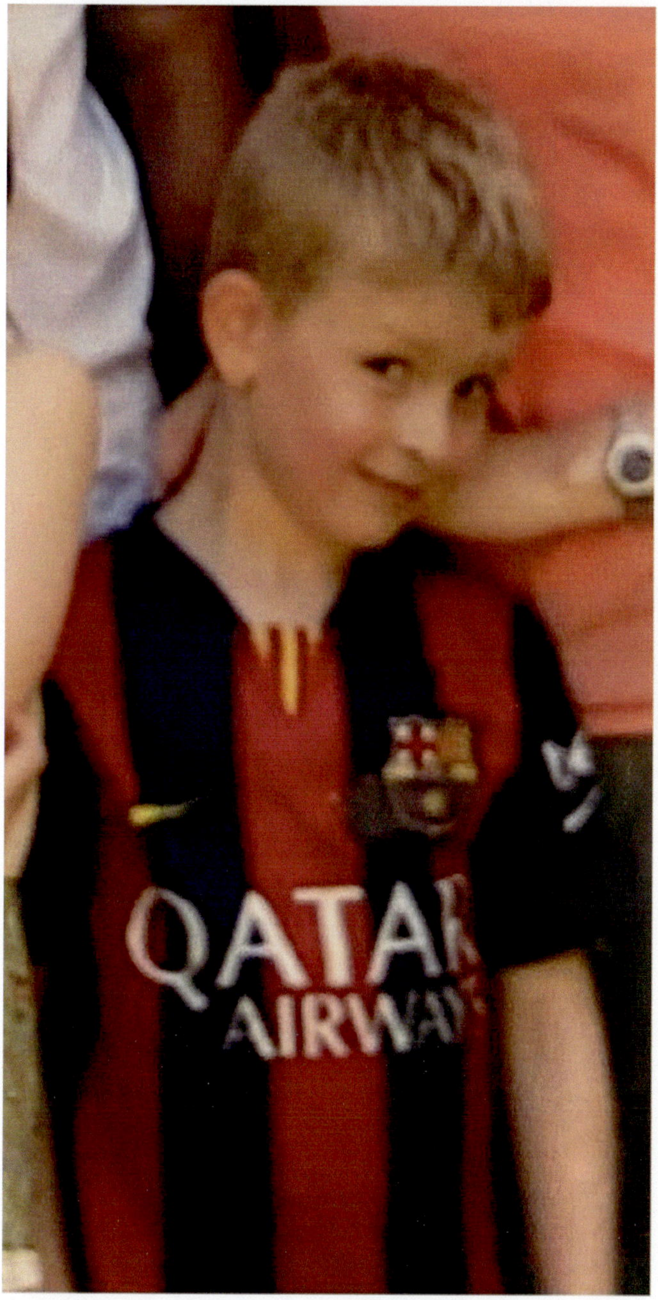

Fig. 4 This young man had a marked AHP since a child (A) which persisted leading to a face turn left and chin down (B). He underwent Kestenbaum surgery for left face turn and inferotransposition one tendon width of all 4 muscles which markedly improved head posture (C)

B.

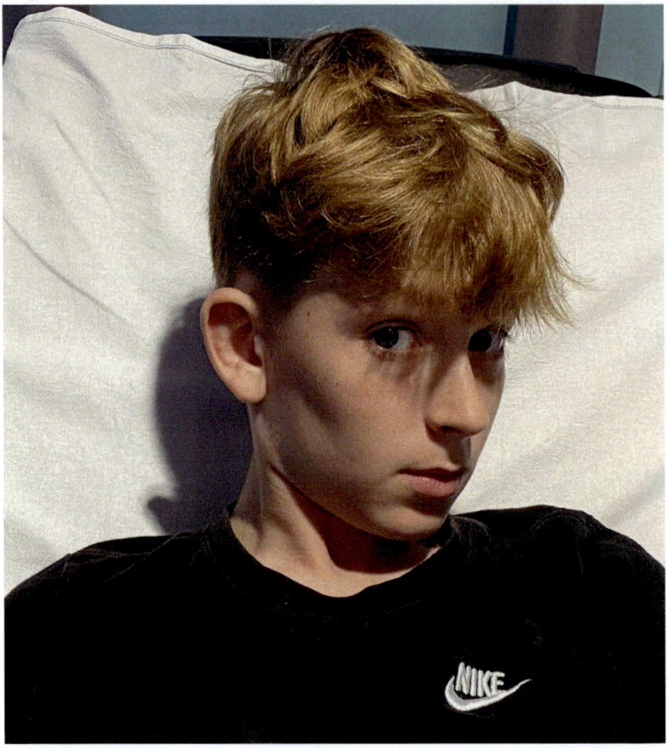

Fig. 4 (continued)

c.

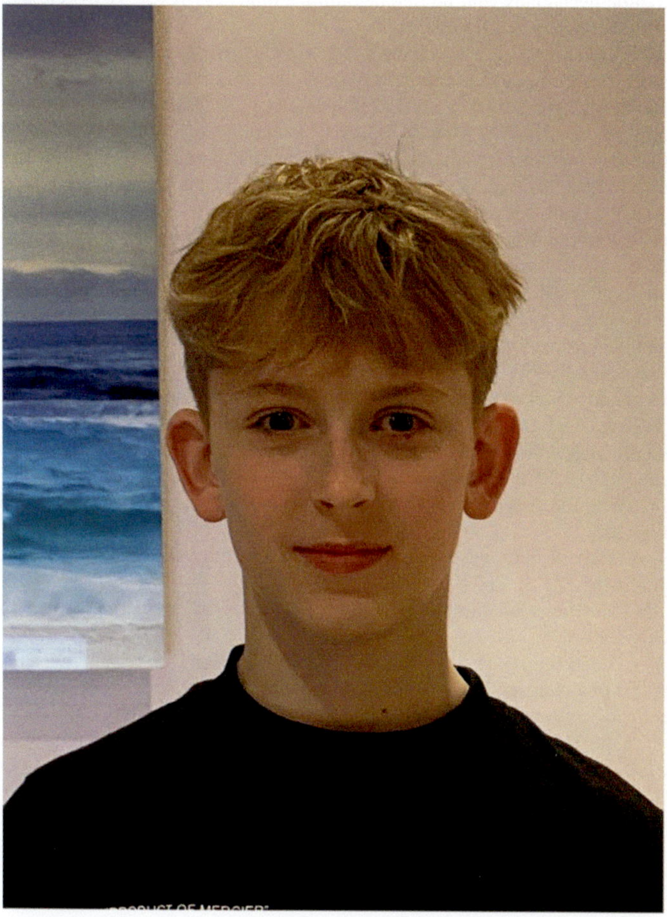

Fig. 4 (continued)

References

1. Kestenbaum A. Nouvelle opération du nystagmus. Bull Soc Ophthamol Fr. 1953;2:1071–8.
2. Anderson JR. Causes and treatment of congenital eccentric nystagmus. Br J Ophthalmol. 1953;37(5):267–81. https://doi.org/10.1136/bjo.37.5.267. PMID: 13042022.
3. Hertle RW, Dell'Osso LF, FitzGibbon EJ, Thompson D, Yang D, Mellow SD. Horizontal rectus **tenotomy** in patients with congenital nystagmus: results in 10 adults. Ophthalmology. 2003;110(11):2097–105. https://doi.org/10.1016/S0161-6420(03)00802-9.
4. https://www.nice.org.uk/guidance/ipg299/chapter/1-Guidance
5. Cham KM, Abel LA, Busija L, Kowal L, Bachar Zipori A, Downie LE. Surgical interventions for infantile nystagmus syndrome. Cochrane Database Syst Rev. 2021;2(2):CD013390.
6. Singh A, Ashar J, Sharma P, Saxena R, Menon V. A prospective evaluation of retroequatorial recession of horizontal rectus muscles and Hertle-Dell'Osso tenotomy procedure in patients

with infantile nystagmus with no definite null position. J AAPOS. 2016;20(2):96–9. https://doi.org/10.1016/j.jaapos.2015.10.021.
7. Hertle RW, Dell'Osso LF. Re: Chang et al.: Surgical treatments to improve visual acuity in infantile nystagmus syndrome: a report by the American academy of ophthalmology (Ophthalmology. 2023;130:331–344). Ophthalmology. 2023;130(8):e29–30.
8. Theodorou M, Quartilho A, Xing W, Bunce C, Rubin G, Adams G, Dahlmann-Noor A. Soft contact lenses to optimize vision in adults with idiopathic infantile nystagmus: a pilot parallel randomized controlled trial. Strabismus 2018;26(1):11–21. https://doi.org/10.1080/09273972.2017.1418394. Epub 15 Jan 2018.
9. McLean R, Proudlock F, Thomas S, Degg C, Gottlob I. Congenital nystagmus: randomized, controlled, double-masked trial of memantine/gabapentin. Ann Neurol. 2007;61(2):130–8. https://doi.org/10.1002/ana.21065.
10. Hertle RW, Felius J, Yang D, Kaufman M. Eye muscle surgery for infantile nystagmus syndrome in the first two years of life. Clin Ophthalmol. 2009;3:615–24.
11. Dell'Osso L, Gauthier G, Liberman G, Stark L. Eye movement recordings as a diagnostic tool in a case of congenital nystagmus. Am J Optom Arch Am Acad Optom. 1972;49(1):3–13.
12. Zheng Y, Holt DG, Law JJ, Morrison DG, Donahue SP. Management of strabismus associated with infantile nystagmus syndrome: a novel classification to assist in surgical planning. Am J Ophthalmol. 2019;208:342–6.
13. Kraft SP, Irving EL. A case of different null zones for distance and near fixation. Am Orthopt J. 2004;54:102–11.
14. Goto N. A study of optic nystagmys by the electro oculogram. Acta Soc Ophthalmol Japn. 1954;58:851–65.
15. Pierse D. Operations on the vertical muscles in cases of nystagmus. Br J Ophthalmol. 1959;43(4):230–3.
16. Chang MY, Binenbaum G, Heidary G, Cavuoto KM, Morrison DG, Trivedi RH, Kim SJ, Pineles SL. Surgical treatments to improve visual acuity in infantile nystagmus syndrome: a report by the American academy of ophthalmology. Ophthalmology. 2023;130(3):331–44.
17. Zheng Y, Law JJ, Holt DG, Morrison DG, Donahue SP. Long-term outcomes following surgery for infantile nystagmus syndrome with abnormal head positioning. Am J Ophthalmol. 2020;210:3–7.

Injectable Treatments for Management of Strabismus

Ian B. Marsh and Katherine Smyth

Abstract This chapter describes the use of non-surgical treatments of strabismus, the evidence available to support this method of managing patients, and discusses the typical conditions that can be treated. Included is a description of setting up a service and the equipment required. Outcomes and complications are discussed.

Keywords Botulinum toxin · Bupivacaine · Esotropia · Exotropia · Electromyogram

1 Introduction

The goal of realignment of the visual axes has been surgical since German ophthalmologist, Johann Friedrich Dieffenbach first reported his technique in 1839. Since that time the operations undertaken have evolved and improved in conjunction with changes in anaesthesia from local to general anaesthetic. In 1973 Scott [1] published his first paper on the use of Botulinum toxin in rhesus monkeys to induce strabismus. He then reported the treatment of strabismus in adults in 1980 [2]. Botulinum toxin was licensed for use in blepharospasm, hemifacial spasm and strabismus by the Food and Drug Administration in the USA in 1989. Since that time many papers have been published regarding its usage in both ophthalmic and non-ophthalmic conditions. Many are aware of its widespread use in the field of cosmetic medicine, smoothing wrinkles, but it is also an important tool in current modern strabismus management.

The use of bupivacaine injections to produce a permanent change in eye position arose from both animal experimental work, to try and produce chemical treatments for strabismus and case reports and subsequent series of unexpected findings of induced

I. B. Marsh (✉)
Royal Liverpool University Hospital, Liverpool, UK
e-mail: ian.marsh2001@gmail.com

K. Smyth
Royal Bolton Hospitals NHS Trust, Bolton, UK

S. Jain (ed.), *Surgical Management of Strabismus*,
https://doi.org/10.1007/978-3-031-80633-9_14

deviation following the use of local anaesthetic injections for other procedures. The evolution of both botulinum toxin and bupivacaine treatments will be discussed in this chapter.

2 Botulinum Toxin Injection Treatment

Botulinum toxin is an exotoxin of Clostridium Botulinum, one of the genus of clostridium bacteria. It produces eight antigenically distinguishable exotoxins (A, B, C_1, C_2, D, E, F and G). All serotypes interfere with neural transmission by blocking the release of acetylcholine, the principal neurotransmitter at the neuromuscular junction, causing muscle paralysis. Recovery of function occurs by neural budding, which regenerates the nerve to muscle or organ connections that have been destroyed. This process takes about 3 months. The most potent botulinum exotoxin is type A and this is the toxin commercially available for medical use. Type B can be obtained for patients who do not get a good response or develop significant antibodies to the type A toxin. Following on from Alan Scott's initial publication on animal and human uses of Botulinum Toxin type A, there have been numerous publications outlining the indications for treatment. There are also published Cochrane reviews of these studies [3–5].

3 Setting Up a Service

Delivery of both botulinum toxin (BT) and local anaesthetic (LA) injections are undertaken in an outpatient setting unless a child requires treatment. For children a theatre setting with appropriate anaesthetic support and recovery facilities is required. There are no specific requirements for a surgically sterile environment.

In both adult and children, the equipment requirements are:

(1) Access to an electromyogram (EMG) suitable to detect the electrical signals from the extra ocular muscles.
(2) The various connectors to enable the EMG to work.
(3) Insulated needles to pick up the electrical signal. These must be insulated down to the tip with only the needle bevel exposed.
(4) Topical anaesthetic drops.

Most muscle botulinum toxin injections are given using this EMG guided technique however some clinicians prefer muscle holding forceps or conjunctival incision techniques to inject the BT under direct vision. These are mainly used under general anaesthesia in children. Repeating the treatment after conjunctival opening can be difficult.

There is no agreed anaesthetic technique for paediatric cases. Some anaesthetists are willing to use intravenous ketamine which produces dissociated anaesthesia where the vestibular ocular response (VOR) is either enhanced or not abolished allowing head movement to induce ocular movement. This movement of the head will cause detectable electrical impulses in the extra ocular muscles. There is some concern about this type of anaesthesia due to the current drug abuse use of ketamine. Some patients may suffer with hallucinations, sleep disorders and bad dreams after this treatment. General anaesthesia abolishes the VOR and so accurate localisation of the extra ocular muscle can be difficult. It is important to leave the needle in the injection site for at least 60 seconds and to sit the patient up as soon as practical after injection to try and prevent ptosis.

The reported possible complications/side effects of BT are:

(1) Ptosis—mild, moderate or severe. The last of these is not common.
(2) Inadequate effect due to failure to deliver the drug to the area of motor endplates.
(3) Overcorrection of the deviation with or without diplopia.
(4) Subconjunctival haemorrhage.
(5) Leakage into an adjacent muscle with induction of an undesired vertical or horizontal deviation.
(6) Perforation of the globe—sometimes a through and through penetration. This is a rare but potentially serious complication which can result in loss of vision.

Apart from globe perforation, all these complications/side effect reverse as the botulinum toxin effect wears off.

There are currently three commercially available preparations of Botulinum toxin type A in the UK (Botox®, Dysport® and Xeomin®). They may be regarded as interchangeable however caution is advised when swapping between the different preparations available. Two of them are equivalent in potency, but the third (Dysport®), appears to be only 50% effective in strabismus usage and requires twice as many units to be injected to produce the same clinical effect. They are also produced in different unit vial sizes and caution with their dilution and use is imperative. Dilution is performed with 0.9% Saline for injection. The use of water will denature and cause the botulinum toxin to be ineffective. Xeomin has no complexing proteins and this property allows repeated treatments at high doses without the development of antibodies.

There is one preparation of Botulinum toxin B available—named Neurobloc® in Europe or Myobloc® in USA and Canada. Its use is very limited and is advised when Botulinum toxin A is no longer effective. To date there are no studies as to efficacy available (Figs. 1 and 2).

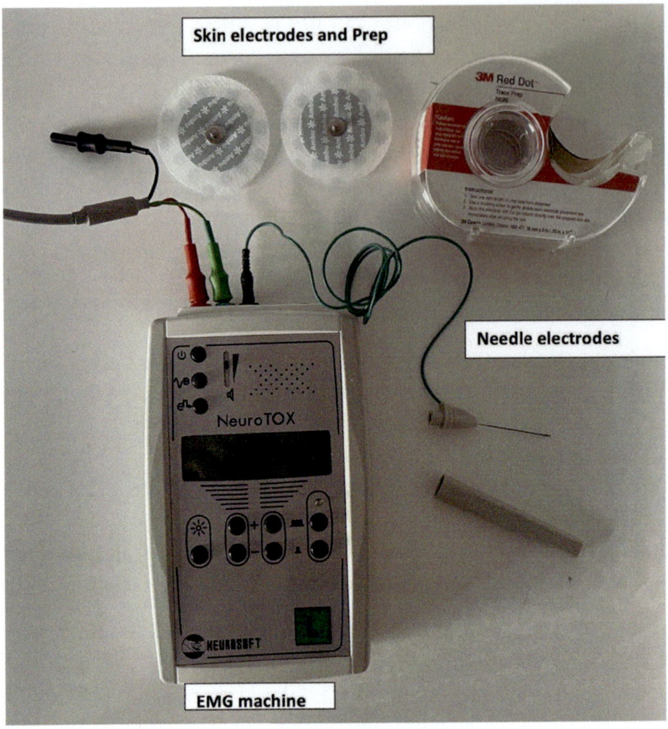

Fig. 1 The author's set up for botulinum toxin and bupivacaine injections

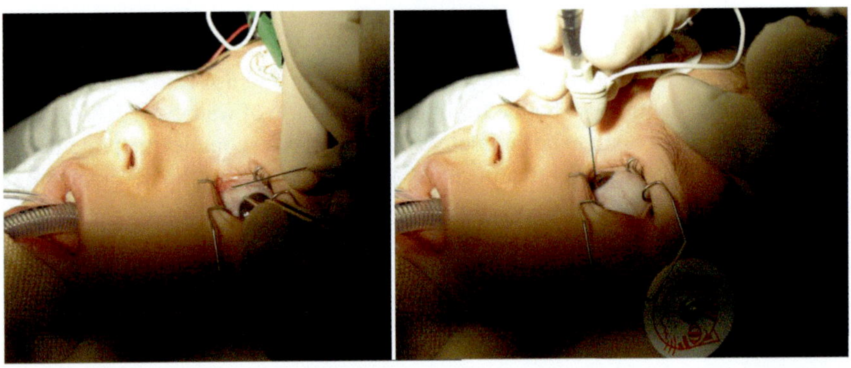

Fig. 2 Injecting botulinum toxin in a child under general anqesthesia. The eye is initially abducted using forceps but otherwise a similar setup to the adults is used. There is no or minimal signal from the EMG unless using Ketamine. The needle should be left in for at least 60 seconds to prevent postoperative ptosis. *Photo courtesy* S. Jain

4 Indications for Use of Botulinum Toxin

There are both diagnostic and therapeutic indications for the use of botulinum toxin

Diagnostic

(1) Assessment of post operative diplopia risk [6]
(2) Paresis or palsy?
(3) Showing patients their possible post operative result
(4) Symptom relief or assessment of causation of symptoms.

Therapeutic

(1) Patients who have had multiple surgeries with an unacceptable appearance. Either patient or surgeon or both are not keen on further intervention. Repeat injections at 3–4 monthly intervals to keep the patients with an acceptable deviation
(2) Unfit for surgery
(3) 6th nerve paresis for possible cure [7]
(4) Decompensated microtropias or phorias [8–10]
(5) Decompensating phorias
(6) Convergence/Accommodative spasm
(7) Congenital/early onset esotropia [11–13]
(8) Acquired nystagmus [14–18].

Post Operative Diplopia Testing

Patients who have had a previous deviation treated by surgery may present with a consecutive deviation. In these cases the original deviation that the operation treated may have reversed. The commonest condition seen in clinical practice is the consecutive divergent deviation in adulthood after childhood surgery for a convergent deviation. During orthoptic assessment, prisms are held in front of one or both eyes to neutralize, under correct and overcorrect the deviation. The patient is then asked to say whether they have diplopia. If double vision is present with prismatic correction, then there is a significant risk of this being present following corrective surgery. In this situation an injection of botulinum toxin, to correct the deviation temporarily, gives the patient the opportunity of experiencing whether double vision would be present post-operatively and if this could be tolerable permanently. If the diplopia is significantly troubling, the patient should be advised of the risks of surgery, surgical intervention should not be undertaken and the patient discharged. This only occurs in the minority of patients, approximately 10%, with a post operative diplopia on prism testing. The others are either able to cope with the two images close together or they do not suffer from diplopia at all. In this situation, surgical intervention can go ahead without concerns. The reaction of the patient to injection of botulinum toxin may give an indication as to whether they would be suitable for adjustable squint surgery. Those who would be happy to have a further injection are generally able to tolerate squint surgery using adjustable sutures, whereas those who have found it traumatic should have conventional or fixed muscle surgery.

Paresis or Palsy

In patients with a lesion of the 6th nerve causing strabismus it can be difficult to ascertain as to whether the lesion has caused complete or partial loss of function of this nerve. Induced paresis of the ipsilateral medial rectus by injection of botulinum toxin will produce abduction of the affected eye beyond the midline in the case of paresis, in which case surgical intervention using a recession and resection technique should allow the patient to obtain either a very large area of binocular single vision (BSV) or in some cases an entirely normal field of BSV, If, however, after the BT injection the eye will only abduct to midline this indicates that there is complete loss of function of the abducens nerve (palsy). Surgical intervention will be to fix the eye in the midline only giving a limited range of SV to the side away from the lesion. Accurate differentiation between paresis and palsy pre operatively enables prognostic information to be given to the patient with regards to outcome of any intervention. Surgery of this condition is discussed in the chapter on disorders of the 6th cranial nerve.

Showing the Post Operative Appearance

In aesthetic or non-functional adult strabismus some patients may request strabismus surgery when the angle of deviation is small and most surgeons would not be inclined to offer intervention. In patients with small inter pupillary distances (IPD), a small angle esotropia is accentuated and may be aesthetically unacceptable. Conversely those with a wider than normal IPD might have an accentuated appearance if a small exotropia is present. Using botulinum toxin to simulate the post operative appearance, will allow the patient to see the surgical effect and might lead the surgeon to have a different target post operative angle than orthotropia.

Symptom Relief or Diagnosis of Causation

Occasionally patients present with symptoms which may not be considered to be ocular in origin (for example headache).or they may have a deviation which is not thought to be related to the symptoms, One option for diagnostic intervention would be monocular occlusion, such that one eye is patched for a short period of time (often the weekend to avoid difficulties in the school or work environment) to see if the symptom under investigation such as headache, eye strain or intermittent diplopia is relieved (alleviated). If this proves to be the case, the problem can then be regarded as a binocular coordination problem and intervention can be offered.

Botulinum toxin can also be useful in those cases where the symptom is intermittent and only occurs rarely, for example the phoria measured is on the edge of normal and intermittent decompensation might be occurring with symptoms. A botulinum toxin injection, which gives 6–12 weeks of effect, will show whether this large phoria is causing the problem.

In situations where the deviation present is not thought to be causative of the symptoms, ocular alignment with botulinum toxin can demonstrate if surgery should be offered or not. Monocular occlusion or correction of the deviation with a temporary prism might help make the diagnosis and suggest the correct course of action. Most patients with these problems are unlikely to require botulinum toxin but it is a useful treatment to have available.

Previous Multiple Surgeries or Poor General Health

Patients with a history of several strabismus procedures to attempt to realign the eyes are often unwilling to undergo more surgery. An example might be a patient with a significant degree of amblyopia who had surgery as a child, became consecutively exotropic due to the inability of the fusion reflexes to keep the eye straight in the long term and following a second exotropia operation may not have achieved a satisfactory appearance. In these situations either a third operation or repeated botulinum toxin injections at three monthly intervals might achieve an acceptable appearance. This can also be used in a patient with acquired loss of sight in one eye.

A significant number of patients presenting for aesthetic strabismus surgery are elderly and may have significant systemic co morbidities which preclude the use of general anaesthetic. These patients may benefit from repeated injections of botulinum toxin which can be used to maintain an acceptable appearance for the patients.

Patients who have already had two rectus muscles moved and therefore operating on a third or fourth one raises the concern of anterior segment ischaemia, may also benefit from using repeated botulinum toxin injections as treatment of choice.

6th Nerve Paresis for Possible Cure

A randomised controlled trial was undertaken where patients, at presentation with a 6th nerve weakness, were allocated either into a treatment arm of immediate botulinum toxin injection to the ipsilateral medial rectus or to the no treatment observation group. Recovery results in either group showed no significant difference. This study is discussed in the chapter on 6th nerve problems. Another retrospective trial disagreed with these findings. The usual management of these patients is observation for recovery with botulinum toxin injection only used when signs of improvement are no longer occurring. If this treatment is given within the first 12 months of onset of the weakness, the outcome can be a complete recovery of lateral rectus function and an effectively full field of BSV.

Decompensated Microtropias or Phorias

Patients with small angle deviations of less that 10 prism dioptres and often with some degree of binocular function are defined as a microtropia. Decompensation of this controlled deviation spontaneously or following a relatively minor head injury can cause a large angle strabismus with or without diplopia. A period of observation may allow these decompensated deviations to recover without treatment. If there is no change in deviation during this period then intervention is required to restore the normal ocular alignment. A minimum of 6 months between onset and action is sensible. If recovery is manifest by the deviation becoming smaller and less symptomatic then continued observation and palliation of symptoms is the sensible way forwards.

If recovery does not occur, then botulinum toxin injection of either medial or lateral rectus, for esotropic or exotropic deviations respectively, can be used. (The muscle to be injected is dependent upon the deviation.)

If the patient obtains an initial overcorrection and then remains straight and controlled 3 months post injection, it is likely that this constitutes a cure and no further treatment will be required. Poorly controlled phorias which are not microtropias can break down into a manifest deviation and botulinum toxin injection can result in a cure for these problems.

Decompensating Phorias

A poorly controlled latent deviation can break down into a manifest deviation in some patients, resulting in symptomatic intermittent diplopia. These tropias are not constant. To aid control, an injection of botulinum toxin into the appropriate muscle can be used. If the prism fusion range is poor, then this effect may only be temporary and surgical realignment or provision of correcting prism may be required in the longer term. Some patients feel that continued intermittent botulinum toxin is preferable to surgery and 3 monthly injections are continued. There are anecdotal reports of permanent 'cure' in these patients after several repeated injections and in addition, there are cases where the time between injections lengthens and eventually discontinued as control improves.

Convergence/Accommodative Spasm

This condition is an extremely difficult problem to manage, and strategies have been suggested including topical cycloplegics and provision of reading glasses. This is recognised to be a functional phenomenon or a processing problem but getting the patient to accept this causation and obtaining an appropriate psychological intervention such as cognitive behaviour therapy may be helpful but may be difficult to access or in some cases impossible where the patient is unwilling to accept the possibility of psychological causation. It is sensible to minimize any ophthalmic intervention to avoid the patient's condition becoming medicalised. Occasionally resetting the eyes straight might be helpful using botulinum toxin but rarely does this cure the condition. The use of this injection in these conditions is somewhat controversial.

Congenital/Early Onset Esotropia

There is no clear consensus on when and how to manage congenital/early onset esotropia. These children often do not have amblyopia and use cross fixation, giving a tripartite field of fixation, and clinically may mimic a bilateral 6th nerve palsy. Binocular vision is absent. Surgical intervention is undertaken either early (within the first 1–3 years of life) or late (after 5–6 years of age). The surgical aim is to produce a good aesthetic appearance for the longer term. It is important to monitor for amblyopia once better ocular alignment has been achieved, particularly in those operated on earlier who are more prone to develop amblyopia, as alternation of fixation can be reduced and preference to one eye use occurs. There has been one published study showing that intervention with botulinum toxin to one or both medial recti produced not only a permanent realignment of the visual axes but also the

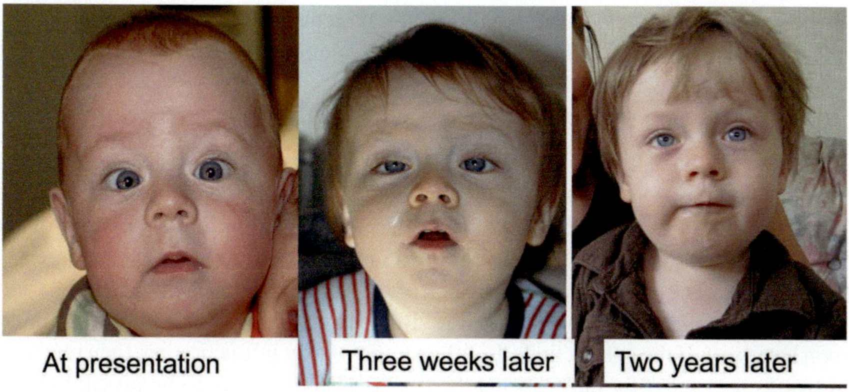

Fig. 3 A 8 month old boy with a large angle infantile esotropia was treated with injections of botulinum toxin (Botox 5U) to each medial rectus. Note the right upper lid ptosis and chin elevation in the middle picture. He remains orthophoric two years following the last injection. *Photo courtesy* S. Jain

development of binocular functions up to and including a high grade of stereopsis (Fig. 3).

Acquired Nystagmus

Patients with neurological disease affecting the visual control pathways can present with acquired nystagmus which is associated with the disabling symptom of oscillopsia. In this situation the world is perceived as constantly moving due to the oscillations of the eyes. The underlying causation is often a chronic progressive neurological condition such as multiple sclerosis which may affect other areas of visual perception. There is no conservative treatment, such as prism, which will ameliorate the symptoms. If the eyes are asymmetrically affected and the 'wobble' is acceptable in the less affected eye with minimal symptoms, then monocular occlusion of the worse eye can be helpful. Pharmacological agents can control symptoms in some patients. The clinician managing the general health of the patient may have tried oral therapies such as Baclofen (a muscle relaxant), Gabapentin (an anti epilepsy medication) Clonazepam (an anti spastic agent) or Memantine (a dementia medication) to treat the nystagmus. All systemic therapies are associated with a side effect profile that the patient might find unacceptable or not tolerated.

Retrobulbar botulinum toxin injections can be of value in managing this problem and symptom however prerequisites for this treatment include

(1) Patients should be confined to a wheelchair. Retrobulbar botulinum toxin interferes with the vestibulo ocular reflex rendering the patient, treated with this technique, unsteady on their feet.
(2) The eye to be treated should have a potentially good level of visual acuity. An MS patient with previous episodes of optic or retrobulbar neuritis and subsequent optic atrophy impacting acuity will find no benefit from the treatment.

(3) As only one eye can be treated, then the patient must accept occlusion of the untreated eye. Diplopia and a mismatch between the two eyes will be present if a patch is not worn.
(4) Acceptance of possible ptosis.

Treatment is usually commenced using 4 times the usual muscle dose and this can be adjusted dependent upon the clinical effect. Delivery is via a retrobulbar needle into the retrobulbar space. Since the reduction of retrobulbar injections to provide ophthalmic anaesthesia, the number of clinicians skilled in this technique has greatly reduced. The risks of this treatment are perforation of the globe, inadequate effect and ptosis which can either be mild or severe. Recovery of this occurs as the botulinum toxin wears off. If the patient finds the effect improves their functioning, then repeated injections at 3 monthly intervals can be given. There appears to be no cumulative effect.

Other Non-strabismus Ophthalmic Uses

Botulinum toxin is also used for non-strabismic indications when it is administered to periocular structures.

Blepharospasm is a condition where the eyelids spasm with repeated involuntary closure and effectively an inability to function normally. There are two types of spasm seen. Classical blepharospasm is where all three parts of the orbicularis oculi muscle are involved and forceable closure occurs which is intermittent. Trigger factors for this closure are sometimes obscure.

Pre tarsal blepharospasm, previously termed apraxia of eyelid opening is limited to the pre tarsal portion of the orbicularis oculi. Gentle lid closure occurs with inability to initiate a lid opening.

Botulinum toxin injections into the periocular skin area and repeated at 3 monthly intervals will help control but not eliminate the spasms in both subtypes of blepharospasm and allow the patient to return to almost normal functioning.

Irritation of the facial nerve will cause involuntary spasms of all the facial musculature innervated by this nerve, a condition termed hemifacial spasm. This can be due to the presence of an aberrant vessel within the cranial cavity touching the facial nerve and a clinical cranial nerve assessment followed by appropriate neuro imaging is required to exclude intra cranial pathology. If an aberrant vessel is identified impinging upon the 7th cranial nerve, decompression of the nerve if patient is fit and suitable for neurosurgery will potentially cure the condition. Alternatively, if there is no touch present or the patient is not suitable for surgery, then repeated injections of botulinum toxin into the periocular area at 3 monthly intervals will reduce the spasms. The lower face will not be affected by this treatment. Although control of the eyelid spasms might be effective the patient might still be bothered by the continuing lower face distortion. Hemifacial spasm can also occur after a Bells palsy when recovery is complicated by excessive contraction of the facial and eyelid muscles. As with all treatments, failure or inadequate effect is always a risk.

Side effects of periocular BT include:

(1) Ptosis which can either be mild, moderate or severe occurs within 2–3 days of injection and tends to disappear within 4–6 weeks. If bilateral, when treating blepharospasm, then the patient might suffer from significant effects on their daily functioning.
(2) Periorbital haematoma can occur but is usually transient and unsightly for the patient but does not have any long-lasting effects, requiring only reassurance.
(3) Leakage of toxin into the orbit can produce diplopia due to paralysis of an extra ocular muscle. Infero-nasal injections might cause an inferior oblique weakness, infero-temporal ones can cause inferior rectus issues. Supero-temporal treatment might leak downwards into the lateral rectus and rarely the supero-nasal site of injection might give a superior oblique weakness. The diplopia due to extra ocular muscle weakness can last longer than that induced by direct therapeutic injection because the dosage of toxin used in the periocular area is higher than that used directly into the intra ocular muscle.

The side effects of periocular botulinum toxin are all local and recover in time as the toxin wears off.
The different preparations of botulinum toxin require different units to be used. Unlike strabismus treatment where the number of units of Dysport require doubling, in periocular treatment the units required are 4 times greater than Botox or Xeomin.

Production of Iatrogenic Ptosis

Injection of BT to the levator complex can be useful in corneal disease to drop the lid to protect the cornea. Examination of the cornea is easier than central tarsorrhaphy. The dose used is usually that for an extra ocular muscle and using minimal doses and topping up if needed is probably sensible.

Loss of Bells phenomenon occurs as superior rectus is affected simultaneously with the levator and so care must be taken to monitor as function recovers.

Cases of inferior rectus overaction secondary to superior rectus weakness have been reported following usage for this indication.

5) Local Anaesthetic Injections in Strabismus

There have been many reports of restrictive eye movement disorders following ocular surgery under local anaesthesia.

- 1993 [19]—4 patients reported who developed inferior rectus restriction after retrobulbar anaesthetic for cataract surgery. Two of the 4 patients had MRI evidence of inferior rectus thickening. Forced duction testing during the corrective strabismus surgery showed marked restriction of elevation of the affected eye. Three out of the four had strabismus surgery with a good outcome.
- 1996 [20]—Following increasing reports of acquired strabismus following local anaesthetic for cataract surgery, 19 patients with this problem were identified. 16 of the 19 patients showed a presumed tight muscle. It was suggested that myotoxicity from a direct injection of local anaesthetic into the extra ocular

muscle causes an initial transient paresis followed by segmental contracture of the injected muscle. The move towards sub-tenons anaesthesia with a blunt cannula was recommended. In both reports, the muscles mainly affected had been the inferior rectus.
- 1997 [21]—A report of 2 cases after retrobulbar anaesthesia for cataract surgery. Abnormal muscle enlargement was seen in both of these patients but in these cases the superior and lateral rectus muscles were involved.
- 2000 [22]—A report of 17 patients who had undergone scleral buckling for retinal pathology and subsequently developed hypotropia. During strabismus surgery there was a positive forced duction test in 14 cases. The authors suggested that local anaesthetic myotoxicity was often the primary cause of strabismus in scleral buckling for retinal detachment.
- 2000 [23]—There was a suggestion that the patient's left eye was predominantly affected due to most surgeons administering anaesthetic being right-handed.

Previous reports had suggested that retrobulbar anaesthesia was the main causation of this issue.

- 2001 [24]—There was a report of 3 cases of diplopia after cataract surgery performed under sub tenons anaesthesia with two patients having inferior rectus restrictions and the third having a medial rectus restriction.
- 2008 [25]—A review article suggested that after retrobulbar and peribulbar anaesthesia there is an initial paresis with diplopia post operatively followed by progressive fibrosis and diplopia in the opposite direction to the initial direction. Recession of the affected muscle is indicated.
- 2013 [26]—There was a first report of inferior rectus recession as a treatment for vertical diplopia after cataract surgery which had been performed under retro bulbar or peribulbar anaesthesia.

Alongside the reported human consequences of local anaesthetic toxicity, there have been papers published on animal experimentation.

- 2004 [27]—A rabbit model was used to study the effect of bupivacaine and ricin on extra ocular muscles. The acute effect on the extra ocular muscle was confined more locally in the bupivacaine injections although recovery of the induced damage was rapid in both cases.
- 2010 [28]—Using the rabbit model again, an investigation of damage and scar formation in injected extra ocular muscles using different concentrations of bupivacaine was reported. The higher concentrations of the drug produced more myonecrosis and scar formation with minimal changes seen in the lower concentrations.
- 2012 [29]—A longer term study in rabbits showed an initial myotoxic changes in the extraocular muscles at one week post injection which resolved by 4 weeks with increased myofiber diameter. This was still present at 8 weeks post injection. The orbital and global layers were affected in this process. Further work addressing the cross-sectional area changes of the myofibrils in rabbits was undertaken in 2018. There was an increase in proportion of the slow muscle fibres and an increase in

the cross-sectional area. This suggests that increased slow fibres has an effect on eye position. These findings were confirmed by a further study in 2020 showing that rabbit superior rectus muscles showed increase in the cross sectional area of the global fibres but not the orbital layer.
- 2022 [30]—Rabbits were used to examine histologically the effect of different concentrations of bupivacaine on the superior rectus muscles. There were two concentrations used (5 mg/ml and 7.5 mg/ml). Both concentrations produced muscle hypertrophy and fibrosis although the higher dose was associated with perimuscular adhesions, conjunctival and scleral oedema and initial muscle atrophy. The lower dose group showed greater conjunctival hyperaemia and muscle hypertrophy. Included in this study were rabbits who had undergone conventional superior rectus resection. The surgical animals had greater conjunctival inflammation and hyperaemia, foreign body reaction (absent in the bupivacaine treated animals) and adhesions. The bupivacaine treated animals had scleral inflammation more frequently than the surgical group. These findings suggest that bupivacaine injections had similar reactions to surgery but possibly less severe consequences.

6) Clinical Use for Strabismus Management

- 2007 [31]—The first clinical report of bupivacaine injection given specifically to treat strabismus. This referenced the animal work showing the cycle of myotoxicity, degeneration, regeneration and hypertrophy of muscle fibres without adverse effects on surrounding tissues. One case was described where 4.5 ml of 0.75% Bupivacaine was injected into the lateral rectus of a patient with diplopia and 14 prism dioptres of esotropia. Paresis of the LR was present for 7 days. At 33 days post injection the patient had a 4 prism dioptre esophoria with resolution of diplopia. The deviation did not return to pre injection levels and was unchanged at 54 days after treatment. Magnetic resonance imaging of the orbit pre and post injection had been performed that showed an increase in the size of the injected muscle by 58% in its posterior portion.
- 2009 [32]—The same group then published a pilot study. There were 6 patients in the study group all having one lateral rectus treated. The bupivacaine volume injected varied from 1 to 4.5 ml and concentration from 0.75 to 3%. MRI was also used to quantify changes in the LR along with measures of alignment. 4 out of 6 showed improved eye alignment with two unchanged. The average alignment change in all patients was 8 prism dioptres and muscle enlargement was 6.2%. One patient suffered a transient retrobulbar haemorrhage without any visual problems.
- 2009 [33]—A further publication from the same group later in the year reported 7 patients treated with both bupivacaine and botulinum toxin. In this situation the muscle to be strengthened was injected with bupivacaine and the ipsilateral antagonist was treated with botulinum toxin. A variety of pathologies causing the initial deviation were present in the treatment group and the dosage of bupivacaine being variable. The ipsilateral antagonist was treated with a half the usual dose of botulinum toxin. The average alignment change was 19.7 prism dioptres which remained stable up to 193 days post injection.

- 2010 [34]—A study of 14 exotropic and 6 esotropic patients treated with bupivacaine alone was published. The dosage used was 4.5 ml of a 0.5% solution. 15 of the 20 patients had improved ocular alignment. Only 40% of the incommitant strabismus patients showed a good response while 86% of the commitant deviations were much better aligned. The conclusion was that denervated muscles did not respond well to treatment with bupivacaine.
- 2013 [35]—There was a further report from the original group regarding 31 comitant horizontal strabismus patients. 19 of these were suffering from esotropia and 12 had exotropia. However this was a mixed group as 16 of the 31 had large angle deviations and were treated with botulinum toxin as well as bupivacaine. 13 patients underwent a second treatment. The follow up period was up to three years and the average was 15.3 months. The original misalignment was reduced by an average of 10.5 prism dioptres. The average reduction with a single bupivacaine injection was 4.7 prism dioptres.

  In the whole group, a residual deviation of 10 prism dioptres or less was present in 53%. Modelling showed that changes in both the agonist and antagonist muscles caused the permanent changes in eye position.

- 2015 [36]—A retrospective review of 30 cases with both eso and exo deviations of less than 20 prism dioptres was published. 11 out of 30 achieved an acceptable eye position at 3 months post injection with an average angle change of between 2.3 and 3.1 prism dioptres for near and distance fixation respectively. A success rate of 37% was quoted.
- 2016 [37]—A report of 55 adults with comitant horizontal strabismus was published. 29 of these were failed surgery. The treatment given in all patients was a combination of bupivacaine or botulinum toxin in combination with bupivacaine. 27 patients required a second treatment for a residual strabismus. Success was defined as a residual deviation of 10 prism dioptres or less. 56% of patients achieved this outcome. If the initial deviation was 25 prism dioptres or less, then the success rate was 66%. In larger initial deviations 40% were corrected successfully. It was suggested that this treatment would be useful to minimize anaesthesia and avoid extra ocular scarring.
- 2019 [38]—Intermittent exotropia of the convergence insufficiency type is difficult to treat surgically. A retrospective study looking at success measured by resolution of symptoms (diplopia, reading difficulties, intermittent blurred vision and headaches, with or without prisms of less than 5 dioptres) found a 6 month and 5 year success rate of 80%. 124 patients were included in the 6 month data and 30 in the 5 year group. 0.75% bupivacaine was used in this study.
- 2020 [39]—Clinical and radiological changes were correlated in a prospective study. The dosage used was 4.5 ml of 0/5% bupivacaine. Between 12 and 17% enlargement of the extra ocular muscle was seen with an average angle change of 7.7 prism dioptres. It was suggested further studies should be performed to evaluate dosages, concentrations to produce a dose response curve.

- 2022 [40, 41]—There were two review articles of bupivacaine treatment published. The first reviewed studies between 1980 and 2021. There were only 8 articles included. The conclusion was that this modality of treatment was useful for treatment of small angle squints but is not recommended for use in cranial nerve palsies or strabismus with atrophy of the extra ocular muscles.

  The second review of bupivacaine with or without botulinum toxin supplementation demonstrated that bupivacaine alone produced 5–8 prism dioptres of deviation change and when used in combination with botulinum toxin the correction was up to 15 prism dioptres. This improvement was unchanged up to 10 years after treatment. The effect was similar in both esotropias and exotropias. It was also stated that as the bupivacaine molecule is small and must be in direct contact with the myofibrils to have an effect. The volume and concentration suggested for use was a minimum of 3mls of a 0.75% solution.

- 2022 [42]—The treatment of convergence insufficiency type intermittent exotropia with bupivacaine to the medial rectus and surgical recession of the lateral rectus. There were 10 patients in the study group and a control group of 20 who had similar pathology but only underwent lateral rectus recession as the primary treatment. The outcome was that the near distance disparity deviation was significantly reduced in the bupivacaine and lateral rectus recession group as compared to the control group.

7) Setting Up a Service for Bupivacaine Muscle Treatment

The same electromyogram, ground and reference electrodes along with the insulated needle electrodes and topical local anaesthetic used for the delivery of botulinum toxin are required for the injection of bupivacaine. Care must be taken if this service is incorporated into the botulinum toxin delivery service. Local protocols should be set and observed to ensure the bupivacaine or botulinum toxin is injected into the correct muscle.

It should be remembered that the muscle injected with bupivacaine will lose function and the deviation being treated will worsen almost immediately. If this causes the eye to move out of its suppression area then diplopia will ensue. Warning the patient in advance about diplopia is sensible and provision of a pad post injection will treat this issue. As the patient will be monocular, then advice not to drive themselves to the appointment should be given. The pad should be kept in place until the diplopia has resolved. This might take up to 2 days. Patients should also be warned about the transient redness and soreness associated with the inflammation caused by the bupivacaine. This is transient and there is no indication for use of topical steroids post injection.

Risks of Treatment

As with botulinum toxin injection, the major risk to vision is perforation of the globe during the process. This can be minimized by ensuring the needle remains tangential to the globe during rotation of the eye. Avoiding excessive pressure on inserting the needle will also mitigate this risk. Inadvertent intravascular injection of bupivacaine is a theoretical risk but attempted aspiration prior to commencing the injection will reduce this possible complication. Ptosis is not likely but some local anaesthetic effect on adjacent extra ocular muscles is possible. Provided case selection is appropriate, the chance of overcorrection is minimal. As previous studies have shown, undercorrection of the deviation is the most common problem encountered with this treatment.

Case Selection

Treatment with bupivacaine alone should be reserved for small angle strabismus patients in which there is no evidence of paresis. Patients suitable would be those who require correction of approximately less than 10 dioptres of squint. Conditions that would benefit from treatment are convergence insufficiency type intermittent exotropia (near exotropia), distance esotropia of ageing and small angle residual deviations. If a greater deviation correction is required then augmentation with botulinum toxin given to the ipsilateral antagonist. This will give up to 15 prism dioptres of deviation change.

Areas Requiring Further Study

(1) Concentration of bupivacaine
(2) Volume of bupivacaine
(3) Dosage of botulinum toxin if used in combination
(4) Timing of botulinum toxin treatment
(5) Is repeat treatment beneficial?

Concentration

There is no consistency in the published papers regarding this In the UK, the only available concentration available commercially is 0.5%. 3 and 4% are produced for use in other areas of medicine but if used in this context, it is an off label and unlicenced medication. The advantage if higher concentrations is the smaller volume injected with more bupivacaine close to the muscle belly, easier injection and higher doses possible. 1ml of 3% bupivacaine will give a dose of 30 mg whereas 5 mls of 0.5% will only give 25 mgs. A study to compare various dosages and the deviation corrected is necessary.

Volume

The higher the concentration the lower the volume required to give the same dose. The smaller the volume is desirable to allow the maximum exposure of the injected muscle to the medication. Larger volumes are also more difficult to inject and less comfortable for the patient. The time taken to inject is also longer in larger volumes.

Dosage of Botulinum Toxin

It has been suggested that only a half normal dose of botulinum toxin should be used in the ipsilateral antagonist muscle but there are no studies supporting this. Further research in this area is needed.

Timing of Botulinum Toxin Treatment

It is suggested that bupivacaine and botulinum toxin should be administered on the same day but there is no evidence to support this. It is possible that botulinum toxin might be delayed until the beginning of myofibril regeneration might give a larger angle change.

Is Repeat Treatment Beneficial?

Some of the studies have patients with repeat treatment but there is no evidence whether repeat injection is cumulative, when it should be given and how often this can be undertaken.

References

1. Scott AB, Rosenbaum A, Collins CC. Pharmacologic weakening of extraocular muscles. Invest Ophthalmol. 1973;12(12):924–7.
2. Scott AB. Botulinum toxin injection into extraocular muscles as an alternative to strabismus surgery. Ophthalmology. 1980;87(10):1044–9.
3. Rowe FJ, Noonan CP. Botulinum toxin for the treatment of strabismus. Cochrane Database Syst Rev. 2009;2.
4. Rowe FJ, Noonan CP. Botulinum toxin for the treatment of strabismus. Cochrane Database Syst Rev. 2017;3(3).
5. Bort-Martí AR, Rowe FJ, Sifre LR, Ng SM, Bort-Martí S, Garcia VR (2023) Botulinum toxin for the treatment of strabismus. Cochrane Database Syst Rev. 2023;3(3).
6. Khan J, Kumar I, Marsh IB. Botulinum toxin injection for postoperative diplopia testing in adult strabismus. J AAPOS. 2008;12(1):46–8.
7. Lee J, Harris S, Cohen J, Cooper K, MacEwen C, Jones S. Results of a prospective randomized trial of botulinum toxin therapy in acute unilateral sixth nerve palsy. J Pediatr Ophthalmol Strabismus. 1994;31(5):283–6.
8. Hatt SR, Gnanaraj L. Interventions for intermittent exotropia. Cochrane Database Syst Rev. 2013;5.
9. Ripley L, Rowe FJ. Use of botulinum toxin in small-angle heterotropia and decompensating heterophoria: a review of the literature. Strabismus. 2007;15(3):165–71.
10. Bansal S, Khan J, Marsh IB. The role of botulinum toxin in decompensated strabismus. Strabismus. 2008;16(3):107–11.
11. Mehner L, Ng SM, Singh J. Interventions for infantile esotropia. Cochrane Database Syst Rev. 2023;1(1).
12. Elliott S, Shafiq A. Interventions for infantile esotropia. Cochrane Database Syst Rev. 2013;7.
13. McNeer KW, Spencer RF, Tucker MG. Observations on bilateral simultaneous botulinum toxin injection in infantile esotropia. J Pediatr Ophthalmol Strabismus. 1994;31:214–9.
14. Ruben ST, Lee JP, O'Neil D, Dunlop I, Elston JS. The use of botulinum toxin for treatment of acquired nystagmus and oscillopsia. J Neuro Ophthalmol. 1994;14(4):2–23.
15. Repka MX, Savino PJ, Reinecke RD. Treatment of acquired nystagmus with botulinum neurotoxin A. Arch Ophthalmol. 1994;112(10):1320–4.

16. Tomsak RL, Remler BF, Averbuch-Heller L, Chandran M, Leigh RJ. Unsatisfactory treatment of acquired nystagmus with retrobulbar injection of botulinum toxin. Am J Ophthalmol. 1995;119(4):489–96.
17. Helveston EM, Pogrebniak AE. Treatment of acquired nystagmus with botulinum A toxin. Am J Ophthalmol. 1988;106(5):584–6.
18. Kosmin AS, Marsh IB, Batterbury M. The use of botulinum toxin injections in the management of acquired nystagmus and oscillopsia. J Clin Rehabil. 1996;10(3):205–9.
19. Hamilton SM, Elsas FJ, Dawson TL. A cluster of patients with inferior rectus restriction following local anesthesia for cataract surgery. J Pediatr Ophthalmol Strabismus. 1993;30(5):288–91.
20. Capó H, Guyton DL. Ipsilateral hypertropia after cataract surgery. Ophthalmology. 1996;103(5):721–30.
21. Ando K, Oohira A, Takao M. Restrictive strabismus after retrobulbar anesthesia. Jpn J Ophthalmol. 1997;41(1):23–6.
22. Salama H, Farr AK, Guyton DL. Anesthetic myotoxicity as a cause of restrictive strabismus after scleral buckling surgery. Retina. 2000;20(5):478–82.
23. Pearce IA, McCready PM, Watson MP, Taylor RH. Vertical diplopia following local anaesthetic cataract surgery: predominantly a left eye problem? Eye (Lond). 2000;14(Pt 2):180–4.
24. Jaycock PD, Mather CM, Ferris JD, Kirkpatrick JN. Rectus muscle trauma complicating sub-Tenon's local anaesthesia. Eye (Lond). 2001;15(Pt 5):583–6.
25. Guyton DL. Strabismus complications from local anesthetics. Semin Ophthalmol. 2008;23(5):298–301.
26. Schild AM, Fricke J, Neugebauer A. Inferior rectus muscle recession as a treatment for vertical diplopia following cataract extraction. Graefes Arch Clin Exp Ophthalmol. 2013;251(1):189–94.
27. Park CY, Park SE, Oh SY. Acute effect of bupivacaine and ricin mAb 35 on extraocular muscle in the rabbit. Curr Eye Res. 2004;29(4–5):293–301.
28. Zhang C, Phamonvaechavan P, Rajan A, Poon DY, Topcu-Yilmaz P, Guyton DL. Concentration-dependent bupivacaine myotoxicity in rabbit extraocular muscle. J AAPOS. 2010;14(4):323–7.
29. Akbari MR, Amoli FA, Alhashemi LH, Ameri A, Jafari AK, Eshraghi B, Bozorgi S. Bupivacaine injection myotoxicity on extraocular muscles. A strabismus alternative treatment: extended histological changes induced in a rabbit model. Binocul Vis Strabolog Q Simms Romano. 2012;27(1):15–22.
30. El-Mofty RMA-M, Kassem RR, Abdel-Salam LO. Histopathological changes in extraocular muscles of rabbits following injection of bupivacaine 5 mg/ml versus 7.5 mg/ml. Cutan Ocul Toxicol. 2022;41(3):210–4.
31. Scott AB, Alexander DE, Miller JM. Bupivacaine injection of eye muscles to treat strabismus. Br J Ophthalmol. 2007;91(2):146–8.
32. Scott AB, Miller JM, Shieh KR. Bupivacaine injection of the lateral rectus muscle to treat esotropia. J AAPOS. 2009;13(2):119–22.
33. Scott AB, Miller JM, Shieh KR. Treating strabismus by injecting the agonist muscle with bupivacaine and the antagonist with botulinum toxin. Trans Am Ophthalmol Soc. 2009;107:104–9.
34. Wutthiphan S, Srisuwanporn S. Bupivacaine injection to treat exotropia and esotropia. Strabismus. 2010;18(4):137–41.
35. Miller JM, Scott AB, Danh KK, Strasser D, Sane M. Bupivacaine injection remodels extraocular muscles and corrects comitant strabismus. Ophthalmology. 2013;120(12):2733–40.
36. Ziahosseini K, Marsh IB. Single injection of bupivacaine for correction of strabismus. Med Hypothesis Discov Innov Ophthalmol. 2015;4(4):157–61.
37. Debert I, Miller JM, Danh KK, Scott AB. Pharmacologic injection treatment of comitant strabismus. J AAPOS. 2016;20(2):106–11.
38. Josephson M, Mathias SA. Treatment of intermittent exotropia of the convergence insufficiency type with bupivacaine 0.75%: 5-year experience and outcomes. J Binocul Vis Ocul Motil. 2019;69(1):3–7.

39. Karaca U, Altinsoy Hİ, Mutlu FM, Ceylan OM. Bupivacaine injection for comitant horizontal strabismus: clinical and radiological results. Arq Bras Oftalmol. 2020;83(3):180–4.
40. Farrelly-Waters M, Smith J, Parmar K. The efficacy of bupivacaine for the treatment of strabismus. Strabismus. 2022;30(1):42–7.
41. Kiarudi MY, Shahri SHG, Es'haghi A, Gharib B, Ansari-Astaneh M-R. Applications of bupivacaine in the non-surgical treatments of strabismus: a review. Strabismus. 2022;30(4):204–8.
42. Tellioglu A, Ocak OB, Inal A, Gurez C, Celik S, Tellioglu DO, Gokyigit B. Treatment of convergence insufficiency type intermittent exotropia with bupivacaine injection to the medial rectus combined with lateral rectus recession. J AAPOS. 2022;26(5):249.

Surgical Treatment of Strabismus Complications

John Bradbury

Abstract Strabismus surgery, while commonly performed and generally safe, carries a spectrum of potential complications that range from minor and self-limiting to severe and sight-threatening. This chapter provides an in-depth overview of these complications, focusing on symptomatic outcomes that often necessitate medical or surgical intervention. Key topics include the definition and incidence of complications, with data from major studies, and a detailed discussion of both mild and severe postoperative issues. These include consecutive deviations, conjunctival and Tenon's complications, globe perforation, infections, lost and slipped muscles, and adherence syndrome. Management strategies and preventative measures are discussed, emphasizing surgical approaches while also considering relevant nonsurgical interventions.

Keywords Strabismus surgery · Surgical complications · Globe perforation · Slipped muscle · Lost muscle · Consecutive deviations · Orbital infection · Pyogenic granuloma

The purpose of this chapter is to outline complications of strabismus surgery emphasising the surgical management whilst discussing relevant nonsurgical solutions.

Some complications can be minor and self-limiting whilst others can be disabling and sight threatening.

J. Bradbury (✉)
Bradford Teaching Hospital, Bradford, UK
e-mail: John.Bradbury@bthft.nhs.uk

S. Jain (ed.), *Surgical Management of Strabismus*,
https://doi.org/10.1007/978-3-031-80633-9_15

1 Definition

Clavien [1] defined complications as ‘any deviation from the normal postoperative course’. This of course is a very broad definition and will include many minor problems which may settle spontaneously or with minimal non-surgical intervention and will not be included in this chapter.

Definitions of complications in strabismus surgery can be tricky and vary between surgeons e.g. is a failure to reach an arbitrary post op angle of say less than 10 PD or post op diplopia in extreme versions a complication?, views may vary. Whereas diplopia in the primary position or reduction in vision is less contentious.

Timescale also may be involved with the definition e.g. Is operating on a patient with consecutive exotropia say 2 years post esotropia surgery a complication or the natural history of patients with poor binocular function.

The emphasis of the chapter will be on those complications which are symptomatic and or require intervention, often surgical, and in the author’s opinion are a direct result of strabismus surgery.

2 Incidence

The incidence of complications in strabismus surgery has been studied in two large studies, which though very different in their methodologies, led to remarkably similar findings (Table 1). The first (the BOSU study) [2] was a nationwide, 2-year prospective survey of severe complications of strabismus surgery carried out by the author through the British Ophthalmic Surveillance Unit. The second (the Moorfields study) [3] was a 5-year prospective audit of 4000 consecutive strabismus operations in a single large teaching hospital [3]. The incidences of complications found by these two studies are shown in Table 1. The key message from these two incidence studies is that for strabismus surgery, there is about a 1 in 400 risk of severe complications (including globe perforation, cellulitis, lost/snapped/slipped muscle); but less than a 1 in 2000 risk of a significant complication (meaning loss of visual acuity or unexpected double vision in the primary position).

2.1 Consecutive Deviations

Consecutive deviations either eso or exo were not included in these publications but are a common outcome of surgical procedures. Consecutive esotropia in the immediate post operative period may not be a complication in many incidences, but be a deliberate outcome in certain types of exotropia e.g. when operating on patients with consecutive exotropia, where a large post operative drift is expected. Therefore

Table 1 Incidence of complications in strabismus surgery

Complication	Bradbury and Taylor [2] incidence figure (%)	Ritchie and Ali [3] incidence figure (%)
Severe complication (any complication with potential to cause poor visual outcome)	0.25 (1 in 400)	0.22 (1 in 455)
Significant complication (poor or very poor visual outcome at 6 months)	0.04 (1 in 2400)	0.02 (1 in 4076)
Globe perforation	0.08	0.07
Snapped/lost muscle	0.02	0.05
Suspected slipped muscle	0.07	0.05
Periorbital infection	0.06	0.07
Scleritis	0.02	0.10

consecutive esotropia may only be considered a complication where it is persistent, cosmetically poor and/or causing symptoms.

Consecutive Esotropia in the immediate post operative period may require intervention if troublesome but in most cases can be watched as this is likely to improve assuming ductions are full enough to rule out a slipped muscle. The diplopia can be managed by a reducing prism or botulinum toxin, rarely is surgery required and maybe indicated if the angle is large, the diplopia is troublesome, a prism is not tolerated, there are significant reduced ductions or a risk of amblyopia.

Consecutive esotropia has a prevalence quoted between 6 and 20% [4] although many improve spontaneously without any intervention. The risks for consecutive esotropia according to Jang [4] include high myopia, amblyopia, near exotropia, lateral incomitance, and unilateral surgery, this was for consecutive esotropia in the 2 weeks following surgery, as I have said many will improve spontaneously especially those types with a large post operative drift such as post op consecutive exotropia patients, poor binocularity usually leads to the exotropia re occurring rather than an esotropia.

Consecutive exotropia is almost never a desired outcome post operatively and so virtually all cases could be considered a complication albiet one that may not require any surgical intervention if small and not causing any symptoms.

The prevalence of consecutive exotropia is quoted between 4 and 29%, [5] with the prevalence increasing, the longer the follow up period. The risks for consecutive exotropia are either mechanical due to limited adduction postoperatively which could be due to an over recessed medial rectus, an over resected lateral rectus or slippage/malanchoring of the medial rectus(pseudotendon of the medial rectus is a common finding in reoperations) or due to poor binocular function post operatively.

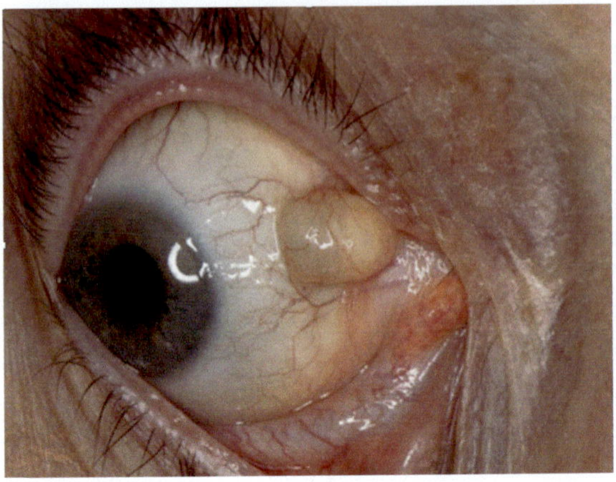

Fig. 1 Conjunctival cyst

Less Severe Complications sometimes requiring Surgical Intervention

Most conjunctival/adenexal tissue complications settle spontaneously or with the help of lubricants or topical steroids, only rarely is surgery required. Here are a few examples.

2.2 *Conjunctival Epithelial Inclusion Cyst Fig. 1*

This rare complication is caused by deposition of conjunctival epithelial cells into deeper tissues. Most are small, but some can be large, especially those at muscle insertions. They enlarge and need surgical removal as in this case. The whole cyst needs to be removed whole without puncturing the cyst to reduce the chance of recurrence.

2.3 *Conjunctival Dehiscence Fig. 2*

If the suturing has been inadequate the conjunctiva may retract exposing the muscle sutures. This in most cases can be left to re epithelialize but if it looks unsightly or the patient is distressed then the conjunctiva may need re suturing.

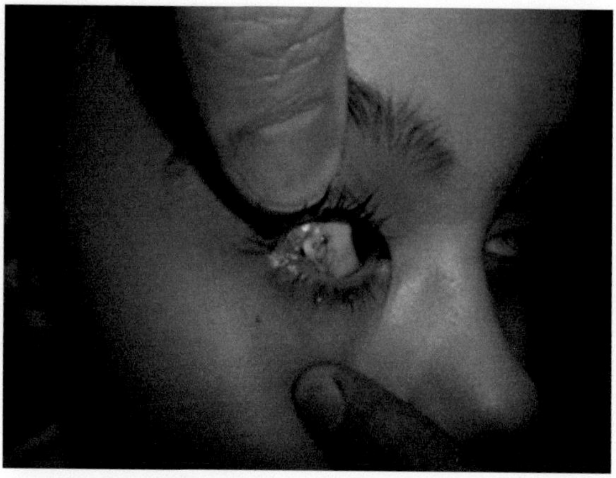

Fig. 2 Conjunctival dehiscence

2.4 *Prolapsed Tenon's Capsule*

This occurs in children and young adults with a prominent Tenon's layer. It is caused by poor conjunctival closure. If the prolapse is large, it may need to be trimmed, but it usually resolves spontaneously.

2.5 *Pyogenic Granuloma Fig. 3*

This is seen more commonly in children. Post operatively patients develop a raised fleshy mass arising from the conjunctival wound edge. This fleshy mass appears a few weeks after surgery and is composed of inflammatory cells and capillary proliferation. It may be confused with a suture granuloma. The lesion may be so large that it still protrudes after lid closure. If small this can settle with topical steroids. If large and unsightly it needs surgical removal. I like to diathermy the base and inject subconjunctival steroid. Rarely it can re occur.

3 Severe Complications

3.1 *Globe Perforation*

Globe perforation is the commonest severe complication of strabismus surgery, reported in 0.13–1% of cases [6]. In the BOSU study, the incidence was 1: 1000. In the BOSU study this was more common in children, possibly due to surgical access, although it did not reach statistical significance. One patient developed endophthalmitis and had to have an evisceration. Although globe perforation is relatively

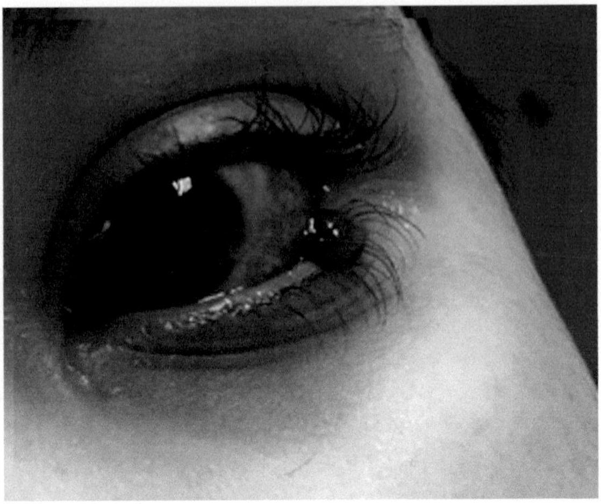

Fig. 3 Pyogenic granuloma

common, a poor or very poor outcome is extremely rare. Complex surgery involving suturing posteriorly such as faden procedures may have a higher incidence of globe perforation.

In the BOSU study, globe perforation sometimes occurred when placing a traction suture. This resulted in some cases of penetration into the anterior chamber and a soft eye, making strabismus surgery difficult. Most cases of posterior segment perforation had immediate treatment, usually cryotherapy or laser. There was one case of retinal detachment in a high myope who had bilateral globe perforation from bilateral Harada–Ito procedures.

The management of globe perforation is not evidence-based. Ninety percent of cases are treated with cryotherapy and/or laser [7]. In children, where globe perforation is more likely, retinal detachment is unlikely as they have formed vitreous. I perform a fundus examination to confirm the diagnosis with the pupil dilated peroperatively by injection of 1 or 2 mL of local anesthetic sub-Tenon's. I do not perform peroperative treatment, but seek a vitreoretinal opinion, if available. In adults, I perform a fundus examination and, in patients with a high risk of retinal detachment (i.e. high myopes), I treat any holes either by laser or cryotherapy and then seek vitreoretinal opinion. I do not treat those at low risk, but seek a later vitreoretinal opinion. All patients have systemic antibiotics to reduce the risk of endophthalmitis. The BOSU study reported one case of endophthalmitis leading to evisceration in a 3-year-old.

Rathod [8] reported two cases of endophthalmitis, two retinal detachments, one suprachoroidal hemorrhage, and one choroidal scar.

Strategies to prevent globe perforation include:

- avoiding suturing in areas with scleral thinning and,
- techniques (i.e. hang-back procedures) that do not involve direct scleral suturing in thinner areas or where access is difficult.

3.2 *Orbital/Periorbital Infection*

Significant infection following strabismus surgery tends to take one of two forms: diffuse orbital cellulitis which rarely requires surgical intervention or localized abscess at the muscle insertion which often does. In the BOSU study there were 13 cases in total, with approximately equal numbers of diffuse orbital infection and muscle insertion abscesses. Three of the muscle insertion abscesses developed a slipped muscle and required surgical exploration to retrieve the muscle. A similar case has been reported with bilateral orbital infection [9]. Management of diffuse orbital infection requires systemic antibiotics (which were curative in all the BOSU cases). A muscle insertion abscess will also require systemic antibiotics but may also need surgical exploration to drain the abscess and make good any muscle slip. The intervention needs to be timely to prevent a lost muscle scenario, any surgeon who has a high index of suspicious that an insertion infection is developing should consider an early surgical intervention to clear any infection and to secure the muscle to the sclera, as watching such infection in an outpatient setting is challenging especially in children.

In a series of 26 cases of endophthalmitis following strabismus in Holland, [10] histological examination of the specimens showed that that infection had tracked into the eye from a postoperative muscle insertion infection. An aggressive approach to muscle insertion infection may therefore be warranted to prevent this. Preseptal cellulitis can also occur following strabismus surgery (0.06% in the Moorfields study) but responds promptly to standard antibiotic protocols. The Dutch study also reported all cases were below age 9 or older than 65 years of age. In children they suggested lacrimal sac massage before surgery.

3.3 *Lost Muscle Fig. 4*

We define this complication as a muscle lost *peroperatively*. In the BOSU study there were a total of six lost muscles. The majority of these were elderly patients, four of whom had had previous strabismus surgery. Four were medial recti and two were lateral recti. Medial rectus is probably the most common muscle lost at the time of surgery. This may be related to how frequently the muscle is operated on but also to anatomical factors; it lacks the attachments to the oblique muscles that the other recti have so it can retract more easily into the posterior orbit. Loss of a muscle often occurs after a muscle snaps—as soon as this happens, it is vital to attempt to secure the proximal end of the snapped muscle with toothed forceps before it retracts.

Should a muscle retract and be lost peroperatively it is better to try to find it at the primary surgery, rather than wait for a later date [11]. A common mistake is to look for the muscle around the surface of the globe when in fact the rectus muscles lie slightly away from the globe, as can be appreciated from axial orbital images. Careful exploration with suitable retractors can usually identify the muscle sheath within

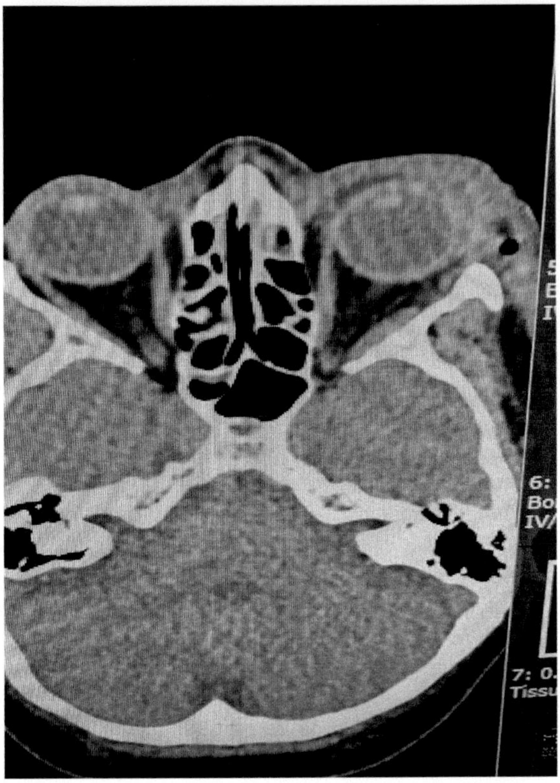

Fig. 4 This patient had a traumatic rupture of her Left Lateral Rectus which has retracted into her orbit. Although this is not a result of a surgical complication it represents where a intraoperative lost muscle may appear on a CT scan

which lies the muscle. Some authors have suggested using the oculocardiac reflex as a way of finding the muscle as pulling on the muscle would slow the heart rate; this is not always reliable. If the muscle cannot be found, one can at least suture the check ligaments and Tenon's which surround the muscle back to the original muscle insertion, allowing some of the muscle action to be transferred through these tissues to the eye. A primary muscle transposition should not be performed as this could lead to the second, totally avoidable complication of anterior segment ischemia. It would be better for an experienced strabismus surgeon to explore at a second operation. MRI and CT scans rarely add much to the surgical reoperation plan as the muscle is not found except in the anticipated location. The exception to this is in cases of previous orbital trauma or congenitally abnormal orbital anatomy. Some authors have advocated an orbital approach for a posteriorly situated muscle either through a lateral orbitotomy or transnasally [12] this will depend on the local availability of orbital surgical expertise.

4 Slipped Muscle

A slipped muscle can be defined as a postop overcorrection, with 50% or more reduction in movement in the action of the operated muscle. Technically, it remains a suspected slipped muscle until it is confirmed at a second operation. In the BOSU study, the incidence was 0.07%. In 3 of the 18 cases these occurred as a result of a postoperative muscle insertion infection. Poor or very poor outcomes were found in 3 out of 18, all of whom were children.

Slipped muscles seem to take two main forms. One is a true slipped muscle, similar to lost muscle in that there was a problem with the sutures or insertion within days to a couple of weeks after the operation. The suture fails and the muscle slips. This is dealt with like the lost muscle scenario. The more common presentation occurs months or even years later with a gross limitation of action of the muscle. Exploration usually reveals that muscle has a large pseudotendon, that is the muscle is attached to the sclera via stretchy, white scar tissue. This may have occurred due to stretching of a poorly inserted muscle over a long period of time. In all cases, one needs to excise the pseudotendon and re-attach the meaty part of the muscle to the globe. Quite often there has been concurrent shortening of the antagonist which will require recession, together with a conjunctival recession. Very rarely, a muscle can slip many years later but as an acute presentation, which can mimic a neurological cause of acute diplopia.

4.1 Adherence Syndrome Fig. 5

This is a restrictive condition, often progressive, caused by orbital fat prolapsing through a surgically disrupted posterior Tenon's. Poorly performed previous surgery to the inferior oblique is often implicated [11]. Occasionally, it is caused by trauma or by lid surgery. To prevent this, care must be taken to visualize the posterior edge of the inferior oblique so only the muscle is hooked at the time of surgery, avoiding damage to Tenon's and fat. Excessive bleeding may interfere with visualization and contributes to the scarring process. If orbital fat prolapses during surgery it can be repositioned or excised and the posterior Tenon's repaired. Often the problem is found postoperatively as the patient develops progressive hypotropia and limitation of elevation. Surgical options are to explore the inferior fornix, excise any scarring and orbital fat, repair the posterior Tenon's capsule defect, and then if necessary recess the inferior rectus, Tenon's, and conjunctiva, followed by an amniotic membrane graft Burton in his series usually performed an extensive conjunctival peritomy over nearly 180 degrees, recessing the conjunctiva while leaving the sclera to re-epithelialise, and in addition recessed the inferior rectus by 2.5–3 mm. Only one patient required an additional operation. Of the 11 patients who had undergone surgery all showed a significant improvement in their symptom. However, none had normal ocular motility post operatively.

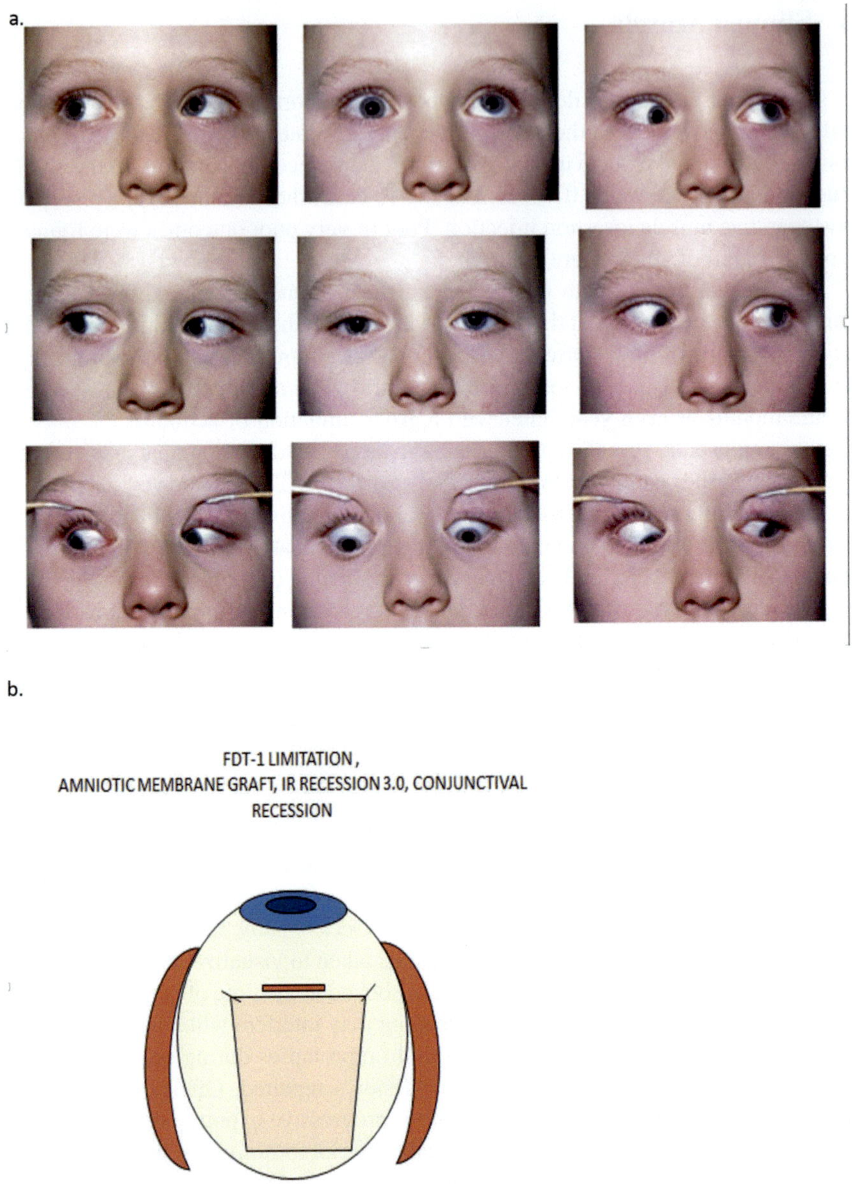

Fig. 5 Inferior fornix adherence syndrome post right inferior oblique surgery (a), preoperative appearance showing limitation of elevation of the right eye, (b) surgical plan and (c) postoperativre appearance

c.

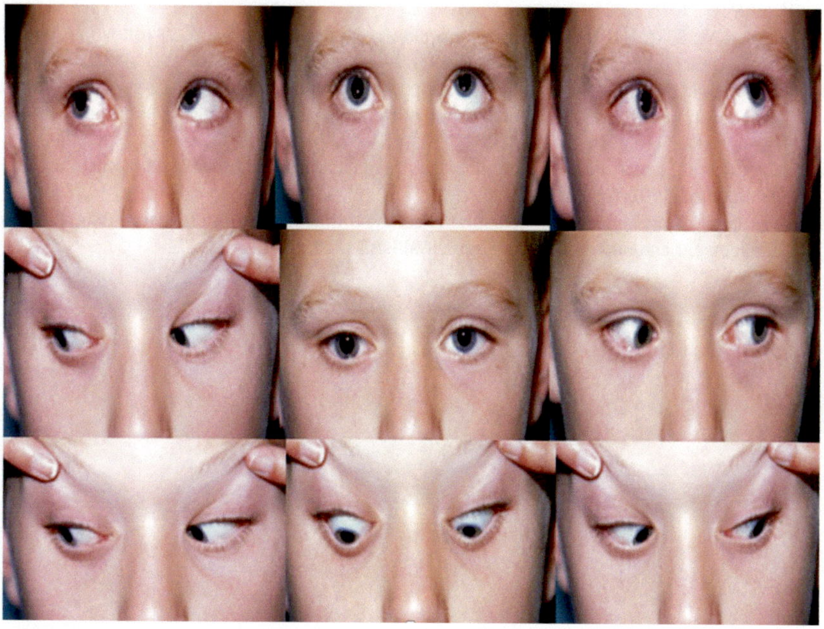

Fig. 5 (continued)

Other severe complications include Endophthalmitis, the management of which is beyond the scope of this chapter and is extensively covered elsewhere and post op scleritis which does not require any surgical intervention but often extensive intervention by a uveitis specialist.

References

1. Ali MZ. Assessment of postoperative complications in abdominal surgeries by Clavein-Dindo classification system in the Indian hospital setting. Acad J Surg. 2021;4:16. https://index.pkp.sfu.ca/index.php/record/view/4271853.
2. Bradbury JA, Taylor RH. Severe complications of strabismus surgery. J AAPOS. 2013;17(1):59–63.
3. Ritchie AE, Ali N. The incidence of complications in 4000 consecutive strabismus operations. J AAPOS. 2019;23(3):140–1.
4. Jang JH, Park JM. Factors predisposing to consecutive esotropia after surgery to correct intermittent exotropia. Graefe's Arch Clin Exp Ophthalmol. 2012;250:1485–90.
5. Bradbury JA, Doran RM. Secondary exotropia: a retrospective analysis of matched cases. J Pediatr Ophthalmol Strabismus. 1993;30:163–6.
6. Noel LP, Bloom JN, Clarke WN, et al. Retinal perforation in strabismus surgery. J Pediatr Ophthalmol Strabismus. 1997;34:115–7.
7. Simon JW. Scleral perforation during eye muscle surgery: incidence and sequelae. J Pediatr Ophthalmol Starbismus. 1992;29:273–5.

8. Rathod D, Goyal R, Watts P. The management of globe perforation during strabismus surgery. J AAPOS. 2010;14:25.
9. Kothari M, Sukri N. Bilateral staphylococcus aureus sub-Tenon's abscess following strabismus surgery in a child. J AAPOS. 2010;14:193–5.
10. Simonsz HJ, Rutar T, Kraft S, et al. Endophthalmitis after strabismus surgery: incidence and outcome in relation to age, operated eye muscle, surgical technique, scleral perforation and immune state. Acta Ophthalmol. 2021;99(1):37–51.
11. MacEwan C, Lee J, Fells P. Aetiology and management of the detached rectus muscle. Br J Ophthalmol. 1992;76:131–6.
12. Burton B, Dawson E, Lee J. Adherence syndrome following inferior oblique surgery: management and outcome of 14 cases. Strabismus. 2004;12(3):169–74.

Teaching Strabismus Surgery

John Ferris

Abstract The aim of this chapter is to provide a practical guide on how to use simulation techniques, with a variety of model eyes, to teach the fundamental building blocks of strabismus surgery, before trainees transition to live surgery. It will also describe how to teach more advanced strabismus surgery procedures and how to help trainees develop from novices into safe, independent and adaptable strabismus surgeons.

Keywords Simulation · OSSCAR · Practice · Phillips Studio · Bioniko · Virtual mentoring · Simulation gallery

1 Introduction

In a training environment where many trainees are preoccupied by their cataract surgical numbers, strabismus surgeons have to work hard to convince trainees that learning the "dark arts" of strabismus surgery is worthwhile. For those trainees who might ask, "Why do I need to learn how to perform strabismus surgery if I am not going to be a paediatric ophthalmologist?" the answer, to any strabismus surgeon, is self-evident. They know that tissue handling, manual dexterity, suturing skills, intra-operative adaptability and the art of surgical planning are all enhanced by an exposure to strabismus surgery and are transferrable skills, which will be of value to any ophthalmic surgeon. Furthermore, being able to dissect through the conjunctiva and Tenons capsule to identify the extent of a scleral laceration/perforation and to be able to hook and secure a rectus muscle on a 6/0 vicryl suture, are essential skills for any ophthalmologist who manages ocular trauma.

Teaching our trainees strabismus surgery is also a chance to demonstrate how rewarding a specialty it is, and in an era where there is an international shortage of paediatric ophthalmologists and strabismus surgeons, this opportunity should not be wasted.

J. Ferris (✉)
Cheltenham General Hospital, Cheltenham, UK
e-mail: johndferris@me.com

S. Jain (ed.), *Surgical Management of Strabismus*,
https://doi.org/10.1007/978-3-031-80633-9_16

Over recent years there have been increasing pressures on surgical training across the world. Shorter training programs, less time in the operating theatre, trainers not having enough time to supervise surgical training and the pressure of long waiting lists, especially in the post-Covid era, are all reducing surgical opportunities for our trainees. The aim of this chapter is to provide a practical guide of how to deliver simulation-based training, which will mitigate these factors and enable trainees to develop into competent strabismus surgeons, in a safe, rewarding and timely fashion.

2 Does Simulation Training Work?

We now have randomised control trial standard evidence that simulation training works. The GLAucoma Simulated Surgical Trial (GLASS) [1] and The Ophthalmic Learning and Improvement Initiative in Cataract Surgery Trial [2] (OLIMPICS) conducted by Will Dean and his co-workers in Southern Africa, proved that trainees who underwent a structured program of simulation training improved their surgical competence threefold (as measured by an OSSCAR matrix), compared to trainees who had not undertaken this structured form of training.

They also performed more operations with fewer complications in the following 12 months and their confidence increased by a factor of two. These RCTs also showed that having watched videos of their own simulated surgery the scores trainees awarded themselves were very similar to those awarded by their trainers. The importance of this is that trainees can accurately chart their progression towards competence.

3 Developing a Culture of Training

Before discussing the practicalities of delivering strabismus simulation training, the importance of developing a culture of simulation training in your training program should be emphasised. The role of the training program is to provide trainees with the resources they need to develop their surgical skills. The trainer should be seen as a facilitator, someone who is there to help trainees develop their surgical competencies in a safe environment. However, it is the trainee who is ultimately responsible for how quickly they progress and how much live surgery they get to perform. For those who engage with simulation training the learning curve is short and steep and they are able to progress to live surgery in a very short period of time. The converse is also true!

Trainees are naturally competitive so when they see colleagues who have embraced this model of training developing surgical skills and performing more live surgery, they are likely to want to follow in their footsteps. So, this culture of simulation training becomes a virtuous circle.

4 Simulation Materials

Strabismus surgeons pride themselves on the low-tech nature of their surgery and this also applies to the materials needed to teach strabismus surgery [3, 4] No expensive virtual reality simulation is required. Although some trainees may have access to a wet-lab where they can perform strabismus surgery simulation on a variety of animal materials, or even access to human cadavers, these forms of simulation, unlike model eyes which can be used anywhere, do not readily lend themselves to the principles of sustained, deliberate practice. This is why this chapter will concentrate on model eye simulation.

The following materials/equipment are all that are required to teach strabismus surgery:

(1) Instruments—one pair of needle holders, toothed forceps, Westcott scissors and a supply of 6/0 vicryl sutures.
(2) Model eyes—any of the following:

- Ping-pong ball model eyes—these cheap realistic model eyes made from ping-pong balls, modelling, foam, and modelling clay are easy to make from materials that can be found anywhere in the world and cost less than $2 (Fig. 1)

  Video 1—**How to make the model eye** https://vimeo.com/manage/videos/529712364.
- Phillips Studio strabismus eyes (https://phillipsstudio.co.uk)—the Basic Strabismus eyes have 4 rectus muscles. The Advanced Strabismus eyes also

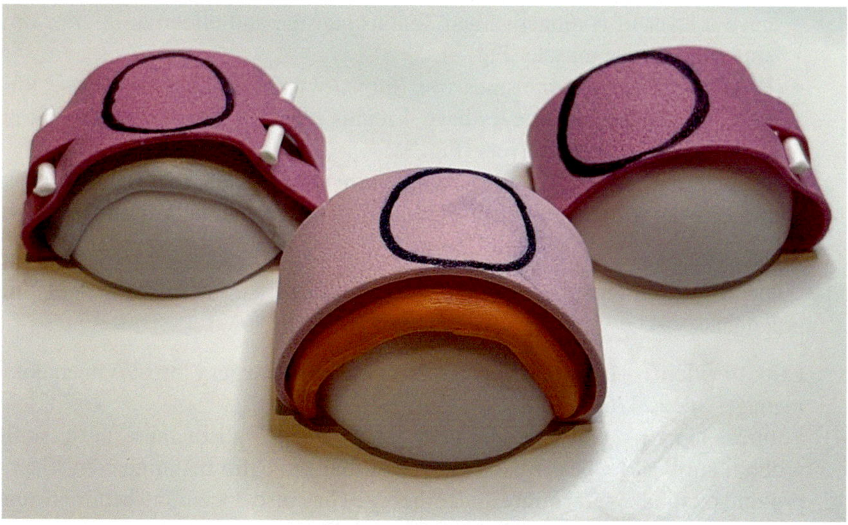

Fig. 1 Ping-pong ball model eyes

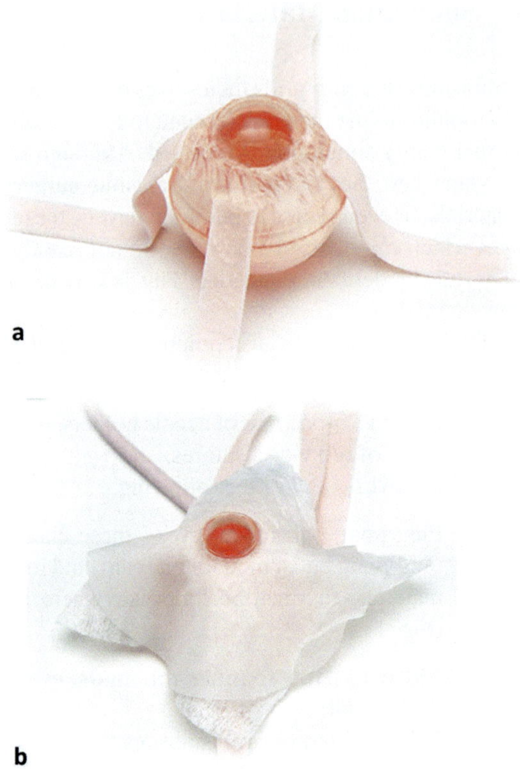

Fig. 2 Phillips Studios Basic (a) and Advanced (b) strabismus eyes

have a layer of conjunctiva and Tenons capsule and either an inferior or a superior oblique muscle (Fig. 2).

- Bioniko EX-ONE strabismus eye (https://www.bioniko.com)—these life-like 3-D printed model eyes have 4 rectus muscles, realistic sclera, but no conjunctiva or Tenons layers (Fig. 3).
- Kenneth Wright and Yi Ning Strube have developed a 3D printed silicone model eyes with very realistic conjunctiva, sclera and rectus muscles [5].

(3) Mobile phone and a selfie stand with a ring light—by using a selfie stand to suspend a mobile phone over the model eyes, trainees can record their simulation practice.

Link to video 2—**How to record your strabismus surgery** https://vimeo.com/manage/videos/476586171.

(4) Surgical loupes—although it is possible to practice all of these basic skills without surgical loupes, I personally feel that the extra magnification loupes provide facilitates safer strabismus surgery. They also encourage better posture and more time spent with the operating light illuminating the surgical field instead of the back of the trainee's head!

Fig. 3 Bioniko—EX-ONE strabismus model

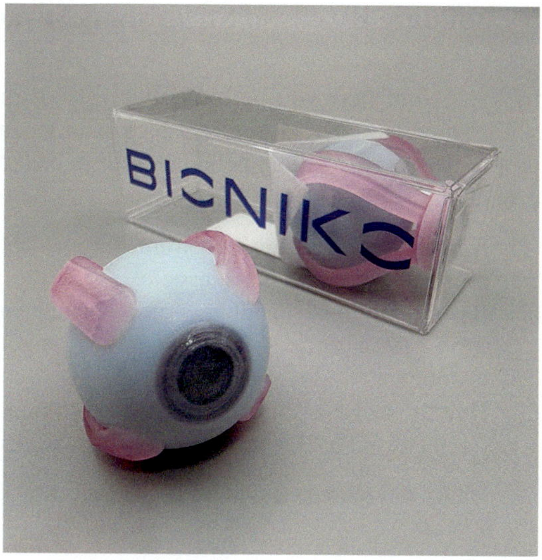

(5) Scoring matrix—Modified version of the ICO's strabismus surgery Ophthalmic Surgical Competency Assessment Rubric (OSCAR) [6] adapted for the basics of strabismus surgery (Fig. 4)

Ophthalmic Simulated Surgical Competency Assessment Rubric - Basic Strabismus Surgery skills

		Novice (score =0)	Advanced beginner (score = 1)	Competent (score = 2)	Score
1	**Technique of holding suture needle in a needle holder**	Loads needle in proper direction for a forehand pass but sometimes loads incorrectly for a backhand pass. Loads too close or too far from swaged end of the needle.	Loads needle correctly for forehand and backhand passes but is inefficient and often requires multiple attempts.	Loads needle correctly and efficiently for forehand and backhand passes.	
2	**Scleral passes**	Does not approach the globe with the needle tangentially. Unable to accurately obtain correct needle depth or length of pass.	Safely approaches the globe with the needle tip directed tangentially to the globe. Scleral passes are frequently too short or of incorrect depth (too shallow or too deep).	Approaches the globe with the needle tip directed tangentially and scleral passes are of the correct depth and length. Regrasps the needle ready to make the next pass.	
3	**Technique of surgical knot tying**	Requires multiple extra hand manoeuvres to make the first throw lay flat / or loosens first throw whilst attempting to perform the second throw.	Is able to tie a flat surgeon's knot first throw without loosening it but second and third throws are inefficient.	Is able to efficiently tie a flat, square surgeon's knot.	
4	**Placement of a continuous suture in a rectus muscle**	Multiple attempts required to load or unload the needle holder. Suture placement is inaccurate (too close or too far from insertion). Locking bites not performed correctly.	Is able to safely secure the muscle but is inefficient. Inefficient performance of locking bites.	Is able to safely, efficiently and accurately secure the muscle with a continuous suture.	

Fig. 4 Basic strabismus surgery skills OSSCAR

5 Building Blocks of Strabismus Surgery

Irrespective of how you perform strabismus surgery, there are a number of core skills which are integral to all strabismus procedures and trainees need to develop these competencies before being allowed to undertake any part of a live strabismus operation:

(1) Knowledge of surgical instruments and sutures—for example the intrinsic properties of a spatulated needle.
(2) Basic instrument handling—how to hold instruments correctly and learning "good table manners" i.e. what you should and should not do with each instrument.
(3) How to make a safe scleral pass of the appropriate depth and length, both forehand and backhand and tangential and perpendicular to the limbus (Fig. 5).

Link to Video 3—**Scleral Passes** https://vimeo.com/manage/videos/218278288.

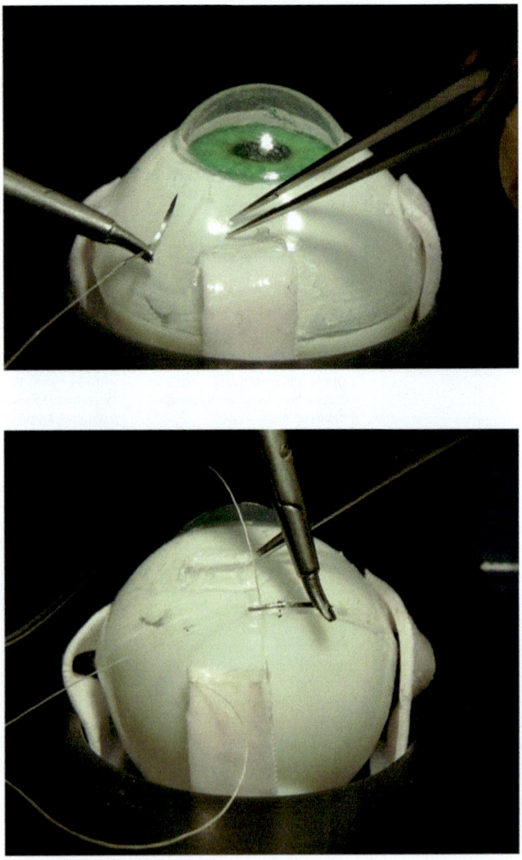

Fig. 5 Scleral passes—Phillips Studios basic strabismus eye

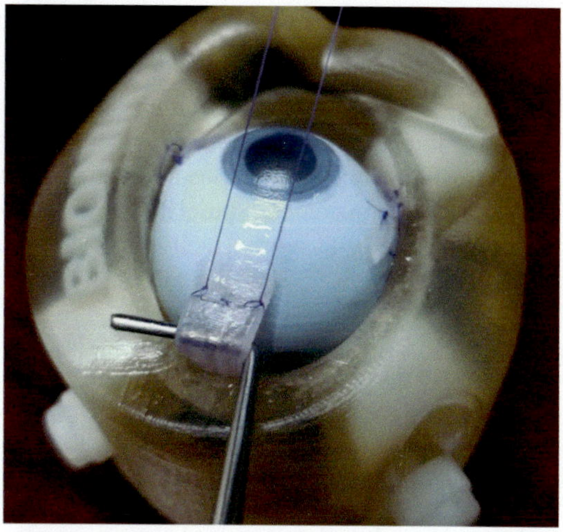

Fig. 6 Rectus muscle secured on a 6/0 vicryl suture—Bioniko EX-ONE strabismus eye

(4) Surgical knot tying—been able to tie a secure surgical (reef) knot in a timely fashion.
(5) How to secure a rectus muscle with a 6/0 vicryl suture (Fig. 6).

Link to video 4—**Rectus muscle recession** https://vimeo.com/manage/videos/476586171.

6 Tips for Starting Training with a Novice Trainee

Historically, simulation training consisted of a trainer demonstrating a technique on a model eye, then observing a trainee attempting to perform the same manoeuvres and repeating them until they had grasped the basics of the technique. The trainee would then practice at home and come back in a week or so to demonstrate their refined technique to their trainer. Although this form of training was very effective it was time-consuming for the trainer.

Now, instead of conducting face-to-face teaching along these lines, trainees can be asked to watch videos of basic scleral suturing skills and knot tying techniques on the Simulation Gallery website (https://gallery.simulatedocularsurgery.com) and then to practice what they had watched on a model eye, before recording their practice on their mobile phones. They can then assess their own progress by scoring their simulation using the modified OSSCAR, before showing their trainer these clips and receive feedback about how their technique could be improved. This training cycle is repeated until the trainer is satisfied that they can make safe scleral passes, secure a rectus muscle with a 6/0 vicryl suture, and are able to tie a secure surgical knot.

Virtual mentoring is also feasible, if a trainee does not have access to a local trainer who is able to supervise their practice and comment on their progress. With the selfie stand and mobile phone set-up illustrated in Video 2, a trainer can observe practice sessions remotely and in real time using Zoom. This approach has been used successfully by WSPOS.

Link to video 5—https://www.youtube.com/watch?v=g8pLBqDrqfI.

Taking this a step further, we have demonstrated that first year ophthalmology trainees, who had no prior exposure to strabismus surgery, are able to develop all of these basic competencies, purely by watching videos of surgical simulation, and without any face-to-face or virtually supervised training [7].

7 Introduction to Live Surgery

7.1 Initial Surgical Exposure

Once a trainee has demonstrated their competence in performing these building blocks of strabismus surgery, they are ready to start performing them during live surgery. Although there are many different ways of introducing trainees to live surgery, I usually teach the following components of strabismus surgery first:

(1) Securing a rectus muscle for a recession or resection with 6/0 vicryl—a lateral rectus muscle is preferable, as there is usually better access to the muscle and the nose does not act as an impediment to suturing.
(2) Making the first scleral passes by the rectus muscle insertion, rather than more posteriorly, where access is more challenging.
(3) Conjunctival closure.

7.2 Active Observation

As well as performing these steps during their initial operations trainees are encouraged to pay close attention to the following:

(1) How conjunctival incisions are performed, be they limbal or fornix-based incisions.
(2) How to dissect into the sub-Tenons space and use the position of the ciliary vessels to identify the location of the rectus muscle insertions.
(3) How to hook the rectus muscle under direct vision, rather than blind hooking and how to perform a pole test, during fornix-based surgery.
(4) How to use sharp and blunt dissection to prepare the rectus muscle for suturing.
(5) How to accurately and consistently measure the amount of recession or resection.
(6) The importance of learning how to be a good assistant, how to improve access to the surgical field by holding instruments correctly and learning to predict what

the primary surgeon is going to do next, so you can provide them with a better view of the surgical field.

(7) The importance of maintaining good illumination of the surgical field, maintaining a good posture and utilising the mobility of the surgical stool/chair to change your position relative to the patient.

7.3 Continued Simulation

Trainees, who can make safe scleral passes and secure rectus muscles on 6/0 vicryl sutures, have developed the instrument and tissue handling skills to move directly to performing the steps above under the direct supervision of their trainer. Although the Phillips Studio advanced strabismus models have conjunctiva and Tenons capsule layers, I have not found that practice with these models is essential for teaching skills 1–5 listed above.

For fornix based surgery, the Advanced Strabismus eyes and Wright-Strube eyes are helpful for practicing how to create a forniceal incision and then how to hook and expose the rectus muscle. Although the rectus muscles on the models are much easier to hook than in real life and they cannot be split (Fig. 7).

Link to video 6—https://vimeo.com/manage/videos/95944234.

If you have the access to freshly defrosted cadaver material, this is perhaps the most realistic way of simulating the creation of a conjunctival incision, identifying, hooking and dissecting a rectus muscle.

Just as a sports person or a musician will spend hours practicing in between performances, we should encourage our trainees to continue practising their muscle suturing and scleral pass skills on the model eyes, in between operating lists. Trainers should give trainees feedback after every operation, with tips for how their technique could be refined so they know what aspects of their surgery they need to focus on during these practice sessions. A single Phillips Studio basic strabismus eye can be

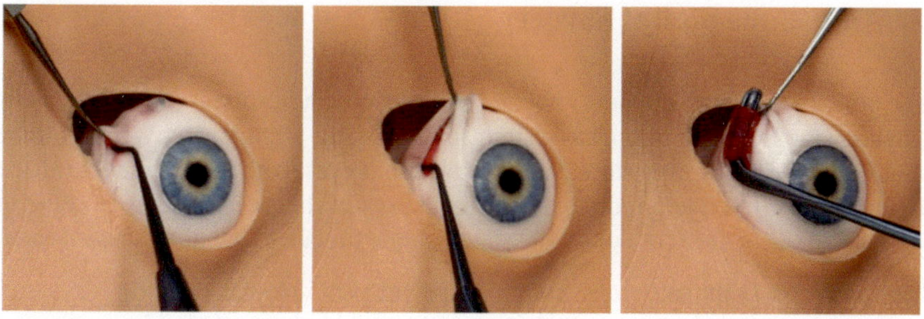

Fig. 7 Hooking a rectus muscle via a fornix based incision—Wright and Strube model eye (Courtesy of Dr. Yi Ning Strube)

used to perform well in excess of 50 recession/resection procedures, by repeatedly re-suturing the rectus muscles back onto the sclera.

Modelling clay can be used to fashion a nose and an orbital rim, to make mimic the difficulties of access to the rectus muscles posed by these natural obstacles, making simulation more realistic. Trainees should also be encouraged to practice suturing with their non-dominant hand, so they can comfortably suture with both hands.

As with cataract surgery training, there will come a point when the trainee is ready to put all of the steps together and perform a complete case. As a trainee's case numbers increase, the fluency and flow of their surgery will improve.

8 Moving Towards Independent Surgery

It always amazes me how reliant most trainees are on the words of instruction and encouragement from their trainer and the help of an experienced scrub nurse, even when they have performed 10 or more strabismus surgeries. So, once a trainee is able to complete entire cases reasonably fluently, the following steps are suggested:

(1) Inform the trainee that although you will be assisting them you will not be offering any form of instruction or comment during the case, unless it is absolutely necessary.
(2) Inform the scrub nurse not to offer any surgical instruments or sutures unless the trainee specifically asks for them.

Initially, most trainees find this very disconcerting as they do not realise how much they have relied on feedback from their trainer and assistance from the scrub nurse. However, they soon begin to take responsibility for the flow of the operation and develop confidence in their own decision making. The next step is for the trainer is to leave the operating theatre and sit in the coffee room, available if required!

9 Adjustable Squint Surgery

The principles of both the bow knot and sliding noose adjustment technique can be taught on the Phillips Studio, basic strabismus eyes, the Bioniko and Wright-Strube strabismus eyes. However, the advanced strabismus eyes, with their conjunctival and Tenons layers, provide a more realistic simulation of these techniques, as some of the inherent difficulties of adjustable squint surgery relate to handling these tissues.

Link to video 7—https://vimeo.com/manage/videos/95846452.

The same principles are applied for teaching more advanced strabismus surgery techniques i.e. ask trainees to watch videos of live and simulated surgery, then practise these techniques and record their practice, before reflecting on their performance and watching these videos with their trainer.

10 Post-operative Adjustment

Trainees can be taught how to advance and how to recess a muscle, with the trainer applying traction on the rectus muscle to mimic the feel of a live adjustment. An extra layer of realism to this simulation can be created by combining KY jelly and red food colouring, or fake blood and placing this under the conjunctiva and Tenons to obscure the adjustable sutures.

11 Other Simulation Scenarios

For truly immersive simulation the following scenarios can be enacted:

(1) Coping with an anxious patient—ask trainees to talk to the "patient" so they learn what phrases to say during the adjustment process. A trainer can play the role of an anxious patient and start to move the model head slightly, and express their discomfort, as the trainee carries out the adjustment. This will test the trainee's ability to deal with this "patient", allaying their fears, at the same time as they carry out the adjustment.
(2) How to deal with a bow knot that has been inadvertently tied off—to simulate this the trainer ties off the bow knot prior to adjustment, without warning the trainee.
(3) How to deal with a snapped suture—the trainer intentionally frays the 6/0 vicryl suture, again without telling the trainee, and then watches how they cope when it snaps during the adjustment process.

This immersive simulation is more akin to that undertaken by airline pilots, who do not know what disaster is about to befall them when they are undertaking flight simulation training, they just have to react to the situation as it evolves.

12 Inferior Oblique Surgery

The Phillips Studio advanced strabismus model eyes have either an inferior or a superior oblique muscle and all of the principle steps of an inferior oblique recession, or myectomy can be simulated with this model eye (Fig. 8):

- The appropriate placement of the fornix incision.
- Dissection through the conjunctiva and Tenons.
- Identifying the inferior oblique tendon and hooking the muscle under direct vision. The inferior oblique cannot be split, but the manoeuvres involved in hooking the muscle can be practised.
- Suturing of the inferior oblique and reattaching it to the sclera.

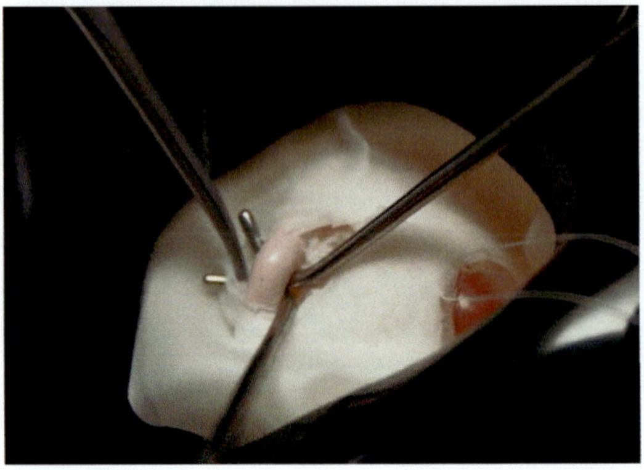

Fig. 8 Exposure of an inferior oblique muscle—Phillips Studio advanced strabismus eye

Link to video 8—https://vimeo.com/manage/videos/95845829.

Freshly frozen cadaver simulation is also an excellent way to practice the steps involved in an inferior oblique recession, if you have access to this material.

Once a trainee is able to complete entire rectus muscle surgeries, has assisted at three or more inferior oblique recessions, they can be talked through the steps of inferior oblique surgery, even without having had prior simulation experience on model eyes or cadaver material.

13 Superior Oblique Surgery

Although superior oblique techniques, such as a superior oblique tuck and a Harada-Ito procedure can be taught on the advanced strabismus model eyes, freshly defrosted cadavers material provides a much more realistic simulation experience. The thin and stretchable superior oblique tendon in the cadaver eyes has almost the same properties as the tendon has in life, enabling surgeons to get a realistic feel for how to identify and hook the superior oblique tendon and place tucking sutures.

14 Summary

Hopefully this chapter will provide a practical framework for how to deliver safe and effective strabismus surgical training. The key messages are:

- Trainers should facilitate simulation training, but it must be led by trainees.
- The basic building blocks of strabismus surgery can be taught with inexpensive model eyes and trainees should only proceed to live surgery when these have developed these competencies.

- Sustained, deliberate, practice, combined with self-directed learning, are the key elements of developing into a competent and then an expert strabismus surgeon.
- The learning curve to competency can be greatly shortened with simulation training.
- Immersive simulation, like that undertaken by pilots, is possible with a little imagination.

Witnessing a trainee's transition from simulated to live surgery, watching their confidence grow as they progress to completing entire cases and seeing them experience the satisfaction of restoring good ocular alignment for their patients is incredibly rewarding. Perhaps more importantly, it enables trainees to experience the profound impact that strabismus surgery has on people's lives and will hopefully inspire some of them to become the strabismus surgeons of the future.

References

1. Dean WH, Buchan J, Gichuhi S, Philippin H, Arunga S, Mukome A, Burton MJ, et al. Simulation based surgical education for glaucoma versus conventional training alone: the GLAucoma simulated surgery (GLASS) trial. A multicentre, multicountry, randomized controlled, investigator-masked educational intervention efficacy trial in Kenya, South Africa, Tanzania, Uganda and Zimbabwe. Br J Ophthalmol. 106(6):863–9. https://doi.org/10.1136/bjophthalmol-2020-318049.
2. Dean WH, Gichuhi S, Buchan JC, Makupa W, Mukome A, Otiti-Sengeri J, Arunga S, Mukherjee S, Kim MJ, Harrison-Williams L, MacLeod D, Cook C, Burton MJ. Intense simulation-based surgical education for manual small-incision cataract surgery: the ophthalmic learning and improvement initiative in cataract surgery randomized clinical trial in Kenya, Tanzania, Uganda, and Zimbabwe. JAMA Ophthalmol. 139(1):9–15. https://doi.org/10.1001/jamaophthalmol.2020.4718.
3. Malik M, Shah N, Kit V, Jain S. Development of a low-cost strabismus surgery simulation model. Eye (Lond). 35(3):805–10. https://doi.org/10.1038/s41433-020-0966-1. Epub 19 May 2020.
4. Adebayo T, Abendroth M, Elera GG, Kunselman A, Sinz E, Ely A, Elkamshoushy A, Soni AJ. Developing and validating a simple and cost-effective strabismus surgery simulator. J AAPOS. 22(2):85–8. https://doi.org/10.1016/j.jaapos.2017.11.006. Epub 10 Mar 2018.
5. Jagan L, Turk W, Petropolis C, Egan R, Cofie N, Wright KW, Strube YNJ. Validation of a novel strabismus surgery 3D-printed silicone eye model for simulation training. J AAPOS. 24(1):1–3.e6. https://doi.org/10.1016/j.jaapos.2019.10.008. Epub 7 Jan 2020. PMID: 31923621.
6. Golnik KC, Motley WW, Atilla H, Pilling R, Reddy A, Sharma P, Yadarola MB, Zhao K. The ophthalmology surgical competency assessment rubric for strabismus surgery. J AAPOS. 16(4):318–21. https://doi.org/10.1016/j.jaapos.2012.04.005. PMID: 22929445.
7. Jones R, Ferris J. Can residents develop basic strabismus surgery competencies without any face-to-face teaching? In: AAPOS annual meeting. New York; 2023.

Management of Incomitant Strabismus

Saurabh Jain

Incomitant strabismus is an ocular deviation that is different in different directions of gaze. Surgically these are some of the most difficult patients to manage as it is almost impossible to get the deviation down to a small enough figure that they are able to fuse in all directions. Therefore, it is very important to manage patient expectations throughout the process and to ensure that realistic goals are set. If the patient can have single or near single vision in primary and downgaze that should suffice for the vast majority of activities of daily living as long as they are prepared to accept diplopia in the other directions of gaze that when necessitate them either adopting head posture.

On the whole, incomitant strabismus tends to be acquired with some notable exceptions like Duane and Browns syndrome. It is therefore also more commonly associated with double vision. These are the common causes of incomitant strabismus in adults:

- Nerve Palsy
- Mechanical Limitation
  - Thyroid eye disease
  - Traumatic (Blow Out Fractures)
  - Myotoxic effect of local anaesthetics
  - Following retinal detachment surgery
- Special Congenital Forms—Duane's, Brown's etc.

When planning surgical management of incomitant strabismus,9 gaze measurements obtained either using prisms in free space or the synoptophore are absolutely essential. There are certain rules that are very useful in deciding which muscles to target first and this chapter highlights these using cases.

S. Jain (✉)
Royal Free Hospital, London, UK
e-mail: Saurabh.jain@nhs.net

S. Jain (ed.), *Surgical Management of Strabismus*,
https://doi.org/10.1007/978-3-031-80633-9_17

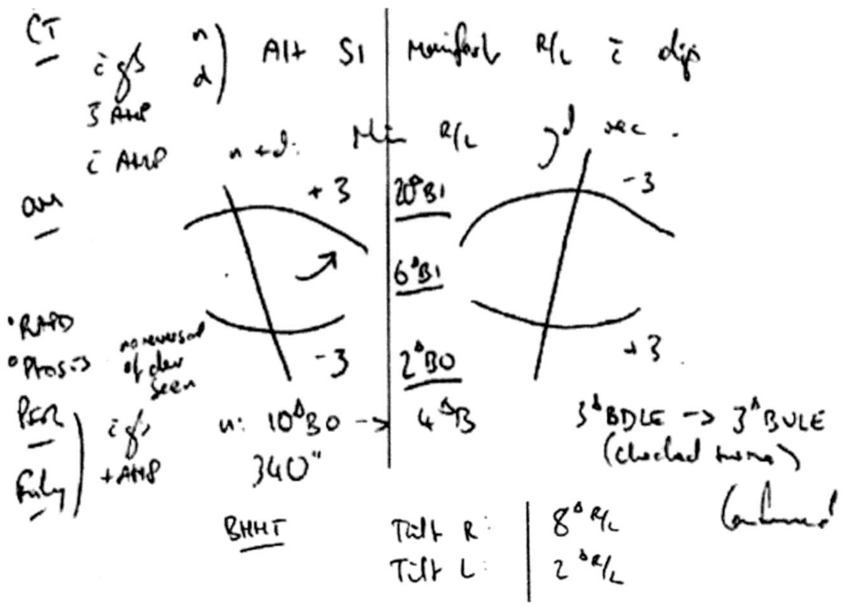

Fig. 1 Orthoptic assessment of case one showing right sided limitation of depression in adduction with corresponding inferior oblique overaction as well as contralateral inferior rectus overaction and superior rectus underaction

Case One

This is a 15-year-old girl who has vertical diplopia as long as she can remember and find it difficult to read for long periods. She's about to go to university and is concerned about this double vision in downgaze. Looking at the ocular motility she has a right sided limitation of depression in adduction with corresponding inferior oblique overaction as well as contralateral inferior rectus overaction and superior rectus underaction (Fig. 1), all suggestive of a long-standing right fourth nerve palsy which is further confirmed on the head tilt test. Her Hess chart also confirms this (Fig. 2).

Looking at the ocular deviations she has a significant right hypertropia that is most in laevodepression associated with excyclotorsion (Fig. 3).

Considering the direction of action of the extra muscles, the two muscles that work in the direction of gaze are the right superior oblique or the left inferior rectus. So she would benefit more from either a right superior oblique tuck or a left inferior rectus recession. As discussed in Chap. 9, a SO tuck by itself is not a very strong procedure so a left IR recession might be a better choice to match the limitation.

Therefore, the first rule of surgical treatment of incomitant strabismus is to target the muscles that move the eye in the direction of maximum deviation.

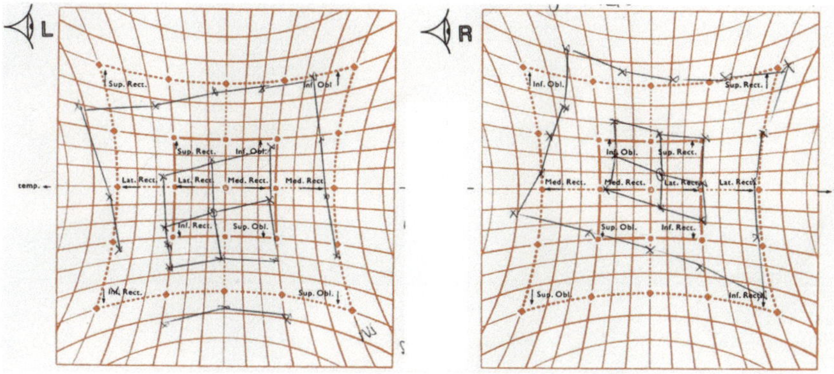

Fig. 2 Hess chart for case one showing right superior oblique underaction and well developed muscle sequelae

4 PD BI 2 R/L 5 degrees excyclo	20 PD BI 7 R/L 5 degrees excyclo	4 PD BI 15 R/L 2 degrees excyclo
4 PD BI 4 R/L 5 degrees excyclo	6 PD BI 9 R/L 5 degrees excyclo	4 PD BI 20 R/L 2 degrees excyclo
8 PD BO 10 R/L 10 degrees excyclo	2 PD B0 6 R/L 9 degrees excyclo	4 PD B0 30 R/L 12 degrees excyclo

Fig. 3 Nine gaze ocular deviation assessment for case one

Case Two

A 62 year old Caucasian woman who is a high myope of—8.5 OD and—4.0 OS. She is now pseudophakic and doing well. She can read comfortably but complains of horizontal diplopia and the distance and is finding it difficult to drive. She has normal visual acuity at 0.00 in each eye with a right to alternating esotropia in the distance of 18 PD BO compared to only 10 PD BO for near (Figs. 4 and 5). She also has some lateral incomitance with the esotropia being worse in right gaze as seen in the 9 Gaze measurements. She was investigated for a possible right sixth palsy, but eventually this was felt to be more likely to be a myopic esotropia.

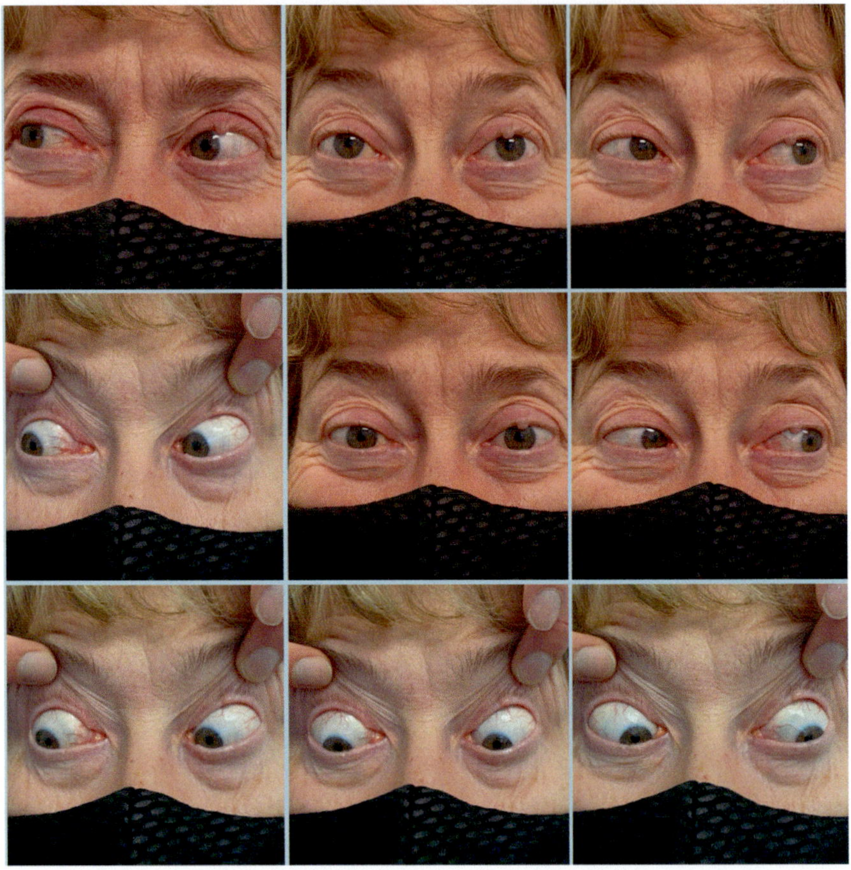

Fig. 4 Ocular motility for case two

Near: 10 PDBO
Distance: 18 PDBO

20 PD B0	10 PD B0	8 PD B0
20 PD B0	10 PD B0	6PD B0
20 PD B0	10 PD B0	6 PD B0

Fig. 5 Nine gaze ocular deviation assessment for case two

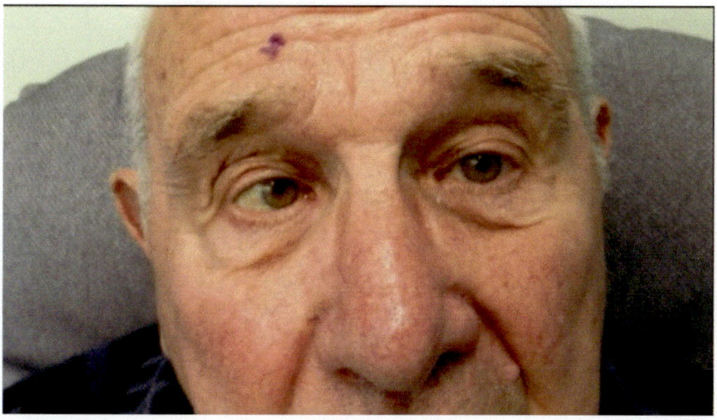

Fig. 6 Clinical photograph for case three demonstrating a right esotropia secondary to sixth nerve palsy

We know that extra muscle surgery has secondary effects. Recession is most effective in the direction of action of the weakened muscle and resection produces a leash which results in greatest effect when the eye rotates away from the operated muscle. These effects can augment or detract from intended aim of surgery.

Here if we recess the MR in the left eye not only will it improve the deviation in primary gaze for both near and distance but when the patient looks to the right, the additional weakening effect of the recession will kick in, leading to a further reduction in the esotropia in right gaze. Conversely a right MR recession or a right LR resection or plication will have the maximum effects in left gaze where the esotropia is already lower. This could therefore induce consecutive exotropia and should be avoided.

Rule number two therefore is to be aware of the secondary effects of surgery on the extra ocular muscles and use them to your advantage.

This is also very important when dealing with patients with thyroid eye disease as a IR recession can lead to reversal of the deviation in down case and therefore should be done only in small controlled amounts and ideally not on adjustable sutures.

Case Three

A 77-year-old Caucasian man has an eighteen month history of double vision which is not improving. He has a history of microvascular risk factors and has normal vision in each eye. Has a right esotropia increasing in right gaze with limitation of right abduction all suggestive of a right sided sixth nerve palsy (Figs. 6 and 7).

Like the case above, he could benefit from the left MR recession but he is not keen on surgery on the good eye.

In cases like this, the LR function is really important to determine. This could be done by either using a force generation test or botulinum toxin to investigate whether the eye can move beyond the midline. If so, he would benefit from a recess resect procedure and if not he needs a transposition as highlighted in Chap. 10 (Fig. 8).

Fig. 7 Nine gaze ocular deviation and ocular motility assessment for case three

28 PD BO	10 PD BO	5 PD BO
30 PD BO	10 PD BO	5 PD BO
25 PD BO	15 PD BO	7 PD BO

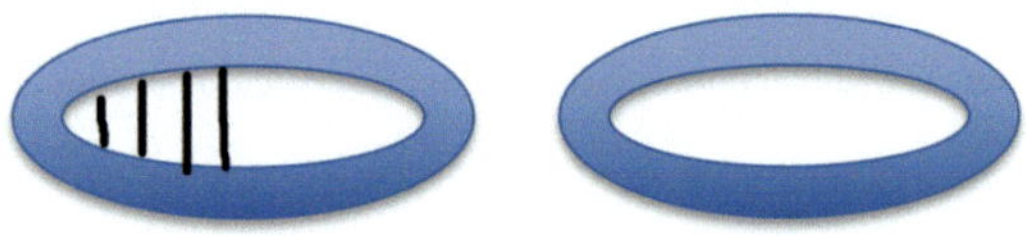

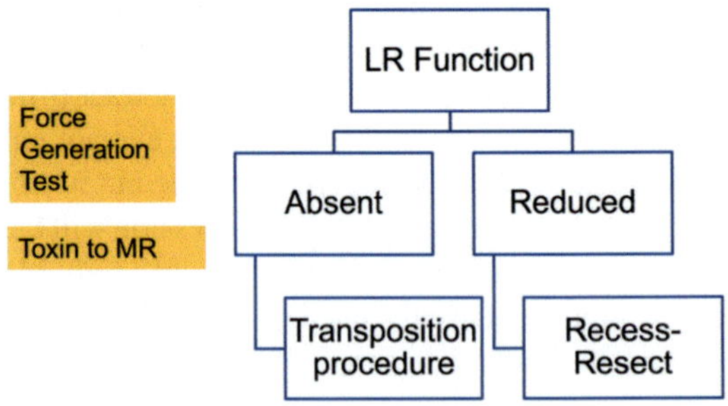

Fig. 8 Decision making flowchart in surgical treatment of sixth nerve palsy

Therefore, rule number three is, if there is no function in a paralysed muscle, borrow one that does work.

Case Four

A 50 year old man underwent an injection of peribulbar local anaesthetic to the left eye prior to retinopexy. Following this he has found he cannot elevate the left eye fully and experiences double vision in upgaze (Figs. 9 and 10).

As both the ocular motility and deviation show he has a left hypotropia that is significantly worse in upgaze. A forced duction test shows the left rectus to be tight due to the myotoxicity caused by the local anaesthetic, possible injected within the muscle belly. Bupivacaine demonstrates specific myotoxicity for muscle fibres, with initial degeneration of myofibrils followed by repair by satellite cell that leads to a hypertrophied muscle complex.

In such a case it is really important to release the restriction prior to planning any other surgery and should be the first port of call. He did well with a small left inferior

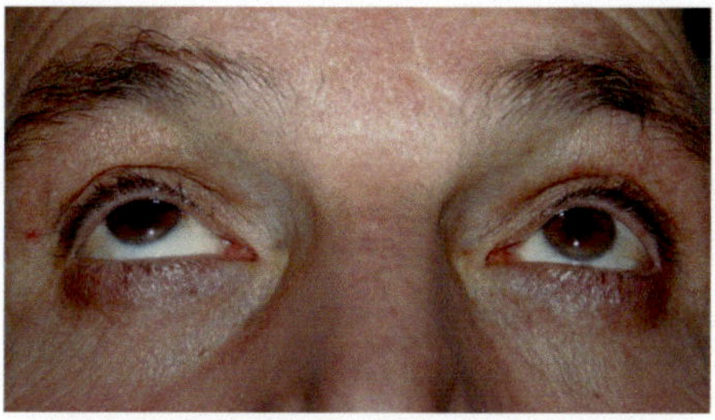

Fig. 9 Clinical photograph of case four demonstrating limited elevation of the left eye

R/L 17 PD	**R/L 14 PD**	**R/L 14 PD**
R/L 4 PD	R/L 6 PD	R/L 4 PD
R/L 13 PD	R/L 14 PD	R/L 16 PD

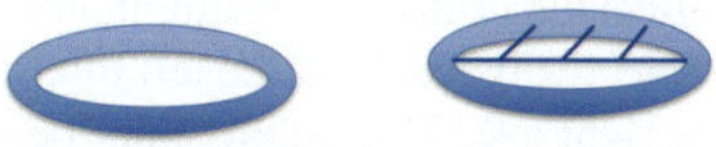

Fig. 10 Nine gaze ocular deviation and ocular motility assessment for case four

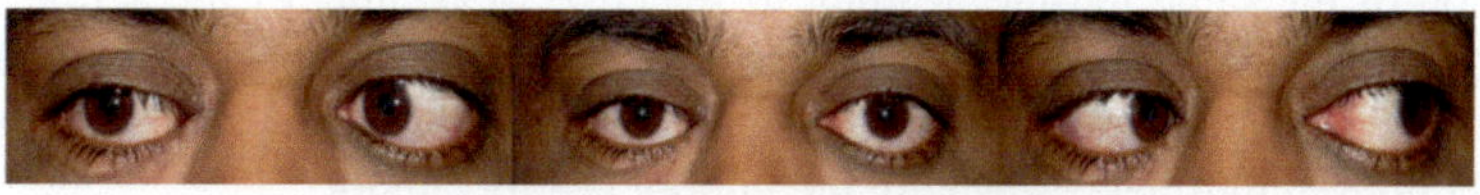

	4 R/L	
18R/L	**14 R/L**	**11 R/L**

Fig. 11 Clinical photograph and ocular deviation measurements for case five demonstrating increasing deviation in downgaze

reactors recession which improved his elevation and got rid of the double vision in primary gaze.

So rule number four is if there is a restriction or mechanical limitation aim to release it if at all possible.

Case Five

Case five is a 40 year old man with thyroid disease who has undergone bilateral orbital decompressions and a right IR recession. He has been left with persistent double vision in downgaze but is asymptomatic in straight gaze (Figs. 11 and 12).

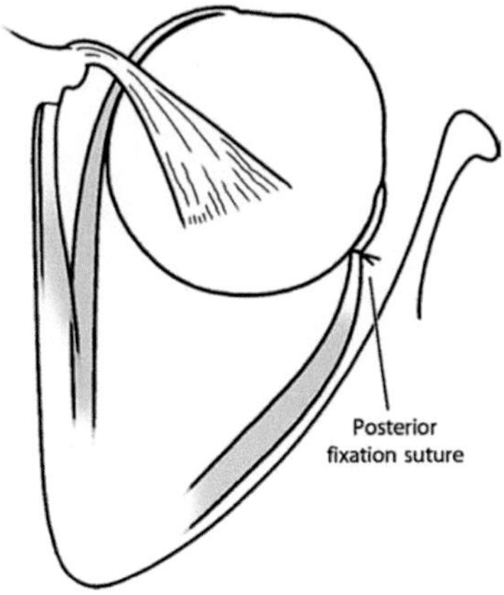

Fig. 12 Text as above- from Strabismus surgery and its complications, Springer 2007. David Coats, Scott Olitsky-rights obtained

In this scenario it is very important that whatever procedure is carried out does not affect the primary gaze alignment. Therefore, he would do well with a procedure that selectively weakens the left inferior rectus to match the limitation in depression of the right eye. This could either be a Faden procedure which is a retro equatorial myopexy on the left IR or a Scott procedure which is a simultaneous recession and resection of the same muscle, leading to selective weakening of the action of the operated muscle in its direction of action without any effect in primary gaze. It also has the advantage of being adjustable although the caveats of using adjustable sutures on tight thyroid muscles, especially the infinity reactors apply.

Therefore, rule number five is if not possible to release the limitation aim to match it in the contralateral eye.

In summary, incomitant strabismus is a surgical challenge and patients need to be counselled appropriately.

Rules for Surgical Management of Incomitant Strabismus

- Target the muscles that move the eyes in the direction where the deviation is the greatest.
- Be aware of the secondary effects of surgery on the extra ocular muscles and use them to your advantage.
- If there is no function in a paralysed muscle, borrow one that does work.
- If there is a restriction or mechanical limitation, aim to release it if possible.
- If not possible to release limitation, aim to match it in the contralateral eye.

Index

S. Jain (ed.), *Surgical Management of Strabismus*,
https://doi.org/10.1007/978-3-031-80633-9

MIX
Papier aus verantwortungsvollen Quellen
Paper from responsible sources
FSC® C105338

If you have any concerns about our products,
you can contact us on
ProductSafety@springernature.com

In case Publisher is established outside the EU,
the EU authorized representative is:
Springer Nature Customer Service Center GmbH
Europaplatz 3, 69115 Heidelberg, Germany

Printed by Libri Plureos GmbH
in Hamburg, Germany